Treatment of Peritoneal Surface Malignancies

Guest Editor

JESUS ESQUIVEL, MD

SURGICAL ONCOLOGY CLINICS OF NORTH AMERICA

www.surgonc.theclinics.com

Consulting Editor

NICHOLAS J. PETRELLI, MD

October 2012 • Volume 21 • Number 4

SAUNDERS an imprint of ELSEVIER, Inc.

W.B. SAUNDERS COMPANY

A Division of Elsevier Inc.

1600 John F. Kennedy Boulevard ● Suite 1800 ● Philadelphia, PA 19103-2899

http://www.theclinics.com

SURGICAL ONCOLOGY CLINICS OF NORTH AMERICA Volume 21, Number 4
October 2012 ISSN 1055-3207, ISBN-13: 978-1-4557-5424-3

Editor: Jessica McCool

Surgical Oncology Clinics of North America (ISSN 1055-3207) is published quarterly by Elsevier Inc., 360 Park Avenue South, New York, NY 10010-1710. Months of publication are January, April, July, and October. Business and Editorial Offices: 1600 John F. Kennedy Blvd., Ste. 1800, Philadelphia, PA 19103-2899. Customer Service Office: 3251 Riverport Lane, Maryland Heights, MO 63043. Periodicals postage paid at New York, NY and additional mailing offices. Subscription prices are $274.00 per year (US individuals), $401.00 (US institutions), $135.00 (US student/resident), $314.00 (Canadian individuals), $498.00 (Canadian institutions), $193.00 (Canadian student/resident), $392.00 (foreign individuals), $498.00 (foreign institutions), and $193.00 (foreign student/resident). Foreign air speed delivery is included in all *Clinics* subscription prices. All prices are subject to change without notice. **POSTMASTER**: Send address changes to *Surgical Oncology Clinics of North America*, Elsevier Health Science Division, Subscription Customer Service, 3251 Riverport Lane, Maryland Heights, MO 63043. **Customer Service: 1-800-654-2452 (US and Canada). 314-447-8871 (outside U.S. and Canada). Fax: 314-447-8029. E-mail: journalscustomerservice-usa@elsevier.com** (for print support); **journalsonline support-usa@elsevier.com** (for online support).

Reprints. For copies of 100 or more, of articles in this publication, please contact the Commercial Reprints Department, Elsevier Inc., 360 Park Avenue South, New York, New York 10010-1710. Tel. 212-633-3813; Fax: 212-462-1935; E-mail: reprints@elsevier.com.

Surgical Oncology Clinics of North America is covered in *MEDLINE/PubMed (Index Medicus)* and *EMBASE/ Excerpta Medica, Current Contents/Clinical Medicine,* and *ISI/BIOMED.*

Printed and bound by CPI Group (UK) Ltd, Croydon, CR0 4YY
Transferred to digital print 2012

Contributors

CONSULTING EDITOR

NICHOLAS J. PETRELLI, MD
Bank of America Endowed Medical Director, Helen F. Graham Cancer Center at Christiana
Care Health System, Newark, Delaware

GUEST EDITOR

JESUS ESQUIVEL, MD, FACS
Director, Peritoneal Surface Malignancy Program, Saint Agnes Hospital, Baltimore,
Maryland

AUTHORS

ITZHAK AVITAL, MD, FACS
Head, Peritoneal Surface Malignancies Center of Excellence; Medical Director, Bon
Secours Cancer Institute, Richmond, Virginia; Assistant Professor, Uniformed Services
University of the Health Sciences, Bethesda, Maryland

DARIO BARATTI, MD
Peritoneal Surface Malignancy Program, Department of Surgery, Fondazione IRCCS
Istituto Nazionale dei Tumori, Milan, Italy

BJÖRN L.D.M. BRÜCHER, MD, FRCS (Engl), FACS
Founder and Director, Theodor-Billroth-Academy®, Munich, Germany

CHANEL H. CHONG, MBBS (UNSW)
Hepatobiliary and Surgical Oncology Unit, Department of Surgery, University of New
South Wales, St George Hospital, Sydney, Australia

TERENCE C. CHUA, BScMed (Hons), MBBS (UNSW), MRCS (Ed)
Hepatobiliary and Surgical Oncology Unit, Department of Surgery, University of New
South Wales, St George Hospital, Sydney; St George Clinical School, University of New
South Wales, New South Wales, Australia

KATHY CROWLEY, CRNA
Chief CRNA, Department of Anesthesiology, Saint Agnes Hospital, Baltimore, Maryland

MARCELLO DERACO, MD
Peritoneal Surface Malignancy Program, Department of Surgery, Fondazione IRCCS
Istituto Nazionale dei Tumori, Milan, Italy

DOMINIQUE ELIAS, MD, PhD
Chief, Department of General Oncologic Surgery, Institut Gustave Roussy, Villejuif, France

ORIETTA FEDERICI, MD
Department of GI Surgery, Regina Elena National Cancer Institute, Rome, Italy

ALFREDO GAROFALO, MD, FACS
Department of GI Surgery, Regina Elena National Cancer Institute, Rome, Italy

GABRIEL GLOCKZIN, MD
Department of Surgery, University Medical Center Regensburg, Regensburg, Germany

DIANE GOÉRÉ, MD
Department of General Oncologic Surgery, Institut Gustave Roussy, Villejuif, France

LUIS GONZÁLEZ-BAYÓN, MD, PhD
Servicio de Cirugía General III, Hospital General Universitario Gregorio Marañón;
Associate Professor, Universidad Complutense de Madrid, Madrid, Spain

SANTIAGO GONZÁLEZ-MORENO, MD, PhD
Chairman, Department of Surgical Oncology; Director, Peritoneal Surface Oncology
Program, MD Anderson Cancer Center, Madrid, Spain

C. WILLIAM HELM, MA, MBBChir
Professor, Division of Gynecologic Oncology, Departments of Obstetrics, Gynecology
and Women's Health, Saint Louis University School of Medicine, St Louis, Missouri

IONUT HUTANU, MD
Department of Surgery, University of Medicine and Pharmacy 'Gr T Popa', Iasi, Romania

SHIGEKI KUSAMURA, MD, PhD
Peritoneal Surface Malignancy Program, Department of Surgery, Fondazione IRCCS
Istituto Nazionale dei Tumori, Milan, Italy

EDWARD A. LEVINE, MD, FACS
Surgical Oncology Section, Department of General Surgery, Wake Forest University
School of Medicine, Winston-Salem, North Carolina

DAVID L. MORRIS, MD, PhD
Hepatobiliary and Surgical Oncology Unit, Department of Surgery, University of New
South Wales, St George Hospital, Sydney; St George Clinical School, University of New
South Wales, New South Wales, Australia

AVIRAM NISSAN, MD, FACS
Chief, Division of Surgical Oncology, Department of Surgery, Rabin Medical Center, Petah
Tikvah, Israel

GLORIA ORTEGA-PÉREZ, MD
Servicio de Cirugía General y Aparato Digestivo, Hospital Universitario de Fuenlabrada,
Fuenlabrada; Honorary Professor, Universidad Rey Juan Carlos, Madrid, Spain

POMPILIU PISO, MD
Professor, Department of Surgery, St. John of God Hospital Regensburg, Regensburg,
Germany

FRANÇOIS QUENET, MD
Department of Surgery, Centre anticancéreux Val d'Aurelle, Montpellier, France

PIERO ROSSI, MD
Dipartimento di Chirurgia D'Urgenza, Senologica e dei Trapianti, Fondazione Policlinico Tor Vergata, Roma, Italy

KENNETH P. ROTHFIELD, MD
Chairman, Department of Anesthesiology, Saint Agnes Hospital; Adjunct Associate Professor, University of Maryland School of Nursing, Baltimore, Maryland

PERRY SHEN, MD, FACS
Surgical Oncology Section, Department of General Surgery, Wake Forest University School of Medicine, Winston-Salem, North Carolina

JOHN H. STEWART IV, MD, FACS
Surgical Oncology Section, Department of General Surgery, Wake Forest University School of Medicine, Winston-Salem, North Carolina

ALEXANDER STOJADINOVIC, MD, FACS
Department of Surgery, Walter Reed National Military Medical Center; GI Cancer Program Leader, United States Military Cancer Institute; Professor of Surgery, Uniformed Services University of the Health Sciences, Bethesda, Maryland; COL, Medical Corps, United States Army

O. ANTHONY STUART, BS
Washington Cancer Institute, Washington Hospital Center, Washington, DC

PAUL H. SUGARBAKER, MD, FACS, FRCS
Program in Peritoneal Surface Malignancy, Washington Cancer Institute, Washington Hospital Center, Washington, DC

MARIO VALLE, MD, FACS
Department of GI Surgery, Regina Elena National Cancer Institute, Rome, Italy

KURT VAN DER SPEETEN, MD, PhD
Department of Surgical Oncology, Ziekenhuis Oost-Limburg, Genk; Department of Medicine, Research Group Oncology, University of Hasselt, Hasselt, Belgium

KONSTANTINOS I. VOTANOPOULOS, MD, PhD, FACS
Surgical Oncology Section, Department of General Surgery, Wake Forest University School of Medicine, Winston-Salem, North Carolina

Contents

The indications for peritonectomy + hyperthermic intraperitoneal chemotherapy (HIPEC) are based on careful assessment of disease extent, but no imaging procedure is accurate enough to identify lesions smaller than 5 mm or extensively diffuse. Video-laparoscopy allows, with minimal surgical trauma, correct staging with a reliable prediction of expected cytoreduction index. Operative laparoscopy is indicated for palliation of neoplastic ascites with chemotherapy, offering encouraging results. Minimally invasive surgery in the treatment of minimal peritoneal carcinomatosis is not yet validated from wide international experience; the procedure is technically possible with strict indications, and combination with intraoperative hyperthermic chemotherapy is strongly recommended.

This article outlines the anesthetic management of patients undergoing cytoreductive surgery with hyperthermic intraperitoneal chemotherapy. This includes a discussion of preoperative evaluation, hemodynamic monitoring, fluid and electrolyte therapy, and temperature management. An understanding of the unique physiologic consequences of this procedure is essential to ensure good outcomes and avoid patient injuries.

Several methods of delivering hyperthermic intraperitoneal chemotherapy (HIPEC) during the course of cytoreductive surgery have been described, but no significant differences in treatment results have been found among them. HIPEC is a safe treatment for the patient and for healthcare workers involved in the procedure provided standard protective and environmental measures are used. This article describes the different techniques in use and the technology available for the administration of HIPEC. Also reviewed are the safety features that must be taken into consideration when performing this procedure. Recommended guidelines to prevent associated occupational hazards are provided.

Cytoreductive surgery (CRS) and hyperthermic intraperitoneal chemotherapy (HIPEC) are complex procedures with a very steep a learning curve (LC). This study evaluates the LC of CRS and HIPEC in a single-center experience of peritoneal surface malignancies (PSMs). Approximately 140 to 150 cases were necessary for the acquisition of competence in CRS and HIPEC with adequate radicality and acceptable safety. Eighty to 100 cases were necessary to assure short-term prognostic gains in rare PSMs. This article highlights how LC and continuous monitoring of surgical performance is critical in evaluating the credibility of emerging and already established PSM centers.

Peritoneal surface malignancy is a common manifestation of intra-abdominal malignancies. Systemic chemotherapy offers no long-term survival and poor quality of life for these patients in their terminal stages of disease. By contrast, cytoreductive surgery combined with perioperative intraperitoneal and intravenous chemotherapy has resulted in encouraging clinical results. Further improvements should come from both clinical phase II/III studies and pharmacologic research. This article reviews the current pharmacologic data and controversies regarding the perioperative intraperitoneal and intravenous application of chemotherapy.

This article focuses on the use of intraperitoneal hyperthermic chemotherapy for the treatment of peritoneal dissemination from appendiceal primary tumors. The first part of the article details patient selection criteria used at the Wake Forest University School of Medicine and the use of preoperative imaging and endoscopic evaluation in the management of this cohort of patients. The second part of the article focuses on clinical outcomes for patients undergoing hyperthermic intraperitoneal perfusion for peritoneal dissemination from appendiceal tumors. Finally, future challenges for the use of hyperthermic intraperitoneal perfusion for appendiceal primary tumors are explored.

Peritoneal carcinomatosis (PC) carries a worse prognosis than other sites of colorectal metastases. If incomplete resection of PC affords no benefit to patients, complete resection of PC is beneficial in selected patients. The combination of complete cytoreductive surgery to treat the visible PC and hyperthermic intraperitoneal chemotherapy (HIPEC) to treat the nonvisible PC is on the verge of becoming the gold standard. The prognostic impact of a complete resection is high, but that of HIPEC per se is more hypothetical. The presence of a few resectable liver metastases associated with PC is not a contraindication to surgery plus HIPEC.

underwent cytoreductive surgery (CRS) plus hyperthermic intraperitoneal chemotherapy (HIPEC), resulting in median survival of 22 to 63 months. However, level I data from prospective randomized trials are limited. Further trials are indicated to identify peritoneal carcinomatosis in at-risk patients early in the natural history of the disease and confirm the efficacy of multimodality therapy (CRS/HIPEC/systemic therapy) in those with CRCPC amenable to CRS in the modern era of novel targeted and cytotoxic systemic therapy.

The benefits that are reported in patients who have carcinomatosis from colorectal cancer increase as the extent of disease within the abdomen and pelvis decreases. To optimize treatments that involve cytoreductive surgery and perioperative chemotherapy, early intervention is necessary. Strategies to improve the results of carcinomatosis treatments include second-look surgery and hyperthermic intraperitoneal chemotherapy in patients at high risk for recurrence. Alternatively, the use of hyperthermic intraperitoneal chemotherapy can be used to treat or prevent carcinomatosis at the time of primary colorectal cancer resection in selected patients.

SURGICAL ONCOLOGY
CLINICS OF NORTH AMERICA

NOW AVAILABLE FOR YOUR iPhone and iPad

Foreword

Treatment of Peritoneal Surface Malignancies

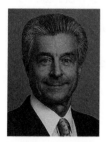

Nicholas J. Petrelli, MD
Consulting Editor

This issue of the *Surgical Oncology Clinics of North America* is devoted to the diagnosis and treatment of peritoneal surface malignancies. The guest editor is Dr Jesus Esquivel from the Department of Surgery at St. Agnes Healthcare Center in Baltimore, Maryland. Dr Esquivel has dedicated his career to the diagnosis and treatment of peritoneal surface malignancies. His training included a fellowship under the mentorship of Paul Sugarbaker, MD at the Washington Cancer Center. Dr Esquivel has put together an international group of expert authors/researchers to discuss these malignancies.

There are 12 articles in this issue of the *Surgical Oncology Clinics of North America*, which run the gamut of the diagnosis and treatment of peritoneal surface malignancies. This starts with Dr Garofalo and associates in the first article, which discusses patient selection for cytoreductive surgery and the role of laparoscopy in the diagnosis, staging, and treatment. Dr Paul Sugarbaker in the twelfth article discusses a plan for individualized care for early intervention for the treatment and prevention of colorectal carcinomatosis, in which he has tremendous experience. An additional interesting article by Sugarbaker and associates discusses the pharmacology of perioperative intraperitoneal and intravenous chemotherapy in peritoneal surface malignant patients. Dr Edward Levine from Wake Forest University discusses the current status and future directions in appendiceal cancer with peritoneal dissemination. Dr Levine leads the peritoneal malignancy program at Wake Forest.

The authors in this issue have devoted their careers to the management of these patients, which requires a multidisciplinary care approach in centers that focus on

Surg Oncol Clin N Am 21 (2012) xiii–xiv
http://dx.doi.org/10.1016/j.soc.2012.07.008
1055-3207/12/$ – see front matter © 2012 Elsevier Inc. All rights reserved.

surgonc.theclinics.com

program development and research. I thank Dr Esquivel for his efforts and congratulate the authors on an excellent issue, and for their commitment to treating these patients.

Nicholas J. Petrelli, MD
Helen F. Graham Cancer Center
4701 Ogletown-Stanton Road
Suite 1213
Newark, DE 19713, USA

E-mail address:
npetrelli@christianacare.org

Preface

Treatment of Peritoneal Surface Malignancies

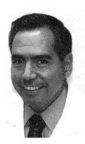

Jesus Esquivel, MD, FACS
Guest Editor

Ten years have gone by since the first issue on the Management of Peritoneal Surface Malignancies by the *Surgical Oncology Clinics of North America*.

As such, I thought it would be appropriate to start this preface with a summary of the comments, challenges, and future directions outlined by Drs Sugarbaker and Petrelli in the first issue. I will follow with a description of the current articles and, finally, this preface concludes with an analysis of where we are now, a decade later, and where we are headed over the next decade in respect to the current challenge for multidisciplinary management of peritoneal surface malignancies.

TEN YEARS AGO

The first issue presented the current state-of-the-art and provided the possible directions for future research over the next decade for peritoneal surface malignancies. Dr Sugarbaker pointed out that there are often disagreements concerning the time at which a clinical research project matures into "standard of practice" but that, in his opinion, cytoreductive surgery (CRS) and hyperthermic intraperitoneal chemotherapy (HIPEC) represented the current standard of practice for patients with *Pseudomyxoma peritonei* of appendiceal origin as well as for patients with malignant peritoneal mesothelioma. In regards to colorectal cancer with peritoneal dissemination, he mentioned the phase III study by Drs Verwaal and Zoetmulder and commented that this unique trial may stand alone as the only randomized study required in this group of patients. He added that perhaps 15,000 colorectal cancer patients in the United States would be candidates for evaluation for this therapy. In regards to gastric and ovarian cancers, he indicated the need to establish the role of hyperthermic intraoperative intraperitoneal chemotherapy.

Surg Oncol Clin N Am 21 (2012) xv–xviii
http://dx.doi.org/10.1016/j.soc.2012.07.006
1055-3207/12/$ – see front matter © 2012 Elsevier Inc. All rights reserved.

surgonc.theclinics.com

He concluded by stating that it may be recognized that a requirement for change in the standard of practice exists in patients with peritoneal surface malignancy and that what is less clear is the proper choice of perfusion techniques and chemotherapeutic options that will optimize these favorable results. More phase III studies are necessary to establish the knowledgeable use of perioperative intraperitoneal chemotherapy in the adjuvant treatment of gastrointestinal and ovarian cancers and Sugarbaker emphasized that quantitative prognostic indicators are extremely important; they will continue to play a role in the refinement of the most important aspect of this treatment to date, proper selection of patients.

Dr Petrelli asked the readers to be careful when distinguishing between standard of care and investigational treatment and recognized that this is sometimes a difficult issue to resolve. He added that what we do know is that the standard of care for patients with peritoneal surface malignancies involves a multidisciplinary team approach. He praised the commitment of all the authors to finding the best treatment for this group of patients and that continued research and development of prospective randomized trials will allow the field to move forward successfully.

He outlined four areas for which there is room for research:

1. The proper choice of perfusion techniques and chemotherapeutic options.
2. The amount of heat necessary for an optimal cell kill, which would result in acceptable morbidity and mortality.
3. A simpler and less costly perfusion apparatus.
4. Finding quantitative prognostic indicators that will allow proper selection of patients for therapy.

TEN YEARS LATER

This second issue represents once more the state-of-the-art description by experts from around the world on the current status and future directions regarding the management of the most common peritoneal surface malignancies. Much has happened in this last 10 years and the readers will witness through these articles the tremendous efforts around the world dedicated to advance this field of peritoneal dissemination from gastrointestinal and gynecological malignancies. We have included articles that focus on patient selection for multimodality treatments that combine cytoreductive surgery to eradicate all visible metastatic disease to the abdomen and pelvis, coupled with HIPEC to eradicate microscopic residual disease, and the different methods to deliver the heated intraperitoneal perfusion. Readers will become familiar with the steep learning curve for this procedure, the anesthetic challenges as a result of induced hyperthermia in the setting of lengthy operations, and the role of laparoscopy in evaluating patients for cytoreductive surgery and treating intractable ascites. Additional articles describe the important contribution of pharmacodynamic and pharmacokinetic data to the science of HIPEC; the need for replacing histological examinations with genetic signatures in order to select patients better for intravenous systemic chemotherapy before, after, or in place of cytoreductive surgery and HIPEC; results from the only prospective randomized study comparing HIPEC versus no HIPEC after cytoreductive surgery in patients with gastric cancer with peritoneal dissemination; the ongoing prospective randomized studies and the incredible frustration with trying to conduct such trials; an excellent article on ovarian cancer, the ultimate biological model to study HIPEC; and, finally, an article with a suggestion for intriguing roles for HIPEC in the prophylactic setting.

ANALYSIS OF 2003 AND 2013

There is no doubt that the number of patients that are experiencing a good long-term result from the treatment of their peritoneal surface malignancy in 2013 is far superior to the number in 2003. Another uncontested statement is the fact that this difference is for the most part due to improvements in CRS and HIPEC regarding patient selection, operative technique, and better ways to deliver the heated perfusion.

That being said, numerous important questions remain unanswered. To return to Dr Petrelli's four points in 2003, there is still tremendous variation when it comes to (1) the proper choice of perfusion techniques and chemotherapeutic options and (2) the amount of heat necessary for an optimal cell kill, which would result in acceptable morbidity and mortality. Progress has been made in (3) simpler and less expensive apparatus to deliver the perfusion and (4) finding quantitative prognostic indicators.

Precise preoperative staging is mandatory in neoadjuvant trials to compare treatments, identify subgroups that will benefit the most, and prevent overtreatment in patients who will not benefit from an aggressive surgical procedure. At the present time, our selection criteria remains ill-defined and the biggest challenge in the treatment of patients with peritoneal surface malignancies may well be moving from demonstrating what can be done to learning what should be done. Many of us have done extensive surgical procedures with multivisceral resections and HIPEC in patients with signet ring cell carcinomas of colorectal origin just to find out that the patients did not benefit at all from our operative intervention.

Also, at the present time, we accept CRS and HIPEC as a package, without knowing what the added benefit of HIPEC is to a complete surgical eradication of metastatic disease to the abdomen and pelvis. While the ongoing French trial (Prodige 7) will answer this question in a highly selected group of patients, it is going to take a long time before we know the results and, in my opinion, it will not show the expected difference in survival because patients are randomized after having cleared too many hurdles: limited disease, good response to neoadjuvant chemotherapy, and the achievement of a complete cytoreduction. In addition, the choice of HIPEC versus no HIPEC becomes even more important in patients with low tumor burden from a tumor with a low level of biological aggressiveness like *P peritonei*.

Almost everybody agrees that we need prospective randomized trials that compare systemic therapy to CRS + HIPEC and trials that compare CRS with and without HIPEC.

During this last 10 years, 2 ACOSOG trials have attempted to answer both questions. The first trial was closed in 2004 before it even started and the second trial closed in 2012 because only 1 patient was accrued to the trial in 18 months. In my opinion, conducting prospective randomized phase III trials that compare HIPEC versus no HIPEC, at least in the United States, is a lesson in human nature and unlikely to contribute to evidence-based medicine.

Rather, what we need to focus on now is collaboration between medical and surgical oncologists in order to discuss the selection criteria and timing to introduce CRS + HIPEC as another therapeutic tool in the individualized, multimodality treatment of colorectal cancer patients with peritoneal dissemination.

The American Society of Peritoneal Surface Malignancies (ASPSM) was created in 2009 to facilitate such a collaboration and to try to do the best that we can with what we have and what we know while trying to answer important questions, preferably under the auspices of a clinical research protocol.

NEXT TEN YEARS

What will happen over the next decade? There will be data on systemic therapy in patients with colorectal cancer with peritoneal dissemination. The Peritoneal Surface Disease Severity Score will become a tool to stratify patients according to the severity of their carcinomatosis. Systemic therapy will continue to improve with numerous ".ibs" and ".abs" coming into the clinical arena; this will increase the number of patients that will be eligible for cytoreductive surgery.

The question of HIPEC or no HIPEC after complete cytoreduction will have to be addressed for each individual histology.

There will be an increased use of laparoscopy not only to score the severity of the peritoneal dissemination but also to perform the cytoreductive surgery in patients with low tumor burden and to do HIPEC in patients at high risk of developing carcinomatosis.

MRI will become the imaging study of choice for patients with mucinous appendiceal neoplasms with peritoneal dissemination.

The ASPSM will continue to increase its membership, currently 144 members from 17 countries, and through scientific research collaboration between medical and surgical oncologists and support personnel, the society will lead the development and conduct of relevant clinical trials that will determine the optimal treatment of patients with peritoneal surface malignancies while maximizing benefits and minimizing side effects.

Areas that we need to work on over the next decade:

1. Pretherapy staging as precise as possible.
2. Standardization of HIPEC delivery.
3. Incorporation of CRS + HIPEC to the treatment armamentarium of patients with peritoneal surface malignancies.
4. Discussions with the medical oncologist regarding timing of CRS + HIPEC.
5. Prospective phase II studies that can lead to expert opinion guidelines.

In conclusion, I think there is a bright future for Cytoreductive Surgery in the treatment of patients with peritoneal surface malignancies. For now, recognizing that even evidence has its limits, the question of whether HIPEC needs to be added to a complete cytoreduction or not needs to be answered on an individual basis; this answer needs to come from a prospective multidisciplinary discussion at a tumor board conference.

Jesus Esquivel, MD, FACS
Peritoneal Surface Malignancy Program
St. Agnes Hospital
900 Caton Avenue
Mail Box 207
Baltimore, MD 21229, USA

E-mail address:
jesquive@stagnes.org

Patient Selection for Cytoreductive Surgery and Hyperthermic Intraperitoneal Chemotherapy, and Role of Laparoscopy in Diagnosis, Staging, and Treatment

Mario Valle, MD, Orietta Federici, MD, Alfredo Garofalo, MD*

KEYWORDS

- Peritoneal carcinomatosis • Staging • Staging laparoscopy • Refractory ascites
- Intraperitoneal hyperthermic chemotherapy

KEY POINTS

- Peritonectomy + hyperthermic intraperitoneal chemotherapy (HIPEC) shows good late results only for patients in whom a complete cytoreductive surgery was performed; the expected completeness of cytoreduction (CC0) is the cornerstone of the indications to the treatment.
- Imaging (computed tomography [CT] and CT/positron emission tomography [PET]) is still considered the first-choice diagnostic test in the workup of peritoneal carcinomatosis, but video-laparoscopic (VLS) staging is the only presidium that allows a correct staging and a reliable forecast of the expected CC0.
- The VLS staging technique is safe and reliable, not presenting major complications and mortality.
- In refractory malignant ascites not suitable for surgery, laparoscopic HIPEC shows encouraging results regarding both the ascites and the improvement in the Karnofsky index.
- VLS peritonectomy might be used in minimal carcinomatosis, confined to 1 or 2 sectors and well-defined histologic types. At present, in the absence of comparative data with open surgery, it is not possible to consider it as a gold standard in minimal carcinomatosis.

INTRODUCTION

The integrated approach to peritoneal carcinomatosis is based on the change of paradigm introduced by Paul Sugarbaker, who considers this abnormality as a locoregional disease in which only the abdominal compartment is involved.[1] Following this

Department of GI Surgery, Regina Elena National Cancer Institute, Via Elio Chianesi 53, Rome 00144, Italy
* Corresponding author.
E-mail address: garofalo@ifo.it

Surg Oncol Clin N Am 21 (2012) 515–531
http://dx.doi.org/10.1016/j.soc.2012.07.005
1055-3207/12/$ – see front matter © 2012 Elsevier Inc. All rights reserved.

approach, and carrying out an accurate assessment of locoregional tumor burden, patients can be selected for treatment with a procedure that combines surgery (peritonectomy) and hyperthermic intraperitoneal chemotherapy (HIPEC).

The first step of selection consists in excluding from the integrated treatment all the patients with hematogenous metastases in the extra-abdominal districts and with nonresectable liver metastases.

Of paramount importance is the qualitative and quantitative assessment of locoregional tumor burden and the forecast of the extent of resection needed to achieve complete cytoreduction; the main purpose of this assessment is to select for treatment those patients who can achieve a real improvement in survival, also carefully evaluating the operative risk.[2]

Peritonectomy + HIPEC, when a complete cytoreduction is accomplished, permits an overall survival (OS) and a disease-free survival (DFS) that cannot be achieved by any other kind of treatment.[3–7]

DIAGNOSIS AND EXCLUSION OF PATIENTS WITH EXTRAREGIONAL DISEASE OR HIGH PERITONEAL CANCER INDEX: IMAGING

The first role of imaging is to rule out the presence of distant metastases in extra-abdominal areas, which is an absolute criterion of exclusion. The lesions pertaining to peritoneal carcinomatosis can be demonstrated directly through ultrasonography, computed tomography (CT), magnetic resonance imaging (MRI), and ^{18}F-fluorodeoxyglucose (FDG) positron emission tomography (PET)/CT.

Ultrasonography is useful in detecting ascites, large abdominal masses, or liver metastases. CT gives valid topographic representation of the abdominal cavity and a precise definition of site, type, and extent of the pathologic process.

The main findings for peritoneal carcinomatosis on CT scan are focal or diffuse thickening of peritoneal folds, appearing as sclerotic, jelly-like, reticular, reticulonodular, nodular, or in large plaques. According to such an appearance, it is possible to identify different types of peritoneal carcinomatosis, namely infiltrative, micronodular (miliary), and macronodular (nodous) forms, with some overlapping among them.

Nodular or plaque lesions can show various levels of enhancement after intravenous injection of contrast media, or even a little attenuation, with cyst-like appearance; sometimes it is possible to see calcification deposits inside the lesions.

Mesenteric involvement is often of the sclerotic type, with thickening and retracted appearance of the single layers. In the greater omentum it is often possible to see reticular/micronodular, or a nodular aspect and/or large plaques, in some cases where a huge and thick neoplastic tissue layer of inhomogeneous density is located between the abdominal wall and the bowel loops ("omental cake").

Chances of identifying nodular lesions depend on the anatomic location; small nodules (<5 mm) are more easily recognized on the surfaces of liver or spleen.

Image visualization on different planes (multiplanar reconstruction sagittal, coronal, oblique) can help in searching for lesions on curved structures such as diaphragm, paracolic gutters, and small-intestine loops.

Small-bowel and large-bowel loops can be warped and attached to each other, capable of causing stenosis and mechanical intestinal obstruction. Ascites is present in more than 70% of cases, free or entrapped; CT scan can demonstrate free ascites if the amount is more than 50 mL. In the upper part of the abdomen the fluids collect first in the hepatorenal space and in the subphrenic right and left spaces; in the lower part the initial collection is in the Douglas pouch, then around urinary bladder and in paracolic gutters.

Primary tumor can also be identified (if it has not yet been surgically removed); if not possible, the synchronous peritoneal lesion can be assumed as primary, or a spread from an extra-abdominal focus (eg, breast cancer, melanoma) might be hypothesized.

In the differential diagnosis, some rare diseases causing similar lesions should be considered: tuberculous peritonitis, mesenteric panniculitis, diffuse peritoneal leiomyomatosis, and extramedullary hematopoiesis.

Pseudomyxoma peritonei can grow close to the original lesions (localized form) or spread to most of the peritoneal surface (diffuse form). CT shows solid, inhomogeneous tissue, mostly hypodense, localized around the peritoneal sides, which usually appears thickened by the irritating action of mucin; ascites is often present. As for peritoneal carcinomatosis, even a pseudomyxoma peritonei fibrotic reaction can cause adhesions with obstruction of the intestinal transit.

CT can help in the evaluation of intra-abdominal metastatic diffusion, and in choosing the best treatment option when involvement of liver or head of pancreas is present and when the mesenteric root is grossly infiltrated; in the preoperative evaluation of the peritoneal cancer index (PCI),[8] it shows 88% sensitivity and 12% accuracy. CT shows low sensitivity in assessing small-bowel lesions (8%–17%), which decreases to 11% for lesions smaller than 5 mm in all quadrants with a significant underestimation of clinical PCI.[1,8]

When the CT scan is positive, mainly in patients with bulky tumors, its specificity reaches 100% in all regions.[9–11] CT is very helpful during the early postoperative period because it can identify complications such as fluid collections, abscesses, perforations, fistulae, and pancreatitis.

Magnetic nuclear resonance shows no advantages when compared with CT in the evaluation of PCI and in the prediction of achievable cytoreduction index.

^{18}F-FDG PET, if used alone, underestimates PC. ^{18}F-FDG PET/CT shows instead 90% sensitivity and preoperative specificity of 77% for degree II and III lesions; nevertheless it underestimates small lesions in all locations, when the size of the nodules is less than 5 mm.[12,13] In the follow-up period, CT can detect early recurrences, even if a differential diagnosis between true relapses and fibrotic scars caused by treatments is often difficult; in these patients ^{18}F-FDG PET/CT can help to make a differential diagnosis.

Usually ^{18}F-FDG PET/CT is positive after completeness of cytoreduction index grade 2 (CC2) to CC3 and negative after CC0 to CC1.[4]

Not all histologic types show good glucose uptake at ^{18}F-FDG PET/CT; it could therefore be advisable to perform a preoperative examination to assess the initial glucose uptake to exclude false negatives in the follow-up period of nonuptaking tumors. Recent studies showed that both CT and ^{18}F-FDG PET/CT were unable to give a correct staging of carcinomatosis. One may conclude that nowadays there is no noninvasive procedure that can correctly evaluate PCI and expected cytoreduction index after treatment, especially if the lesions are small (**Figs. 1** and **2**).[12,13]

INDICATIONS FOR INTEGRATED TREATMENT: LOCOREGIONAL STAGING

The first attempt at defining locoregional staging of peritoneal carcinomatosis was conducted by the Japanese, after the first studies completed in the 1990s about the association of surgery and locoregional chemotherapy for the treatment of locally advanced gastric cancer.

A staging format for carcinomatosis from gastric cancer was proposed:

- P1 (few nodules above the mesocolon)
- P2 (moderate amount of nodules even below transverse mesocolon)
- P3 (many spread nodules)

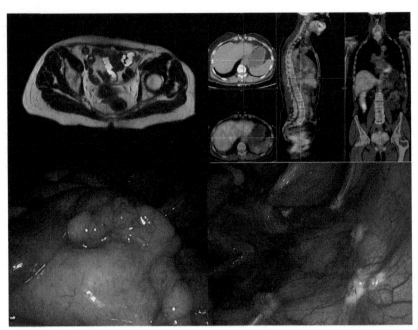

Fig. 1. Peritoneal carcinomatosis from duodenal cancer with negative MR and CT/PET imaging. The staging laparoscopy shows: PCI = 21, with positivity in sectors 9, 10, 11, and 12.

This classification is simple, shows a good prognostic value, with a 2-year survival rate that falls from 21% for P1 to 4% for P3 and, with slight modifications, can be used even for different forms of carcinomatosis; notwithstanding, it is not accurate enough concerning the distribution and localization of neoplastic lesions.

Gilly's classification is also very simple, but more modern:

- Stage 0: no macroscopic signs of disease
- Stage I: nodules smaller than 5 mm, confined to one abdominal region
- Stage II: nodules smaller than 5 mm, disseminated through the abdomen
- Stage III: size of nodules between 5 mm and 2 cm
- Stage IV: lesions larger than 2 cm

Even so, this classification is not detailed enough about the distribution of the lesions.

Sugarbaker's classification is more useful for both prognosis and research, and is based on the PCI (**Fig. 3**). The abdomen is divided into 9 sectors and the small bowel

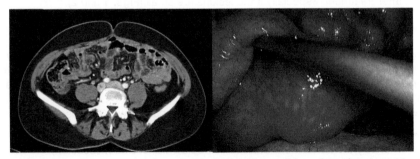

Fig. 2. Negative CT scan; staging laparoscopy highlights small bowel involvement.

Peritoneal Cancer Index

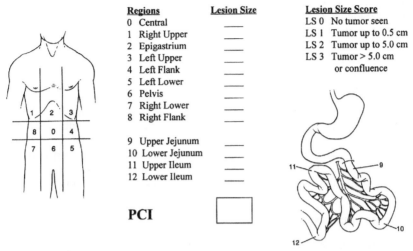

Regions	Lesion Size	Lesion Size Score
0 Central	____	LS 0 No tumor seen
1 Right Upper	____	LS 1 Tumor up to 0.5 cm
2 Epigastrium	____	LS 2 Tumor up to 5.0 cm
3 Left Upper	____	LS 3 Tumor > 5.0 cm
4 Left Flank	____	or confluence
5 Left Lower	____	
6 Pelvis	____	
7 Right Lower	____	
8 Right Flank	____	
9 Upper Jejunum	____	
10 Lower Jejunum	____	
11 Upper Ileum	____	
12 Lower Ileum	____	

PCI

Fig. 3. Peritoneal cancer index. (*From* Harmon RL, Sugarbaker PH. Prognostic indicators in peritoneal carcinomatosis from gastrointestinal cancer. Int Semin Surg Oncol 2005;2(1):3; with permission.)

into 4 more parts; for each sector a score is assigned (Lesion Size score [LS]) related to the actual disease:

- LS 0: no macroscopic evidence
- LS 1: maximum diameter of the lesions up to 0.5 cm
- LS 2: maximum diameter up to 5 cm
- LS 3: maximum diameter larger than 5 cm or confluent nodules

The total of the scores for all sectors gives the PCI.

Stage P1 to P2 of the Japanese classification is equivalent to Gilly's Stage I to II and to Sugarbaker's PCI of less than 13.

The expected achievement of CC0 remains, however, the main prognostic factor[14]: patients who achieve CC1 cytoreduction have a markedly worse outcome, whereas those classified as CC2 to CC3 show very poor results.

If one has to consider Peritonectomy + HIPEC as a curative treatment of peritoneal carcinomatosis, patients who cannot be classified as expected CC0 should be excluded from the procedure. CC1 cases (residual lesions between 0.25 and 2.5 mm) in HIPEC-responder patients can also be considered CC0 after cytoreduction. In CC1 HIPEC nonresponders, CC2, and CC3, the integrated treatment offers limited increase in OS but a marked improvement in quality of life; it can therefore be considered as advanced palliative surgery.

Histology of the primary tumor plays a crucial role in the selection of patients affected by peritoneal carcinomatosis, because it noticeably modifies the cutoff value of PCI during the decision-making process. Selection of patients cannot therefore leave out of consideration the following factors:

- PCI
- Histology of the primary tumor
- Expected CC index

These factors must be related to:

- Age
- Karnofsky Index
- Comorbidities (cardiovascular, respiratory)
- Carcinomatosis-related complications at the time of surgery (intestinal obstruction, ascites)
- Active infections
- Previous systemic chemotherapy, chemoresistance, toxicity
- Disease-free interval from previous surgery

Previous evaluation of resectable hepatic metastases and of possible involvement of other organs, such as pancreas, is mandatory, because an eventual pancreatic resection greatly increases morbidity.

Infiltration of small bowel and its mesentery by lesions that cannot be reduced to CC0 even after HIPEC (and therefore requiring surgical resection) can be treated, providing the remaining healthy small-bowel length is at least one-third of the total.[15–20]

ROLE OF STAGING LAPAROSCOPY

Video-laparoscopy (VLS) is considered an excellent diagnostic procedure, but its wide application in peritoneal carcinomatosis has been discouraged, the objections to this technique being related to:

- Difficulty of trocar positioning in the presence of abdominal wall tumor masses or adhesions from previous surgery
- Skepticism about the reliability and efficacy of the procedure in the staging phase
- Fear of neoplastic contamination of the port sites, supported by the finding of 52% of recurrences for pseudomyxoma peritonei along the surgical scar[21]

Notwithstanding the aforementioned considerations, in their extensive experience the authors have documented a possibility of trocar positioning near 100% (even in patients with multiple previous surgery), the absolute reliability of VLS staging, and the complete absence of neoplastic contamination of the abdominal wall around the port sites, if trocars are inserted using a standardized technique.[20,22,23]

Since the beginning of their experience in 2000, the authors have related the information from VLS staging with PCI with the possibility of obtaining complete cytoreduction. Using this methodology, almost one-half of the patients were excluded from the treatment, many of them being submitted to a second staging laparoscopy after systemic neoadjuvant chemotherapy.

LAPAROSCOPY IN THE STAGING OF PERITONEAL CARCINOMATOSIS

Main aim of laparoscopic staging is to carefully assess the patient's prognosis and the surgical feasibility, considering that the simple surgical exploration is often dangerous in such patients: in advanced abdominal tumors treated with laparotomy alone morbidity from 12% to 23% and mortality from 20% to 36% have been reported.[2]

Diagnostic imaging (CT and CT/PET) is still considered the first and mandatory diagnostic test for peritoneal carcinomatosis: when imaging-based PCI is in favor of enrolling the patient for treatment, VLS staging allows assessment of the true PCI, granting a correct selection of patients according to the expected CC index and a cost/benefit assessment in terms of DFS, OS, and quality of life.

Surgical Technique

The Hasson trocar is introduced and the ascites completely sucked out of the peritoneal cavity, taking care not to contaminate the port sites.

Considering the high incidence of adhesions both from previous surgery and from tumor masses infiltrating the midline, the choice is to avoid median or paraumbilical access; the authors prefer a trocar positioned in the right or left flank or iliac fossa on the mid-axillary line after carrying out clinical evaluation and ultrasound scan of the considered quadrants.

This access allows for a better exposure of the small bowel and its mesentery even in presence of a large omental cake; it also offers the possibility of improving visualization by inserting a second trocar (5 mm) beneath the first one or in the contralateral iliac fossa.

A 30° scope is routinely used; division of adhesions should be kept to a minimum to avoid the risk of lesions to abdominal organs, but should be enough for a complete evaluation of the PCI. In case of tenacious adhesions or neoplastic infiltrations of the median line, it is advisable to explore the right and left sections separately and to carry out a second open access to view the quadrants of the opposite side.

Cytology samples should be taken under direct view. Highly mucinous carcinomatosis sometimes requires a 10-mm trocar in port II to admit insertion of a larger suction cannula. In peritoneal surface malignancies where the pathologic findings are unknown or doubtful, it is important to collect multiple biopsy specimens from the parietal, omental, and pelvic cavity lesions. Diaphragmatic biopsies can cause perforation and infiltration of the muscular wall and should be avoided. When liver metastases or the involvement of major hepatic veins are suspected, as in diaphragmatic lesions larger than 2 cm, VLS ultrasound imaging can be helpful.

To accomplish the laparoscopic definition of PCI, which is determined on the basis of the distribution and size of the tumor nodules, the operating table has to be moved into at least 4 positions: steep anti-Trendelenburg left tilt, steep anti-Trendelenburg right tilt, steep Trendelenburg left tilt, and steep Trendelenburg right tilt.[20]

Personal Experience and Results

The authors' group performed 351 diagnostic VLS procedures in patients with peritoneal surface malignancies (**Table 1**). The average time needed for a diagnostic and staging VLS procedure was 30 minutes (range 15–45 minutes). In one patient the access to the abdominal cavity was impossible because of thick cancerous adhesions between the small-bowel loops and the abdominal wall: this patient underwent midline laparotomy, which confirmed the impossibility of reaching into the abdominal cavity because of massive involvement of the small-intestine loops tightly adherent to the abdominal wall.

In 335 cases, 2 trocars (10 mm and 5 mm, respectively) were enough to carry out the procedure, whereas in 13 cases a third 10-mm trocar was necessary to gain a full view of the abdominal cavity.

In 121 patients the primary tumor was ovarian, in 76 gastric, in 73 recurrent colorectal, in 10 recurrent pancreatic, in 8 cancer of the uterine cervix, and in 1 prostatic; 24 patients had pseudomyxoma peritonei syndrome from appendiceal adenocarcinoma, 14 were affected by mesothelioma, 6 by abdominal sarcomatosis, and 2 by intra-abdominal desmoplastic small round cell tumors. In 15 patients carcinomatosis was the peritoneal progression of a primary breast tumor.

In 5 cases (1.42%) VLS understaged the carcinomatosis (1 mesothelioma, 2 gastric cancers, 1 pseudomyxoma, and 1 ovarian tumor) and, at laparotomy, massive infiltration of the pancreas was detected in gastric cancer and mesothelioma, which resulted in a CC2 peritonectomy. In the pseudomyxoma and ovarian cancer the value of VLS PCI

Table 1
Personal experience of staging laparoscopy in peritoneal surface malignancy

Pathology	Cases	Diagnostic	Unfeasible	Understaging	2-Trocar	3-Trocar	Site Infection	Bleeding	Bowel Perforation	Diaphragm Perforation
Ovary	121	121		2	120	1			1	
Stomach	76	75	1	1	70	8	1			1
Colon-rectum	73	73			71	3	1	1		
Appendix cancer	24	24		1	24					
Breast	15	15			15					
Mesothelioma	14	14		1	14					
Pancreas	10	10			1	9				1
Uterus	8	8			8					
Sarcoma	6	6			6					
DIRCT	2	2			2					
Prostate	1	1			1					
Duodenum	1	1			1					
Total	351	350	1	5	333	21	2	1	1	1
%	100	99.72	0.28	1.42	94.87	6.02	0.57	0.28	0.28	0.28

Abbreviation: DIRCT, desmoplastic intrabdominal round cells tumor.

was lower than open-surgery PCI, but it was nonetheless possible to carry out a CC0 cytoreduction.

In 244 cases (69.5%) advanced carcinomatosis was found with PCI greater than 17: in 62 cases PCI was in the range 0 to 13, in 22 between 14 and 16, in 87 between 17 and 23, in 95 between 24 and 33, and in 85 between 34 and 39. One hundred four patients were excluded from surgical exploration because of massive infiltration of the small bowel or its mesentery basis detected by VLS.

Of patients on whom a diagnostic VLS procedure was performed, 250 of 351 (71.22%) had had at least one previous laparotomy. One hundred seventy-six (50.1%) patients were treated with peritonectomy and HIPEC. Four (2%) patients, who were not eligible for a peritonectomy because of massive infiltration of the small bowel and occlusion, underwent a VLS decompressive ileostomy.

Regarding morbidity, in VLS surgical exploration 5 complications were observed (1.4%), 2 of which (0.56%) were intraoperative: one was a perforation of the diaphragm during biopsy, sutured with laparoscopic technique, whereas the other patient sustained early postoperative bleeding treated by a blood transfusion. Of the remaining 3, 2 (0.56%) showed delayed postoperative infections of the trocar site, treated by topical antibiotic therapy; 1 patient (0.28%) had a small-bowel perforation that was sutured through the port site. No neoplastic seeding was detected at the trocar sites, and all patients who underwent peritonectomy showed negative results regarding port-site metastasis 10 to 40 days after the procedure. No mortality was observed.

Points of Strength

- Evaluation of the small-bowel mesentery (superficial lesions and retractions) (**Fig. 5**)
- Evaluation of all the sectors according to the PCI scoring system (**Fig. 4**)
- Evaluation of small-bowel lesions on the antimesenteric margin (see **Fig. 5**)
- Evaluation of the omental bursa, pelvic cavity, diaphragm, and abdominal wall
- Possibility of peritoneal washing and biopsies for defining the histology of the primary tumor
- Predictive evaluation of the CC index following peritonectomy

Points of Weakness

- Evaluation of the thickness of lesions of the diaphragm
- Evaluation of pancreatic involvement

These issues have been overtaken by coupling VLS examination with VLS ultrasonography.

Indications

- Staging of a carcinomatosis already diagnosed via imaging technology (CT, MRI)
- Staging of a carcinomatosis of unknown origin (biopsy)
- Restaging following neoadjuvant chemotherapy
- Restaging during follow-up in case of dubious imaging
- Restaging following adjuvant chemotherapy

The use of VLS staging as a second look for patients who have already undergone a peritonectomy is not easy, because the presence of adhesions might not allow for a comprehensive evaluation of an eventual relapse nor a good evaluation of all abdominal quadrants. Nevertheless, the presence of ascites often facilitates the insertion of the trocars, provided that ^{18}F-FDG PET/CT gives sufficient information about the origin and entity of the relapse and its possible treatment.

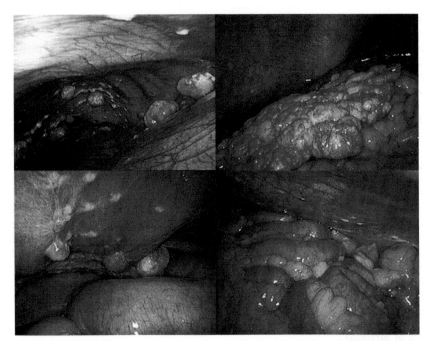

Fig. 4. Complete staging laparoscopy: peritoneal carcinomatosis from colonic cancer.

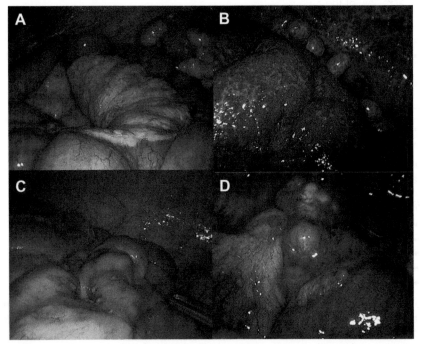

Fig. 5. Small bowel involvement. (*A*) Massive mesenterial infiltration. (*B*) Micronodular infiltration antimesenteric margin. (*C*) Micronodular infiltration of bowel mesentery. (*D*) Macronodular infiltration of bowel mesentery.

Algorithm of the Decision-Making Process for a Correct Indication for Radical Cytoreductive Surgery Based on Laparoscopic Staging

Step 1: Rule out the absolute criteria of exclusion

- Mesenteric root infiltrated or not liable to a complete cytoreduction
- Pancreatic capsule massively infiltrated, not liable to a complete cytoreduction, or requiring major pancreatic resections
- Expected small-bowel resection for more than one-third of the whole length
- Liver metastases: more than 3 on the same lobe, or multiple bilateral, unresectable

Step 2: Determination of relative inclusion criteria

- Ratio between PCI and histology (natural history of the primary)
- Possibility of downstaging by line of systemic chemotherapy

Step 3: Final decision about the possibility of reaching CC0 based on the following:

Ruling out Absolute Exclusion Criteria

+

Relative Inclusion Criteria (ratio between PCI and histology of the primary)

=

Possibility of reaching CC0

The "Small Bowel Factor"

A critical review of the authors' experiences allows some conclusions to be reached.

In the sectors 0 to 8, notwithstanding 59,049 possible combinations of scores of the single sectors, it is theoretically almost always possible to achieve stage CC0 even with the highest PCI (lesions larger than 2.5 cm or merging lesions).

The situation changes when sectors from 9 to 12 (those pertaining to the small bowel in Sugarbaker's classification) are analyzed. Drawing on a mathematical model that considers cytoreduction chances for these 4 sectors, the authors obtained 256 possible combinations. Among all these, only in 68 groups (27%) will it be possible to achieve CC0; in 106 (41%) it will only be possible to achieve CC1 or CC2; while in the remaining 82 combinations (32%) only CC3 will be achieved, or surgery will be impossible.

Because it is possible to reach CC0 only in fewer than 30% of cases in the sectors 9 to 13, the degree of involvement of small bowel turns out to be the true cutoff point about chances to achieve CC0; once pancreatic infiltration and multiple nonresectable hepatic metastases are excluded, the correct evaluation of lesions of the small bowel and its mesentery remains the main goal.[24]

If one considers that imaging techniques show low specificity in the evaluation of these sectors, VLS can be considered essential to the achievement of the correct indication to peritonectomy + HIPEC and the only way to have a correct forecast of the expected degree of cytoreduction.

LAPAROSCOPY IN THE TREATMENT OF PERITONEAL CARCINOMATOSIS
Operative Laparoscopy

Recent studies describe the treatment of a small number of patients with minimal carcinomatosis by laparoscopic peritonectomy + HIPEC,[25,26] showing that it is possible to use this procedure in carefully selected cases. The authors are of the opinion that the methodology deserves further studies in larger series of patients, with special attention paid to the association of cytoreductive surgery to HIPEC because, at least theoretically, the spread of neoplastic cells at the induction of pneumoperitoneum could be wide, resulting in a higher risk of diffusion of a minimal carcinomatosis.

Laparoscopy in the Treatment of Refractory Ascites

Laparoscopy in the restaging of peritoneal carcinomatosis allows the use of a peritonectomy procedure in responders to adjuvant and neoadjuvant chemotherapy; on the other hand, a reevaluation of nonresponders brought to consideration a group of patients with debilitating intractable ascites, with a very poor quality of life. Thirty-three patients underwent hyperthermic intraperitoneal chemotherapy for the palliation of ascites through a minimally invasive approach.[27–30]

Methods

A Hasson trocar was inserted in the right or left pararectal area through a 1-cm incision, taking care not to contaminate the abdominal wall with ascites. The ascites was completely sucked out of the peritoneal cavity through the trocar before insufflation with CO_2. After positioning the 30° 5-mm scope under direct vision, a second 5-mm trocar was introduced in the contralateral iliac fossa. When deemed necessary, release of adhesions was performed to grant free access to the abdominal cavity. If extended adhesiolysis was considered too dangerous, only few adhesions were divided to ensure communication between all abdominal quadrants and to allow free contact of the hyperthermic chemotherapy with all the peritoneal surfaces. Then 3 additional 5-mm trocars were sequentially placed on the right and left side into the free iliac fossa.

A 5-mm grasper was passed out from the peritoneal cavity through the 5-mm trocar to place closed-suction drains into the pelvic cavity and into the right and left subdiaphragmatic spaces. These 3 suctioning drains were connected together to provide a single outflow. The 5-mm trocars were removed and an infusion trocar was placed directly through the 10-mm site where the camera had been inserted. To make the peritoneal space watertight, all drains were secured with a purse-string suture to the skin and connected to the perfusion machine, which was set at an inflow temperature of 43° to 44°C. The aim was to achieve an average temperature of 42°C in the whole peritoneal cavity (**Fig. 6**). The temperature of the infusion was measured by 2 probes, located at the inflow site and at the junction between the 3 outflow drains. The patient's body temperature was monitored by 3 additional probes placed over the skin, in the external ear canal, rectum, and bladder. The average length of laparoscopic preparation was 45 minutes, with a range of 30 to 120 minutes depending on the extent of adhesiolysis.

To allow the spread of the chemotherapy solution throughout the whole peritoneal surface, the tilt of the operating table was changed at 15-minute intervals during perfusion as follows:

1. Straight
2. Trendelenburg + left tilt
3. Trendelenburg + right tilt
4. Straight
5. Reverse Trendelenburg + left tilt
6. Reverse Trendelenburg + right tilt[31]

After a 90-minute perfusion, the chemotherapy agent was recovered and washed out with 2000 mL of 1.5% dextrose. The drains were connected to gravity bags and

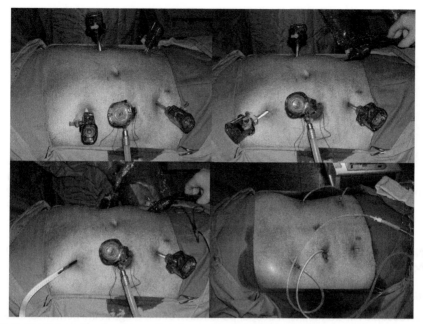

Fig. 6. Treatment of refractory ascites. Laparoscopic HIPEC procedure.

removed postoperatively, when the amount drained was small enough. After removing all drains, the patient was discharged from the hospital.

The drugs used were cisplatin, 50 mg/m^2 and doxorubicin, 15 mg/m^2 for ascites due to ovarian cancer, peritoneal mesothelioma, or breast cancer. In ascites from rectal colon and stomach cancer mitomycin, 12.5 mg/m^2, was used. The volume of perfusion given was 2000 mL and consisted of a peritoneal dialysis solution containing 1.5% dextrose. Fresh frozen plasma (1200 mL) was infused during perfusion. Furosemide was administered along with intravenous fluids to maintain a diuresis of 400 mL/h.[28]

Results
Among the 33 patients treated, the cause of malignant ascites was untreatable peritoneal carcinomatosis from gastric cancer in 12 cases, colon cancer in 7, breast lobular cancer in 5, ovarian cancer in 6, and mesothelioma in 3. In all cases a complete disappearance of the ascites within 9 days after the procedure was observed. The average postoperative increase in the Karnofsky index was 20 points. Even though the treatment was palliative, the disappearance of the refractory ascites had an impact on average survival rate, which in this series averaged 152 days (range 21–796 days). The longest survival times were observed in 3 of 5 cases of breast lobular cancer (807, 736, and 216 days) and in a case of mesothelioma (726 days) (**Fig. 7**), whereas the shortest survival times were observed in patients with gastric cancer. Follow-up ultrasonography or CT 1 month after the laparoscopic HIPEC revealed complete resolution of ascites in 31 of the 33 patients; 1 patient died on the 21st postoperative day, free from ascites. In one case a CT scan 1 year later showed a small, clinically undetectable, fluid effusion in the pelvis. In 2 cases of coexisting neoplastic intestinal obstruction, a laparoscopic ileostomy was performed before the hyperthermic intraperitoneal chemotherapy procedure.

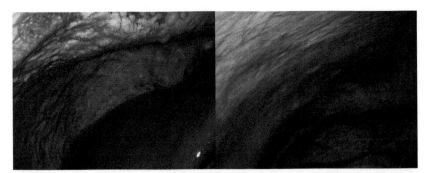

Fig. 7. Mesothelioma patient with PCI = 39, with recurrent ascites 359 days after laparoscopic HIPEC; the patient underwent a second procedure and is still alive after 726 days. The nodular lesions switched to confluent thin plaques, with unchanged PCI, but without signs of disease progression.

No intraoperative or postoperative complications and no mortality related to the procedure were observed.[32,33]

Rationale of Palliative Treatment of Refractory Ascites with HIPEC

Laparoscopic HIPEC results in deeper penetration of the drugs in the peritoneal layers and tumor nodules. In the absence of cytoreductive surgery, during the palliative laparoscopic HIPEC procedures one can assume that the direct cytotoxic effect of this single chemotherapy instillation will be limited: heated chemotherapy is able to eradicate only some layers of cancer cells, with penetration on all the peritoneal surface. As a result of this process a thin layer of fibrosis may develop, which directs the cancerous fluid into the capillary bed and, from there, into the systemic circulation, determining a resolution of the problematic collection of ascites.[27–30,34]

Peritoneal sclerosis and induction of dense adhesions are possibly the major factor regarding the effectiveness of this technique. Ozols and colleagues,[32,35] in their phase I study, reported sclerotizing peritonitis and subsequent pain at the dose-limiting factor of 18 μM when performing intracavitary chemotherapy with doxorubicin in patients with advanced ovarian cancer. The absence of major complications and treatment-related mortality in the patients studied herein suggests that laparoscopic HIPEC is a safe technique. Such treatment is to be considered palliative for untreatable ascites and must be performed exclusively on patients with peritoneal carcinomatosis who are not eligible for peritonectomy with HIPEC.

The treatment's goal is to improve the Karnofsky index, ultimately having some impact on the patient's quality of life. With this perspective in mind, even some patients affected by peritoneal carcinomatosis from lobular breast cancer were treated.

SUMMARY

In the treatment strategy of peritoneal carcinomatosis, VLS is located at the beginning of a critical path of analysis to classify the patient and provide a correct indication for integrated treatment. The technique is safe and reliable, does not lead to major complications and mortality, and is the only presidium that allows for correct staging of peritoneal carcinomatosis and a correct forecast of the expected CC0.

Laparoscopic peritonectomy might be used in minimal carcinomatosis, with PCI confined to 1 or 2 sectors and well-defined histologic types (carcinoma of appendix).

At present, there are no comparative data with open surgery; it is not yet possible, therefore, to consider the former as a gold standard in minimal carcinomatosis.

The use of laparoscopy as treatment is indicated in refractory malignant ascites not suitable for surgery by HIPEC. This method shows encouraging results regarding both the ascites and the improvement in the Karnofsky Index.

REFERENCES

1. Sugarbaker PH. Surgical treatment of peritoneal carcinomatosis: Du Pont Lecture. Can J Surg 1989;32:164–70.
2. Esquivel J, Farinetti A, Sugarbaker PH. Elective surgery in recurrent colon cancer with peritoneal seeding: when and when not to proceed. G Chir 1999;20(3):81–6 [in Italian].
3. Glehen O, Bakrin N, Passot G. Peritoneal carcinomatosis from appendiceal cancer: early adequate therapeutic management for long-term survival. Ann Surg Oncol 2011;18(6):1522–3.
4. Sugarbaker PH. Second-look surgery for colorectal cancer: revised selection factors and new treatment options for greater success. Int J Surg Oncol 2011; 91:5078.
5. Cavaliere F, Valle M, De Simone M, et al. 120 peritoneal carcinomatoses from colorectal cancer treated with peritonectomy and intra-abdominal chemohyperthermia: a S.I.T.I.L.O. multicentric study. In Vivo 2006;20(6A):747–50.
6. Cavaliere F, De Simone M, Virzì S, et al. Prognostic factors and oncologic outcome in 146 patients with colorectal peritoneal carcinomatosis treated with cytoreductive surgery combined with hyperthermic intraperitoneal chemotherapy: Italian multicentric study S.I.T.I.L.O. Eur J Surg Oncol 2011;37(2):148–54.
7. Glehen O, Kwiatkowski F, Sugarbaker PH, et al. Cytoreductive surgery combined with perioperative intraperitoneal chemotherapy for management of peritoneal carcinomatosis from colorectal cancer: a multi-institutional study. J Clin Oncol 2004;22(16):3284–92.
8. Harmon RL, Sugarbaker PH. Prognostic indicators in peritoneal carcinomatosis from gastrointestinal cancer. Int Semin Surg Oncol 2005;2(1):3.
9. Esquivel J, Chua TC, Stojadinovic A, et al. Accuracy and clinical relevance of computed tomography scan interpretation of peritoneal cancer index in colorectal cancer peritoneal carcinomatosis: a multi-institutional study. J Surg Oncol 2010;102:565–70.
10. Koh JL, Tristan DY, Glenn D, et al. Evaluation of preoperative computed tomography in estimating peritoneal cancer index in colorectal peritoneal carcinomatosis. Ann Surg Oncol 2009;16:327–33.
11. Denzer U, Hoffmann S, Helmreich-Becker I, et al. Minilaparoscopy in the diagnosis of peritoneal tumor spread: prospective controlled comparison with computed tomography. Surg Endosc 2004;18(7):1067–70.
12. Pfannemberg C, Koenisgrainer C, Aschoff P, et al. Carcinomatosis for cytoreductive surgery and hypertonic intraperitoneal chemotherapy. Ann Surg Oncol 2009; 16:1295–303.
13. Passot G, Glehen AB, Pellet O, et al. Pseudomyxoma peritonei: role of 18-FDG PET in preoperative evaluation of pathological grade and potential for complete cytoreduction. Eur J Surg Oncol 2010;36(3):315–23.
14. Elias D, Honoré C, Dumont F, et al. Results of systematic second-look surgery plus HIPEC in asymptomatic patients presenting a high risk of developing colorectal peritoneal carcinomatosis. Ann Surg 2011;254(2):289–93.

15. Pisa P, Dahike MH, Ghali N, et al. Multimodality treatment of peritoneal carcinomatosis from colorectal cancer: first results of a new German centre for peritoneal surface malignancies. Int J Colorectal Dis 2007;22(11):1295–300.

16. Capone A, Valle M, Proietti D, et al. Postoperative infections in cytoreductive surgery with hyperthermic intraperitoneal intraoperative chemotherapy for peritoneal carcinomatosis. J Surg Oncol 2007;96(6):507–13.

17. Yan TD, Links M, Fransi S, et al. Learning curve for cytoreductive surgery and hyperthermic intraperitoneal chemotherapy for peritoneal surface malignancy. A journey to becoming a nationally funded peritonectomy centre. Ann Surg Oncol 2007;14(8):2270–80.

18. Sugarbaker PH. Reported impact of cytoreductive surgery and hyperthermic intraperitoneal chemotherapy on systemic toxicity. Ann Surg Oncol 2008;15(6):1800–1.

19. Zappa L, Sugarbaker PH. Compartment syndrome of the leg associated with lithotomy position for cytoreductive surgery. J Surg Oncol 2007;96(7):619–23.

20. Valle M, Garofalo A. Laparoscopic staging of peritoneal surface malignancies. Eur J Surg Oncol 2006;32(6):625–7.

21. Zoetmulder FA, Sugarbaker PH. Pattern of failure following treatment of pseudomyxoma peritonei of appendiceal origin. Eur J Cancer 1996;10:1727–33.

22. Garofalo A, Valle M. Staging video laparoscopy of peritoneal carcinomatosis. Tumori 2003;89(Suppl 4):70–7.

23. Valle M, Garofalo A. Video laparoscopic staging of peritoneal surface malignancies: a new technique of PCI (Peritoneal Cancer Index) definition. 80 consecutive cases: result. 4th International Workshop on peritoneal surface malignancies Madrid. 2004.

24. Benizri EI, Bernard JL, Rahili A, et al. Small bowel involvement is a prognostic factor in colorectal carcinomatosis treated with complete cytoreductive surgery plus hyperthermic intraperitoneal chemotherapy. World J Surg Oncol 2012;10:56.

25. Esquivel J, Averbach A. Combined laparoscopic cytoreductive surgery and hyperthermic intraperitoneal chemotherapy in a patient with peritoneal mesothelioma. J Laparoendosc Adv Surg Tech A 2009;19(4):505–7.

26. Esquivel J, Averbach A, Chua TC. Laparoscopic cytoreductive surgery and hyperthermic intraperitoneal chemotherapy in patients with limited peritoneal surface malignancies: feasibility, morbidity and outcome in an early experience. Ann Surg 2011;253(4):764–8.

27. Valle M, Garofalo A, Federici O, et al. Laparoscopic intraperitoneal antiblastic hyperthermic chemoperfusion in the treatment of refractory neoplastic ascites. Preliminary results. Suppl Tumori 2005;4(3):5122–3.

28. Garofalo A, Valle M, Garcia J, et al. Laparoscopic intraperitoneal hyperthermic chemotherapy for palliation of debilitating malignant ascites. Eur J Surg Oncol 2006;32(6):682–5.

29. Valle M, Van Der Speeten K, Garofalo A. Laparoscopic hyperthermic intraperitoneal peroperative chemotherapy (HIPEC) in the management of refractory malignant ascites: a multi-institutional retrospective analysis in 52 patients. J Surg Oncol 2009;100(4):331–4.

30. Facchiano E, Risio D, Kianmanesh R, et al. Laparoscopic hyperthermic intraperitoneal chemotherapy: indications, aims and results: a systematic review of the literature. Ann Surg Oncol 2012. [Epub ahead of print].

31. Garofalo A, Valle M. Laparoscopy in the management of peritoneal carcinomatosis. Cancer J 2009;15(3):190–5.

32. Di Giorgio A, Naticchiami E, Biacchi D, et al. Cytoreductive surgery (peritonectomy procedures) combined with hyperthermic intraperitoneal chemotherapy

(HIPEC) in the treatment of diffuse peritoneal carcinomatosis from ovarian cancer. Cancer 2008;113(2):315–25.

33. Rasmussen PC, Laurberg S. New treatment of peritoneal carcinomatosis from colorectal cancer. Cytoreductive surgery and hyperthermic intraperitoneal chemotherapy. Ugeskr Laeger 2007;169(38):3179–81.

34. Facchiano E, Scaringi S, Kianmanesh R, et al. Laparoscopic hyperthermic intra-peritoneal chemotherapy (HIPEC) for the treatment of malignant ascites secondary to unresectable peritoneal carcinomatosis from advanced gastric cancer. Eur J Surg Oncol 2008;34(2):154–8.

35. Ozols RF, Young RC, Speyer JL, et al. Phase I study and pharmacological studies of adriamycin administered intraperitoneally to patients with ovarian cancer. Cancer Res 1982;42:4265–9.

Anesthesia Considerations During Cytoreductive Surgery and Hyperthermic Intraperitoneal Chemotherapy

Kenneth P. Rothfield, MD[a,b,]*, Kathy Crowley, CRNA[a]

KEYWORDS

- Cytoreductive surgery • Heated intraperitoneal chemotherapy
- Anesthestic management • Goal-directed fluid therapy • Hemodynamic monitoring
- Colloids • Crystalloids • Third spacing

KEY POINTS

- Cytoreductive surgery with hyperthermic intraperitoneal chemotherapy (HIPEC) is an extensive, invasive procedure that presents unique physiologic challenges.
- During the HIPEC portion of the surgery, patients develop a hyperdynamic state.
- A balanced approach to fluid management, which incorporates both crystalloids and colloids, is encouraged.
- Hemodynamic monitoring with estimation of cardiac output is useful for optimizing organ perfusion while preventing fluid overload.
- To avoid renal injury by chemotherapeutic agents, urine output should be maintained at a high rate during that phase of the procedure.
- Thoracic epidural anesthesia improves analgesia and facilitates early mobilization of patients.

INTRODUCTION

Cytoreductive surgery with hyperthermic intraperitoneal chemotherapy (HIPEC) plays an increasingly important role in the management of patients with a variety of malignancies. These complex procedures subject patients not only to the usual physiologic challenges associated with major surgery, but also to the thermal stress induced by the

Conflict of interest: Dr Rothfield: Speakers Bureau: Hospira, Inc, and Cheetah Medical, Inc. Ms. Crowley: Nil.
[a] Department of Anesthesiology, Saint Agnes Hospital, 900 Caton Avenue, Baltimore, MD 21229, USA; [b] University of Maryland School of Nursing, Nurse Anesthesia Program, 655 West Lombard Street, Baltimore, MD 21201, USA
* Corresponding author. Department of Anesthesiology, Saint Agnes Hospital, 900 Caton Avenue, Baltimore, MD 21229.
E-mail address: krothfiel@stagnes.org

intraperitoneal instillation of heated chemotherapeutic solution. The surgery is complex, and not without complications.[1,2] Safety is therefore the primary goal. The formation of a specialized team, with close communication among anesthesia providers and surgical staff, enhances patient outcomes.[3,4] This article outlines an approach that has evolved over the past 6 years in more than 500 patients at our center, and provides an overview of the management of the surgical patient during the HIPEC procedure.

PREOPERATIVE EVALUATION

In addition to the usual preoperative evaluation of patients undergoing major abdominal surgery, special attention should be paid to a few conditions that may present additional challenges for the anesthesia provider. A thorough preoperative airway evaluation should be performed to avoid unexpected difficulty. Patients may have significant abdominal distention because of various combinations of tumor, mucus, and ascites; 10 to 15 L of pathologic fluid accumulation may be present. Increased abdominal volume and pressure decreases functional residual capacity, predisposing patients to both rapid oxygen desaturation and aspiration of gastric contents after induction of anesthesia.

Cardiac Risk

Because induced hyperthermia results in increased myocardial oxygen demand,[5] patients with preexisting coronary artery disease, heart failure, or other cardiac pathology may be at risk for hemodynamic decompensation. Similarly, patients with depressed left ventricular function may not be able to tolerate aggressive intraoperative volume therapy, which may precipitate pulmonary edema. For these reasons, cytoreductive surgery with HIPEC should be considered as a procedure that presents elevated cardiac risk. For patients with known cardiac disease or other risk factors, preoperative cardiac evaluation per American Heart Association guidelines is recommended.[6]

INTRAOPERATIVE MANAGEMENT
Induction

As previously noted, many patients presenting for HIPEC surgery are at risk for both oxygen desaturation and aspiration of gastric contents. Accordingly, rapid sequence induction is the preferred approach in this setting. In our institution, videolaryngoscopy is commonly used as a first-line technique for endotracheal intubation, and has greatly simplified airway management, even in the setting of anticipated difficult intubation.[7] Meticulous attention to patient positioning and padding of potential pressure sites is performed to decrease the risk of injury during these frequently lengthy procedures.

Hemodynamic Monitoring

In addition to routine monitors, a radial arterial line is placed for both hemodynamic monitoring and blood gas analysis. Our group, however, has recently reconsidered the necessity and utility of central venous monitoring. Central venous and pulmonary artery pressures are static measures, which do not accurately reflect volume status or volume responsiveness.[8,9] Furthermore, central venous lines expose patients to potential mechanical injury and serious infection, and are a well-recognized source of risk to patients undergoing HIPEC.[1] The routine placement of central venous lines, therefore, is no longer performed at our institution, unless indicated for vascular access.

Concerns regarding the safety and utility of invasive hemodynamic monitoring have spurred interest in less-invasive solutions. More recently, our group has used both minimally invasive pulse contour analysis (LiDCO Rapid, LiDCO, Ltd, Cambridge, England)

and noninvasive bioreactance devices[10,11] (NICOM, Cheetah Medical, Tel Aviv, Israel) for hemodynamic monitoring.

Pulse contour analysis monitoring has been previously described in the setting of HIPEC surgery.[12] Analysis of the arterial waveform obtained via a pressure transducer is used to generate estimates of stroke volume and cardiac output.[13] The NICOM (noninvasive cardiac output monitor) uses 2 pairs of electrodes placed around the heart to transmit and receive a 75-kHz signal placed across the thorax. Phasic blood flow in the descending thoracic aorta results in changes in reactance (the combined effect of inductance and capacitance) and phase angle shifts in the received signal. The electrical changes caused by aortic blood flow are translated using a computer algorithm to yield real-time estimates of stroke volume and cardiac output.

Both pulse contour and bioreactance estimates of cardiac output have acceptable clinical accuracy compared with pulmonary artery catheter, and may in fact be more responsive to sudden changes in loading conditions.[14,15] The accuracy of pulse contour analysis, however, may be impaired in patients with septic shock, vasoconstriction, or vasodilation, as changes in peripheral arterial tone may not reflect changes in aortic blood flow.[16]

Beat-to-beat changes in stroke volume induced by positive-pressure ventilation can be used as an estimate of volume responsiveness.[17] In the normal heart, positive-pressure ventilation causes changes in preload, which are exaggerated in the setting of hypovolemia.[18,19] Stroke volume variation (SVV) in the 12% to 13% range may reflect volume responsiveness.[16] Low stroke volume variation usually signifies euvolemia; however, there is substantial technical heterogeneity among the available hemodynamic monitors, and the true significance of elevated SVV may be questionable in some cases.[20] In some studies, pulse-pressure variation has been a more reliable indicator of preload responsiveness that SVV.[16] Additionally, patients with impaired systolic function tend to be more afterload than preload dependent, and may not exhibit increased stroke volume variability in the setting of hypovolemia. With the aforementioned caveats, the addition of dynamic measures of cardiac performance has enabled so-called goal (or flow) directed fluid therapy.

Management During Chemotherapy Infusion

Unique aspects of HIPEC surgery include hemodynamic alterations owing to induced hyperthermia, as well as the potential for nephrotoxicity secondary to the use of chemotherapeutic agents. Appropriate management of intravenous fluid therapy is critical for maintaining optimal end-organ perfusion, and avoiding renal injury. Attention must also be paid to electrolyte balance, coagulation, and the potential need for transfusion.

Hemodynamic Changes During HIPEC

During the intraperitoneal infusion of heated chemotherapeutic agents, patients develop a hyperdynamic, vasodilated circulatory state that is characterized by steady increase in heart rate and cardiac output that reaches its maximum between 70 to 80 minutes of the 90-minute heated chemotherapy phase. As the body temperature decreases after completion of the heated therapy, the hyperdynamic state begins to normalize, but may remain above baseline 10 minutes after the chemotherapeutic lavage is concluded.[21] When the closed abdomen technique is used, increased intra-abdominal pressure may decrease venous return, and further aggravate hemodynamic lability.

The details of these hemodynamic responses have described previously. Using esophageal Doppler to estimate cardiac output, Esquivel and colleagues[21] documented the effect of thermal stress with subsequent development of hyperdynamic circulatory state with increased cardiac output, decreased systemic vascular resistance, increased heart rate, and increased carbon dioxide production (**Box 1**). Although there may be a component of increased myocardial contractility, increases in cardiac output appear to be driven primarily by increased heart rate. Not surprisingly, perioperative complications may be related to acute change in body temperature and increased abdominal pressure.[5]

The use of long-acting antihypertensives is avoided because of the dynamic nature of the procedure. Heart rate is generally maintained at lower than 90 beats per minute. A cardioselective beta-blocker such as metoprolol administered in small increments provides adequate heart rate control without significant vasodilation. In accordance with recommendations by the American College of Cardiology and American Heart Association, patients on preoperative beta-blockers receive these medications perioperatively as well.[22]

Goal-Directed Fluid Management

Although it is tempting to assume that patients undergoing HIPEC surgery will require "massive" crystalloid replacement, it is perhaps more appropriate to substitute the word "meticulous." Fluid overload sets the stage for a variety of postoperative complications, notably pulmonary edema and adult respiratory distress syndrome.[1,23] Crystalloid restriction has been demonstrated to improve outcomes after major gastrointestinal surgery.[24] Our approach to fluid administration has gradually evolved from a traditional "cookbook" approach focused on aggressive, central venous pressure (CVP)-guided replacement of surgical "third-space" losses with crystalloids, to a more goal (flow)-directed strategy in which continuous measurement of cardiac index guides interventions, with a balance of colloids and crystalloids administered for specific therapeutic end points.[25] A recent meta-analysis of fluid management strategies in the setting of major surgery has demonstrated the superiority of goal-directed management over liberal fluid administration in promoting good perioperative outcomes.[26]

In addition to insensible losses (which are typically low) and hemorrhage, surgical patients may develop pathologic fluid accumulations, such as ascites and pleural effusions. Nonpathologic fluid accumulations associated with surgery are less well defined, although the concept of surgical "third spacing" is part of the conventional wisdom in both surgery and anesthesiology. The notion that tissue trauma creates a fluid-consuming third space is so basic a concept that it is presented at the introductory textbook level.[27] Indeed, in our early management strategies for HIPEC surgery, crystalloid administration of 10 to 15 mL/kg/h was routine. The validity of the concept of third spacing, however, has been recently challenged. Experimental preparations demonstrating the existence of the third space rely on radioactive tracer methodology. A review of these studies has revealed substantial flaws in this methodology, calling into question the existence of the "third space."[28]

Box 1
Hemodynamic changes associated with HIPEC

1. Increased cardiac output

2. Decreased systemic vascular resistance

3. Increased heart rate

4. Increased end-tidal CO_2

Unlike the third space, the volume-expanding effects of crystalloid solutions are well characterized. After 1 hour, only 200 mL of a 1-L crystalloid bolus remains in the intravascular space, with the remainder in the interstitium. This extravascular fluid has no volume-expanding effect, and may impair pulmonary function, and interfere with the healing of gut anastomoses. In extreme cases, perioperative weight gain secondary to crystalloids may be linked to increased mortality.[29] Finally, it should be noted that the administration of large volumes of any type of intravenous fluids may cause dilution of platelets and coagulation factors, resulting in clinically significant coagulopathy.

Currently at our institution, continuous noninvasive cardiac output monitoring, as well as urine output, is used to guide fluid administration throughout the procedure. The noninvasive nature of this monitoring confers several advantages. Baseline stroke volume index may be obtained before the induction of anesthesia, and volume responsiveness can be established by performing a passive leg raise test (PLR).[30,31] PLR causes an endogenous fluid challenge of approximately 200 mL, by moving blood normally sequestered in the calf veins into the central circulation. Patients with a 10% increase in cardiac index owing to position change are considered volume responsive. No response to PLR signifies euvolemia, or possibly depressed left ventricular function. During surgery, decreases in stroke volume index may occur because of hypovolemia, venodilation, blood loss, or decreases in venous return from mechanical causes. Fluid responsiveness is also suggested by increases in SVV. Initial therapy in this setting is generally a 500-mL colloid bolus with either 5% albumin or third-generation hydroxyethyl starch (Voluven, HES 130/0.4, Hospira, Inc, Lake Forest, IL, USA).[32] Transfusion with packed red blood cells is rarely necessary. In our experience, typical estimated blood loss averages 300 to 500 mL.

Both human derived and synthetic colloids provide 1:1 volume-expanding effects for several hours. Voluven is favored over first-generation hydroxyethyl starches (Hespan, Hextend) for a variety of reasons. Voluven is a small molecule that is more freely filtered by the kidney, resulting in substantially less plasma and tissue accumulation, and risk of nephrotoxicity.[33] In addition, its effect on Factor VIII and von Willebrand appear to be clinically insignificant.[34] Patients with substantial ascites or who require extensive surgical debulking are at risk for clinically significant protein losses.[35] Because of this, such patients may benefit from volume expansion with albumin as opposed to hydroxyethyl starch.

Renal Protection

Because some chemotherapeutic agents are nephrotoxic, maintenance of steady urine output is encouraged. Unfortunately, it is not known to what degree urine output must be maintained, and the link between intraoperative urine output and postoperative creatinine elevation is unclear.[36] At our institution, the goal is to maintain 100 mL every 15 minutes of urine output for the duration of the hyperthermic perfusion. In some patients, urine output of 50 to 75 mL every 15 minutes may be acceptable. In addition to ensuring euvolemia with administration of both colloid and crystalloids, low-dose dopamine infusion is initiated 15 to 30 minutes before infusion of mitomycin C, and is infused only for the 90 minutes of heated perfusion. Dopamine is a nonselective DA1 and DA2 agonist with multiple dose-related effects. Although dopamine may not afford additional renal protection per se, renal perfusion may be enhanced secondary to increased cardiac output, perfusion pressure, and renal blood flow.[37] Stimulation of DA1 receptors causes renal vasodilation as well as inhibition of active sodium transport in the proximal tubule, leading to natriuresis and dieresis, which is clinically reassuring.[38] Furosemide should be administered only when urine output is inadequate despite confirmation of adequate intravascular volume and renal perfusion.

Temperature Management

The infusion of heated chemotherapy solution causes a gradual rise in core temperature. The temperature and urine output must be documented every 15 minutes and communicated to the surgeon and perfusionist. At some institutions, core temperature is controlled using a combination of cooling and warming regimens at the various stages of the surgery.[39] The surgeon or perfusionist should decrease the temperature of the perfusate when the core temperature approaches 39°C. Of note, there may be disparity of temperature measurements depending on the temperature probe site. In our experience, rectal temperature may exceed nasopharyngeal temperature, possibly owing to local intraperitoneal heat transfer.[40] Additional heat transfer to the patient should be avoided during the chemotherapy phase. At a minimum, fluid warmers must be turned off and forced air warmers should be set to ambient temperature. A strategy used in our institution is to allow patient temperature to drift to 35.5°C before the start of HIPEC.

Electrolyte Management

A variety of acid-base and electrolyte disturbances have been reported in the setting of HIPEC surgery, and may vary with the type of chemotherapeutic agents used.[41,42] Oxaliplatin may predispose patients to lactic acidosis, hyperglycemia, and hyponatremia. Cisplatin may aggravate low magnesium levels, culminating in cardiac dysrhthmias.[43] Approximately 15 minutes before the start of heated chemotherapeutic infusion, a set of laboratory studies is obtained, including chemistries, arterial blood gas, and hemoglobin. Many patients will require electrolyte replacements, most commonly calcium, magnesium, and potassium. Therefore, rechecking electrolytes after the chemotherapy phase of the procedure is prudent. In our experience, the development of acidosis is rare, particularly if adequate cardiac output is maintained. A checklist provides a useful strategy for ensuring that key tasks are accomplished before starting HIPEC (**Box 2**).

Analgesia

Patients undergoing HIPEC via laparotomy incision undergo placement of a thoracic epidural catheter before induction. Proper placement is confirmed with a standard test dose of lidocaine with epinephrine. If excessive vasodilation and hypotension are encountered, the continuous infusion of bupivicaine with fentanyl may be delayed until the chemotherapy infusion is completed.[44] Postoperatively, a pain-controlled

---

Box 2
Checklist 15 minutes before starting hyperthermic perfusion

1. Fluid warmers off
2. Forced air warmer temperature set to ambient
3. Laboratory studies obtained
4. Low-dose dopamine infusion initiated
5. Crystalloid infusion rate sufficient to support urine output 100 mL/15 minutes
6. Temperature communicated to surgical team every 15 minutes
7. Repeat antibiotics as indicated
8. Maintain nominal stroke volume index with 250 to 500-mL colloid boluses as needed

analgesia pump programmed with both a continuous basal infusion and patient demand dose is provided. Intensive analgesia has been helpful at our institution, as well as others,[45] in facilitating early extubation and mobilization. Most of our patients are extubated promptly at the conclusion of surgery, while still in the operating room, instead of several hours later in the intensive care unit. Epidural anesthesia has been used successfully as part of a "fast-track" program for HIPEC at other centers.[46]

SUMMARY

Cytoreductive surgery with HIPEC is an important adjunct in the therapy of peritoneal surface malignancies. Anesthetic management of these cases is enhanced by an understanding of the unique physiologic challenges presented by this procedure. Development of a specialized perioperative group is encouraged for building a team environment that maximizes patient outcomes.

REFERENCES

1. Sugarbaker PH, Alderman R, Edwards G, et al. Prospective morbidity and mortality assessment of cytoreductive surgery plus perioperative intraperitoneal chemotherapy to treat peritoneal dissemination of appendiceal mucinous malignancy. Ann Surg Oncol 2006;13(5):635–44.
2. Kavanagh M, Ouellet JF. Clinical practice guideline on peritoneal carcinomatosis treatment using surgical cytoreduction and hyperthermic intraoperative intraperitoneal chemotherapy. Bull Cancer 2006;93(9):867–74 [in French].
3. Smeenk RM, Verwaal VJ, Zoetmulder FA. Learning curve of combined modality treatment in peritoneal surface disease. Br J Surg 2007;94(11):1408–14.
4. Gonzalez-Moreno S, Gonzalez-Bayon LA, Ortega-Perez G. Hyperthermic intraperitoneal chemotherapy: rationale and technique. World J Gastrointest Oncol 2010;2(2):68–75 [PMCID: 2999165].
5. Kanakoudis F, Petrou A, Michaloudis D, et al. Anaesthesia for intra-peritoneal perfusion of hyperthermic chemotherapy. Haemodynamic changes, oxygen consumption and delivery. Anaesthesia 1996;51(11):1033–6.
6. Fleisher LA, Beckman JA, Brown KA, et al. ACC/AHA 2007 guidelines on perioperative cardiovascular evaluation and care for noncardiac surgery: executive summary: a report of the American College of Cardiology/American Heart Association task force on practice guidelines (writing committee to revise the 2002 guidelines on perioperative cardiovascular evaluation for noncardiac surgery): developed in collaboration with the American Society of Echocardiography, American Society of Nuclear Cardiology, Heart Rhythm Society, Society of Cardiovascular Anesthesiologists, Society for Cardiovascular Angiography and Interventions, Society for Vascular Medicine and Biology, and Society for Vascular Surgery. Circulation 2007;116(17):1971–96.
7. Aziz MF, Healy D, Kheterpal S, et al. Routine clinical practice effectiveness of the glidescope in difficult airway management: an analysis of 2,004 glidescope intubations, complications, and failures from two institutions. Anesthesiology 2011; 114(1):34–41.
8. Marik PE, Baram M, Vahid B. Does central venous pressure predict fluid responsiveness? A systematic review of the literature and the tale of seven mares. Chest 2008;134(1):172–8.
9. Osman D, Ridel C, Ray P, et al. Cardiac filling pressures are not appropriate to predict hemodynamic response to volume challenge. Crit Care Med 2007; 35(1):64–8.

10. Keren H, Burkhoff D, Squara P. Evaluation of a noninvasive continuous cardiac output monitoring system based on thoracic bioreactance. Am J Physiol Heart Circ Physiol 2007;293(1):H583–9.

11. Squara P, Denjean D, Estagnasie P, et al. Noninvasive cardiac output monitoring (NICOM): a clinical validation. Intensive Care Med 2007;33(7):1191–4.

12. Schmidt C, Moritz S, Rath S, et al. Perioperative management of patients with cytoreductive surgery for peritoneal carcinomatosis. J Surg Oncol 2009;100(4): 297–301.

13. Thiele RH, Durieux ME. Arterial waveform analysis for the anesthesiologist: past, present, and future concepts. Anesth Analg 2011;113(4):766–76.

14. Squara P, Rotcajg D, Denjean D, et al. Comparison of monitoring performance of Bioreactance vs. pulse contour during lung recruitment maneuvers. Critical Care (London, England) 2009;13(4):R125.

15. Marque S, Cariou A, Chiche JD, et al. Comparison between Flotrac-Vigileo and Bioreactance, a totally noninvasive method for cardiac output monitoring. Critical Care (London, England) 2009;13(3):R73.

16. Marik PE. Noninvasive cardiac output monitors: a state-of the-art review. J Cardiothorac Vasc Anesth 2012. [Epub ahead of print].

17. Hofer CK, Senn A, Weibel L, et al. Assessment of stroke volume variation for prediction of fluid responsiveness using the modified FloTrac and PiCCOplus system. Critical Care (London, England) 2008;12(3):R82.

18. Michard F. Changes in arterial pressure during mechanical ventilation. Anesthesiology 2005;103(2):419–28 [quiz: 49–5].

19. Rooke GA, Schwid HA, Shapira Y. The effect of graded hemorrhage and intravascular volume replacement on systolic pressure variation in humans during mechanical and spontaneous ventilation. Anesth Analg 1995;80(5):925–32.

20. Pinsky MR. Probing the limits of arterial pulse contour analysis to predict preload responsiveness. Anesth Analg 2003;96(5):1245–7.

21. Esquivel J, Angulo F, Bland RK, et al. Hemodynamic and cardiac function parameters during heated intraoperative intraperitoneal chemotherapy using the open "coliseum technique." Ann Surg Oncol 2000;7(4):296–300.

22. Fleischmann KE, Beckman JA, Buller CE, et al. 2009 ACCF/AHA focused update on perioperative beta blockade: a report of the American College of Cardiology Foundation/American Heart Association task force on practice guidelines. Circulation 2009;120(21):2123–51.

23. Wilson G, Schumann R, Wurm H. Anesthesia for cytoreductive surgery: a case series. American Society of Anesthesiologists Annual Meeting. New Orleans, October 17-21, 2009.

24. Joshi GP. Intraoperative fluid restriction improves outcome after major elective gastrointestinal surgery. Anesth Analg 2005;101(2):601–5.

25. Chappell D, Jacob M, Hofmann-Kiefer K, et al. A rational approach to perioperative fluid management. Anesthesiology 2008;109(4):723–40.

26. Corcoran T, Rhodes JE, Clarke S, et al. Perioperative fluid management strategies in major surgery: a stratified meta-analysis. Anesth Analg 2012;114(3):640–51.

27. Stoelting R, Miller R. Basics of anesthesia. 5th edition. China: Churchill Livingstone; 2007.

28. Brandstrup B, Svensen C, Engquist A. Hemorrhage and operation cause a contraction of the extracellular space needing replacement—evidence and implications? A systematic review. Surgery 2006;139(3):419–32.

29. Lowell JA, Schifferdecker C, Driscoll DF, et al. Postoperative fluid overload: not a benign problem. Crit Care Med 1990;18(7):728–33.

30. Monnet X, Teboul JL. Passive leg raising. Intensive Care Med 2008;34(4):659–63.
31. Monnet X, Rienzo M, Osman D, et al. Passive leg raising predicts fluid responsiveness in the critically ill. Crit Care Med 2006;34(5):1402–7.
32. Westphal M, James MF, Kozek-Langenecker S, et al. Hydroxyethyl starches: different products—different effects. Anesthesiology 2009;111(1):187–202.
33. Jungheinrich C, Scharpf R, Wargenau M, et al. The pharmacokinetics and tolerability of an intravenous infusion of the new hydroxyethyl starch 130/0.4 (6%, 500 mL) in mild-to-severe renal impairment. Anesth Analg 2002;95(3):544–51.
34. Kozek-Langenecker SA. Effects of hydroxyethyl starch solutions on hemostasis. Anesthesiology 2005;103(3):654–60.
35. Raspe C, Piso P, Wiesenack C, et al. Anesthetic management in patients undergoing hyperthermic chemotherapy. Curr Opin Anaesthesiol 2012;25(3):348–55.
36. Owusu-Agyemang P, Arunkumar R, Green H, et al. Anesthetic management and renal function in pediatric patients undergoing cytoreductive surgery with continuous hyperthermic intraperitoneal chemotherapy (HIPEC) with cisplatin. Ann Surg Oncol 2012;19(8):2652–6.
37. Bailey JM. Dopamine: one size does not fit all. Anesthesiology 2000;92(2):303–5.
38. Lokhandwala MF, Amenta F. Anatomical distribution and function of dopamine receptors in the kidney. FASEB J 1991;5(15):3023–30.
39. Fagotti A, Paris I, Grimolizzi F, et al. Secondary cytoreduction plus oxaliplatin-based HIPEC in platinum-sensitive recurrent ovarian cancer patients: a pilot study. Gynecol Oncol 2009;113(3):335–40.
40. Rothfield KP, Crowley K, de Julio A. Accuracy of the DeRoyal nasopharyngeal temperature probe in patients undergoing heated intraperitoneal chemotherapy. Anesth Analg 2011;112:S-222.
41. Raft J, Parisot M, Marchal F, et al. Retentissements hydroelectrolytiques et acid-obasiques de la chimiohyperthermie intraperitoneale. Ann Fr Anesth Reanim 2010;29(10):676–81.
42. De Somer F, Ceelen W, Delanghe J, et al. Severe hyponatremia, hyperglycemia, and hyperlactanemia are associated with intraoperative hyperthermic intraperitoneal chemoperfusion with oxaliplatin. Perit Dial Int 2008;28(1):61–6.
43. Thix CA, Konigsrainer I, Kind R, et al. Ventricular tachycardia during hyperthermic intraperitoneal chemotherapy. Anaesthesia 2009;64(10):1134–6.
44. de la Chapelle A, Perus O, Soubielle J, et al. High potential for epidural analgesia neuraxial block-associated hypotension in conjunction with heated intraoperative intraperitoneal chemotherapy. Reg Anesth Pain Med 2005;30(3):313–4.
45. Schmidt C, Steinke T, Moritz S, et al. Thoracic epidural anesthesia in patients with cytoreductive surgery and HIPEC. J Surg Oncol 2010;102(5):545–6.
46. Cascales Campos PA, Gil Martinez J, Galindo Fernandez PJ, et al. Perioperative fast track program in intraoperative hyperthermic intraperitoneal chemotherapy (HIPEC) after cytoreductive surgery in advanced ovarian cancer. Eur J Surg Oncol 2011;37(6):543–8.

Hyperthermic Intraperitoneal Chemotherapy
Methodology and Safety Considerations

Santiago González-Moreno, MD, PhD[a],*,
Luis González-Bayón, MD, PhD[b,c], Gloria Ortega-Pérez, MD[d,e]

KEYWORDS

- Hyperthermia • Safety • Intraperitoneal chemotherapy • Peritoneal neoplasms

KEY POINTS

- Several methods of delivering HIPEC have been described but no significant differences in treatment outcomes, morbidity, or safety have been found among them. The ultimate choice is left to individual preference or institutional criteria.
- Administration of HIPEC is safe for operating room personnel; chemotherapy exposure during the procedure is negligible provided universal precautions, individual protection measures, and environmental safety guidelines are followed.
- Proper education of operating room staff about the essentials of HIPEC and on the proper handling of chemotherapy is the first safety requirement.

INTRODUCTION

Selected patients with peritoneal surface malignancies benefit from a radical thera-peutic approach consisting of cytoreductive surgery combined with perioperative intraperitoneal chemotherapy (PIC), which may be complemented by systemic chemo-therapy. Numerous studies have shown the efficacy of this strategy, which has led to survival results unknown to date, even in the era of last-generation chemotherapy and biologic agents.[1–3] Its clinical application is fully developed and well-established in specialized centers.[4]

The authors have no conflicts of interest to disclose.
[a] Peritoneal Surface Oncology Program, Department of Surgical Oncology, MD Anderson Cancer Center, Calle Arturo Soria 270, Madrid 28033, Spain; [b] Servicio de Cirugía General III, Hospital General Universitario Gregorio Marañón, C/Dr Esquerdo 46, Madrid 28007, Spain; [c] Universidad Complutense de Madrid, Facultad de Medicina, Plaza de Ramón y Cajal, Ciudad Universitaria, Madrid 28040, Spain; [d] Servicio de Cirugía General y Aparato Digestivo, Hospital Universitario de Fuenlabrada, Camino del Molino 2, Fuenlabrada, Madrid 28942, Spain; [e] Universidad Rey Juan Carlos, Facultad de Ciencias de la Salud, Avda, de Atenas, s/n, Alcorcón, Madrid 28922, Spain
* Corresponding author.
E-mail address: sgonzalez@mdanderson.es

Surg Oncol Clin N Am 21 (2012) 543–557
http://dx.doi.org/10.1016/j.soc.2012.07.001
1055-3207/12/$ – see front matter © 2012 Elsevier Inc. All rights reserved.

The ultimate purpose of PIC is to kill in situ microscopic cancer cells or minute tumor nodules left behind after the performance of (complete) cytoreductive surgery. The specific contribution of PIC to the oncologic outcomes observed for the combined procedure remains to be elucidated, and is currently being addressed by the ongoing French randomized trial PRODIGE-7.[5]

PIC may be administered with hyperthermic intraperitoneal chemotherapy (HIPEC) during the course of cytoreductive surgery, in the first 4 or 5 days after surgery in normo-thermic conditions (EPIC), or as a combination of both. Randomized controlled studies have not been performed to formally assess which modality of PIC is more advantageous. A few retrospective comparative studies are available showing a trend for or even an advantage for HIPEC alone over HIPEC followed by EPIC or EPIC alone, in terms of morbidity (fistula formation), although not in terms of survival,[6,7] but these conclusions need to be interpreted with caution. A recent small retrospective case-control Swedish study[8] reports a survival advantage of HIPEC over sequential postoperative intraperito-neal chemotherapy after complete cytoreduction in colorectal carcinomatosis. It can be stated without a doubt that HIPEC is nowadays the primary method of PIC used by every surgical team treating peritoneal surface diseases and that EPIC (combined with HIPEC or on its own) has a more limited penetration among them.

The acronym HIPEC, coined by the group from the Netherlands Cancer Institute, became the standardized nomenclature for this procedure as a result of the experts' consensus achieved during the Fourth International Workshop on Peritoneal Surface Malignancy (Madrid, 2004).[9] HIPEC combines the pharmacokinetic advantage inherent to the intracavitary delivery of certain cytotoxic drugs, which results in regional dose intensification, with the direct cytotoxic effect of hyperthermia. Hyper-thermia exhibits a selective cell-killing effect in malignant cells by itself, potentiates the cytotoxic effect of certain chemotherapy agents, and enhances the tissue penetra-tion of the administered drug.[10]

This article describes the different techniques in use and the technology available for the administration of HIPEC. Also reviewed are the safety features that must be taken into consideration when performing this procedure. Recommended guidelines to prevent associated occupational hazards are provided.

HIPEC METHODS
Description

HIPEC is delivered in the operating room (OR) after the cytoreductive surgical proce-dure is finalized if a complete cytoreduction has been achieved (CC-0/CC-1). There are two main methods for intraperitoneal administration of hyperthermic chemo-therapy: open abdomen technique and closed abdomen technique. Over the years mixed methods (semiopen or semiclosed) have been reported.

The open method is usually performed by the "coliseum technique," as described by Sugarbaker (**Fig. 1**).[11] After the cytoreductive phase has been finalized, four closed suction drains are placed through the abdominal wall and made watertight with a 3/0 monofilament purse-string suture at the skin. These drains remain in place for the postoperative period. An inflow line is placed over the abdominal wall into the peri-toneal cavity and may be secured by a silk tie at the retractor frame. A different number of temperature probes may be used for intraperitoneal temperature monitoring; at least one in the in-flow line or under the right diaphragm and another one at a distance from this point (pelvis) are used, but a more intensive monitoring may be used. Probe tips may be secured with a silk tie to the tip of the corresponding drains to prevent migra-tion. The skin edges of the abdominal incision are suspended up to a self-retaining

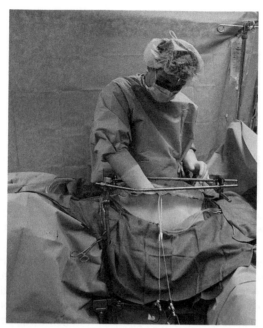

Fig. 1. Open method for the delivery of HIPEC (coliseum technique). The surgeon manipulates the perfusate with proper personal protection. Note the transparent smoke evacuator hose reaching the coliseum on the left. By S González-Moreno; *From* Oruezabal Moreno, M (ed). Oncología Digestiva, Algoritmos Diagnósticos y Terapéuticos. Chapter 7, Fig 7-5, page 52; © 2012; reproduced with permission from Editorial Médica Panamericana.

retractor whose frame has previously been elevated 15 to 20 cm over the patient, thus creating an open space in the abdominal cavity. This is done by a running monofilament number 1 suture. A plastic sheet is incorporated into this suture to prevent chemotherapy solution splashing from occurring. A slit in the plastic cover is made to allow the surgeon's double gloved hand access to the abdomen and pelvis. Impervious gown and protection goggles are mandatory. A smoke evacuator is placed under the plastic sheet to clear chemotherapy vapors or small droplets that may be liberated during the procedure. During the 30 to 90 minutes of perfusion, all the anatomic structures within the peritoneal cavity and the laparotomy incision are uniformly exposed to heat and chemotherapy by continuous manual stirring of the perfusate performed by the surgeon.

A variation of the open technique described and mainly used in Japan uses a device called "peritoneal cavity expander" (PCE). The PCE is an acrylic cylinder containing inflow and outflow lines that is secured over the laparotomy wound. When filled with heated perfusate, the PCE can accommodate the small bowel, allowing it to float freely and be manipulated within the perfusate. After HIPEC is completed, the perfusate is drained, and the PCE is removed. Fujimura and colleagues[12] and Yonemura and colleagues[13] reported about HIPEC with a PCE in carcinomatosis from various malignancies. The use of the PCE is very limited (if any) at the present time and has rarely been used outside Japan. Its interest in this paper is somewhat historical.

In the closed method catheters and temperature probes are placed as described previously, but the laparotomy skin edges are sutured watertight, so that perfusion is done in a closed circuit (**Fig. 2**). The abdominal wall is externally agitated during

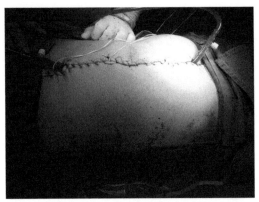

Fig. 2. Closed method for the delivery of HIPEC. An inflow line, an outflow line, and two temperature probes emerge through the temporarily closed midline laparotomy wound.

the perfusion period to promote uniform perfusate and heat distribution, because pooling of these possibly leading to subsequent morbidity is a reasonable concern in this method.[14] A larger volume of perfusate is generally needed to establish the circuit compared with the open technique, and also a higher abdominal pressure is achieved during the perfusion, which may facilitate drug tissue penetration.[15,16] After perfusion, the abdomen is reopened and the perfusate is evacuated. Appropriate anastomoses are performed and the abdomen is closed in the standard fashion. Other teams perform anastomoses and proceed with a definitive closure of the abdomen before HIPEC is started.

The mixed methods (semiopen or semiclosed) have been developed at a later time as an evolution of an open method, to further reduce the chance of OR staff exposure to chemotherapy and prevent heat loss. Rat and colleagues[17] use a latex sheet (abdominal cavity expander) water-tight sutured to the skin edges and then secured to the retractor frame, allowing a controlled overflow of the perfusate and allowing its level to reach well above the skin edges with no spillage. A transparent methacrylate cover with a laparoscopy hand port in its center is placed over the retractor's frame and the latex piece hermetically closing the abdominal cavity. Sugarbaker[18] also reported the use of a closed acrylic device with a lid, mounted on top of the coliseum to provide perfusate containment while allowing manual access to the peritoneal cavity for manipulation.

Comparative Analysis and Choice of HIPEC Method

Each HIPEC method has its own advantages and disadvantages, as shown in **Table 1**. It should be noted that, to the authors' knowledge, no formal prospective controlled comparison of HIPEC methods has been performed. Elias and colleagues[14] performed an early phase trial in which they successively tested seven HIPEC procedures. The authors concluded that closed methods were not satisfactory and that the open technique with traction of the skin upward was superior in terms of technical feasibility, thermal homogeneity, and perfusate distribution. Ortega-Deballon and colleagues[19] recently published a comparative experimental study in a small number of pigs concluding that intraperitoneal hyperthermia can be achieved with both techniques and that the open technique had higher systemic absorption and abdominal tissue penetration of chemotherapy (oxaliplatin) than the closed technique.

The panel of experts assembled for the 2006 Consensus Conference in Milan, after review of scientific evidence, discussion, and voting using the Delphi methodology,

Table 1
Comparative analysis of the different methods used to deliver HIPEC

Feature	Open	Closed	Mixed (semiopen/semiclosed)
Heat and chemotherapy distribution	More uniform[a]	Uneven[b]	More uniform[a]
Heat dissipation	More[b]	Less[a]	Improved (less) compared with open[a]
Time to achieve target temperature	Longer[b]	Shorter[a]	Shorter compared with open[a]
Direct contact of surgeon with chemotherapy (with protection)	Yes[b]	No[a]	Yes[b]
Risk of chemotherapy exposure by operating room staff	Theoretically increased[b]	Minimized[a]	Minimized[a]
Risk of thermal injury	Minimized[a]	Possible[b]	Minimized[a]
Complexity in assembling	Some (more complex if using peritoneal cavity expander)[a]	None[a]	More complex (expander, metacrylate cover, hand port)[b]

[a] Contains possible advantages.
[b] Contains possible disadvantages.

concluded that there is no evidence to establish the superiority of one method over the others regarding patient outcomes, morbidity, or surgical staff safety.[20] A call for future studies to definitively answer this question was made but has not been answered. Therefore, any of the methods listed previously may be used for the delivery of HIPEC.

The criteria that may be taken into consideration when choosing a HIPEC method by emerging treatment programs are mostly subjective: (1) the perceived risk of environmental chemotherapy exposure (the real risk is negligible if proper safety measures are followed, as described later); (2) concerns on possible differences in the uniform distribution of chemotherapy or heat throughout the peritoneal cavity that may result in visceral thermal injury; and (3) possible differences in dosaging and perfusate volume inherent to the closed method.

Each program should use the method that best fits its institutional needs or demands in terms of operational features, safety, and occupational hazard regulations, becoming used to deal with its own advantages and disadvantages. Safety standards and considerations for the administration of HIPEC are addressed in detail later in this article. Undoubtedly, as for any surgical technique, previous experience with one of them (eg, during a training period) has an impact on the choice; however, some teams have changed their method of choice over time, even after extensive experience with one technique.

TECHNOLOGY FOR THE DELIVERY OF HIPEC

Regardless of the method used, an external device that heats the chemotherapy perfusate and continuously circulates it in and out of the patient to keep a target

temperature and volume within the peritoneal cavity is always needed. Key components of this apparatus are as follows:

- A single-use circuit tubing that incorporates in most cases a reservoir where to
  withdraw the perfusate in case of an emergency or keep it before the perfusion
  starts
- A heat source
- A heat exchanger, where the perfusate is actually heated
- A roller pump that forces the perfusate from the reservoir into the patient
- A return method from patient to reservoir, which could be a second roller pump or
  a vacuum source
- Several temperature monitors (heat source, heat exchanger, inflow line, various
  points in the peritoneal cavity)

All these components, except for the single-use circuit tubing that comes inside its own
sterile box, are assembled together creating a machine. Most of these devices also incor-
porate a computerized continuous recording of thermal data that may be displayed in situ
for monitoring during the procedure and then exported or printed with different formats.
This adds security and comfortability to the procedure, avoiding the need to create
written records and also allowing efficient data recording for clinical research.

The first HIPEC machines had to be improvised by putting together all these individual components, in a home-made fashion (**Fig. 3**). Commercially available compact
HIPEC machines have been developed since the late 1990s, and the number of

A   **B**

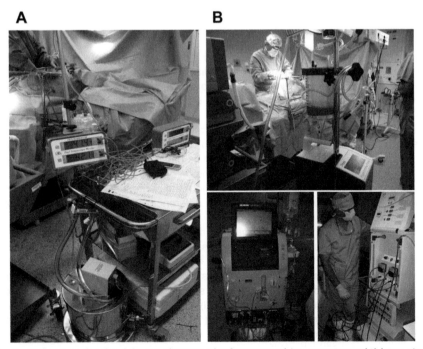

Fig. 3. Technology for the delivery of HIPEC. The former machine prototypes (*A*) have given
way to commercially available, certified compact HIPEC devices (*B*). In *A*, two roller pumps
are mounted on a metallic cart; heater apparatus and heat exchanger lie to the left of
the cart. Temperature registration is manual on a paper sheet. *B* shows three of the devices
listed in **Table 2**.

companies manufacturing them has gradually increased over the years (**Table 2**); this may be regarded as an indirect sign of the acceptability and applicability of HIPEC in clinical practice. This was also a step forward in the regulatory field, because these machines must be approved specifically for HIPEC use by the appropriate regulatory agencies (Food and Drug Administration in the United States, bearing CE marking in Europe), which definitely addresses any institutional medicolegal concerns about the use of this technology in humans.[21] However, availability of HIPEC machines for purchase may bring the opportunity to perform surgical treatment of peritoneal carcinomatosis in suboptimal conditions, without the appropriate training and knowledge, under the false assumption that "the machine does the work." The peritoneal surface oncology community and these companies must work together to warn against and prevent this opportunistic approach, which may result in unacceptable morbidity and suboptimal treatment results. This would eventually bring negative connotations toward the technique, potentially questioning the efforts developed over many years.

The choice of a specific HIPEC apparatus is certainly a subjective issue. Several factors may be taken into account in this decision: ability to achieve adequate hyperthermia in a short time period, adjustable flow rate, user-friendliness, ease of assembling the circuit for the surgical support staff, easy reading and continuous registration of temperatures, availability of technical support, and pricing of the machine itself and of the disposable circuit tubing kits. Testing different options in one's own OR is advisable before making a final decision.

In a HIPEC procedure using one of these devices the roller pump forces the chemotherapy solution into the abdomen through the inflow line and pulls it out through the drains, with a flow rate around 1 L per minute (**Fig. 4**). The instillate's temperature reaches 43°C to 45°C after passing through the heat exchanger, so that the intraperitoneal fluid is maintained at 41°C to 43°C. The perfusate may be first recirculated between the reservoir and the heat exchanger so that it can be heated to an adequate temperature. At this point, full closed-circuit circulation of the perfusate in and out of the peritoneal cavity is established until a minimum intraperitoneal temperature of 41.5°C is achieved and maintained. The drug is then added to the circuit and the timer for the perfusion is started. In bidirectional chemotherapy protocols the intravenous infusion of the appropriate drugs may be started at this time point, although some authors advocate doing it 1 hour before the initiation of HIPEC.

Table 2
Nonexhaustive, alphabetical order list of commercially available devices approved for the delivery of HIPEC

Name	Company	Country	Food and Drug Administration Approved	CE Marking
Belmont Hyperthermia Pump	Belmont Instrument Company	United States	Yes	Yes
Cavitherm	EFS	France	No	Yes
Exiper	Medica S.p.A.	Italy	No	Yes
Gamida Tech	Sunchip	France	No	Yes
Performer	Rand Corporation	Italy	No	Yes
ThermoChem-HT	Thermasolutions	Netherlands/ United States	Yes	Yes

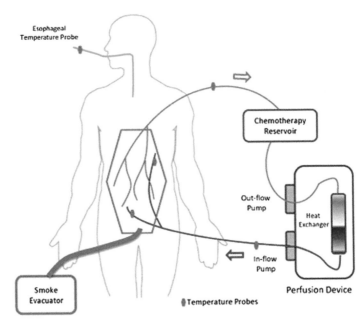

Fig. 4. Schematic representation of the circuit and elements used for the administration of HIPEC.

An original alternative to the use of a closed-circuit external apparatus to deliver HIPEC has been recently described by Ortega-Deballon and colleagues,[22] from Dijon. Their method uses a heat source placed directly in the peritoneal cavity. It consists of two 17-m long electric heating cables insulated with a silicon wrapping. Each cable is connected to a 24-V transformer and then to a 220-V electric outlet. One cable is distributed in the supramesocolic area and the other in the inframesocolic area and between the bowel loops. Although it has been developed and used only in an experimental pig model to date, preliminary data show a favorable safety profile with no direct heat damage to the viscera, efficacy, and technical feasibility that warrant further studies to investigate its application in the human patient. The advantages of this technology in terms of cost, operating time, and simplicity are obvious.

SAFETY CONSIDERATIONS

OR staff faces occupational risks daily, such as blood-borne pathogens, anesthetic gases, or radiation exposure, and are used to dealing with these risks. However, the introduction, handling, and management of chemotherapy in the OR that comes with HIPEC necessarily determine a change in surgical personnel habits and may bring a biased, unrealistic perception of added danger. As for any of the risks mentioned previously, the staff involved in the procedure must be fully aware of its meaning and associated hazards to avoid unnecessary potential health problems or an irrational opposition to their participation in the program.

Education as a Safety Factor: Influence on Behavior

Ignorance may be the most dangerous health risk in the OR. Appropriate education about cytoreductive surgery and HIPEC is a first, mandatory safety factor that must be observed by all personnel involved in the procedure.[23] The surgical oncologist leading the team should take responsibility to provide such education and training as needed. Monographic cancer hospitals might already have in effect educational programs for nurses and ancillary staff about chemotherapy essentials and cytotoxic drug handling procedures and guidelines; in this regard, cancer hospitals have some advantage over general hospitals.

The educational program should cover the surgical technique; the intraperitoneal chemotherapy perfusion; the cytotoxic agents used; the effects of hyperthermia on these drugs and on the patient; and the indications, rationale, and results of the procedure. Then, staff needs to be educated on routes of exposure and risks of low-dose occupational exposure to cytotoxic agents. Additionally, they should be made aware of the potential risks associated with an increased amount of surgical smoke produced during cytoreductive surgery. Finally, personnel have to be trained on how to avoid these exposure hazards and how to perform a safe procedure.

It is well known from a behavioral standpoint (Health Belief Model) that, even with the proper education, it is the individual who ultimately does or does not adhere to self-protective measures, influenced by his or her perception of susceptibility, severity, benefits, and efficacy of the barriers used.[24] "Unrealistic optimism" by which healthcare workers cannot believe they will become ill as a result of hazardous exposures should be avoided.

Surgical Smoke Exposure

Cytoreductive surgery uses high-voltage electrosurgery for visceral dissection and resection and for the electroevaporation of tumor nodules. The amount of smoke generated during this procedure exceeds that created during a regular surgical operation (eg, for colorectal cancer).[25] This fact added to the length of the operation (10–12 hours) may result in cumulative exposure. Contrary to the exposure to chemotherapy, surgical staff tends to underappreciate the risks of electrosurgical smoke and the need to use protective measures.

Just by its physical effects, surgical smoke may produce headache, nausea, and eye and respiratory tract irritation to healthcare workers in the OR. It also hampers the correct visualization of the surgical field. Surgical smoke contains ultrafine particles, whose increase in the environment is related to lung dysfunction, cardiovascular changes, and mortality. Some dangerous substances have been identified in these ultrafine particles, such as benzene, toluene, furfural, and polycyclic aromatic hydrocarbons, some of which are carcinogenic or may cause ischemic heart disease. Additionally, smoke particles can bear viable microorganisms. In a recent Swedish study the amount of ultrafine particles detected during cytoreductive surgery was comparable with that in second-hand (sidestream) smoke of cigarettes. No single or cumulative values of polycyclic aromatic hydrocarbons in this context exceeded the occupational exposure limits.[25,26]

Investigations done by work-safety agencies in Europe and the United States have shown that it is possible to control air contamination from electrosurgical smoke by keeping the OR well ventilated and by using at all times a smoke evacuator.[27,28] Air conditioning should be continuously working throughout the surgical procedure, reaching a slightly higher air pressure in the OR in relation to the surrounding area. Filters of the air conditioner should be high-efficiency particulate air and should be verified once a month for fungal contamination. Doors should be closed during the operation with hermetic closures.[23] These are usually standard OR ventilation procedures, already in effect regardless of the type of surgery.

A smoke evacuator should be ready for use from the beginning of the operation. This device must have a suction unit, an absorbent high-efficiency particulate air filter, and a disposable tube for smoke conduction with a rigid end.[29] Although several options are commercially available, this apparatus is unfortunately not among the regular equipment available in every OR. Filters have a filling indicator; they should be changed frequently, and disposed of as biologic hazardous material. The tip of the smoke evacuator tubing may be handled by the scrub nurse and kept about 5 cm from the origin of the smoke to catch every contaminating substance. Suction must work always while the smoke is being produced; synchronization of the smoke evacuator with the electrosurgical generator is of great help in this regard. Air suction with this device under the plastic sheet is also used as a protective measure during the administration of HIPEC by the coliseum technique.

Additionally, individual protective measures against surgical smoke may be used. High-power filtration mask (FFP-3) with a good fit to nose and mouth is recommended wear for personnel at the OR during cytoreduction and HIPEC. These "healthcare respirators" offer high filtration of submicron particles and protect against concentrations of solid and nonvolatile liquid particles. They do not protect against gases or vapors. It should be noted that, although included in most safety guidelines, breathing through this kind of mask is neither comfortable nor easy and some persons just cannot stand them for prolonged periods of time. The consequences of not wearing them on the health of surgical workers if smoke evacuation and adequate ventilation are reinforced have not been assessed. Additionally, because no study to date has detected chemotherapy particles in the OR air during the administration of open HIPEC[30–32] the need to wear such a mask instead of a regular surgical mask is debatable. Eye protection should be worn as a mechanical barrier not just for the smoke, but also for cytostatic agents and bodily fluid exposure, as part of a universal precaution protocol.

Chemotherapy Exposure

The cytotoxic agents used in HIPEC are cell-cycle independent drugs, whose effects are amplified by heat. The drugs usually used are mitomycin C, cisplatin, doxorubicin, and oxaliplatin. During HIPEC chemotherapy is always diluted, never pure, and absolute doses of drugs are in micrograms, so that it is not possible to have a major spill (defined as <5 g or 5 mL of undiluted cytotoxic agent by the US Occupational Safety Health Administration). Although toxicity of these agents is well described for therapeutic dosages, long-term effects of prolonged, repeated occupational exposure to low doses remain unknown. For this reason, all precautions and guidelines for chemotherapy handling should be observed.[33]

The routes of exposure to chemotherapy during HIPEC are mainly direct contact and inhalation of aerosols or vapors, because accidental injection and ingestion are to be regarded as anecdotal in this context. Direct contact of cytotoxic agent with skin or mucous membranes produces irritation or dermatitis. If absorption of drugs happens and exposure to low doses is frequent, systemic effects could theoretically be possible (bone marrow toxicity, gastrointestinal toxicity, hair loss, and so forth), but this has not been proved. Inhalation of aerosols could happen if vaporization of cytotoxic drugs induced by hyperthermia occurs. The use of the smoke evacuator under the plastic sheet during HIPEC administration using the coliseum technique or the advent of the acrylic covers used in the semiopen methods minimize this route of exposure.

Stuart and colleagues,[30] from the United States, were the first to evaluate the safety of OR personnel during HIPEC. They administered mitomycin C using the coliseum technique. Urine from members of the operating team was assayed for chemotherapy levels. Air below and above the plastic sheet also was analyzed. Finally, sterile gloves commonly used in the OR were examined for permeability to chemotherapy. All assessments of potential exposures were found to be negative, in compliance to established safety standards. Schmid and colleagues,[31] from Germany, arrived at the same conclusions regarding mitomycin C detection levels and glove permeability assays. More recently, a Swedish study reported by Andréasson and colleagues[32] during HIPEC with oxaliplatin using the coliseum technique failed to detect any platinum in the urine or blood of the surgeon or the perfusionist involved in the procedure.

These studies confirm that, even in the method with a higher chance for surgical staff chemotherapy exposure, delivery of HIPEC is a safe procedure from the occupational risk standpoint provided adequate, standard protective measures are observed.

RECOMMENDED GUIDELINES FOR THE SAFE ADMINISTRATION OF HIPEC

Individual protective measures and environmental measures to minimize chemotherapy exposure during HIPEC have been described before and are summarized in **Table 3**.[23] This is a list of generally recommended items but it is ultimately up to every institution and treatment program to define and reinforce their own safety guidelines. Further safety considerations include OR staff selection and health checks, the management of chemotherapy spills, and the cleaning of the OR after an HIPEC procedure.

Staff Selection and Health Checks

Any association between participation in an HIPEC program and the chance of future newborn congenital defects, worsening of a blood dyscrasia, or even developing any health problem in the future should be avoided. Therefore, limitations for participation in the program must be established, among them:

- Pregnant or nursing women
- History of abortions or congenital malformations
- Individuals actively pursuing pregnancy (men and women)

Table 3 Recommendations for a safe administration of HIPEC	
Surgical field	• Use of impervious, disposable drapes. Do not use textile cloth
Lap pads	• A correct lap pad count should be obtained before initiation of HIPEC
Operating room	• Doors should be closed • Signs placed outside the operating room advising that HIPEC is in progress • Restriction of personnel circulation • Absorbent towels on the floor around surgical table for possible spills
Personal protective measures: universal precautions	• Disposable impervious gown (closed front, long sleeves, and closed cuffs) • Disposable impervious shoe covers • Double powderless latex gloving, outer one elbow length; change outer glove every 30 min • Eye protection (goggles) • High-power filtration mask (FFP-3) (debatable)
Environmental measures	• Proper ventilation • Smoke evacuator used continuously over surgical field (under plastic drape in coliseum technique)
Residue management	• Leak-proof rigid containers labeled "cytotoxic agents" should be used for every material or bodily fluid to be discarded during or after HIPEC (and during the following 48 h)

- Hematologic or teratogenic disease history
- Previous chemotherapy or radiotherapy treatments
- Usual work with radiographs or radiation therapy
- Active immunosuppressive treatment
- Allergy to cytotoxic drugs or latex
- Severe dermatologic disease

Regular health checks for healthcare workers involved in the delivery of HIPEC must be performed. These should be done every 6 to 12 months, collecting information on the frequency of exposure to the procedure; any incident (eg, spillage, skin contact) during HIPEC; and new symptoms (especially in skin, mucous membranes, gastrointestinal tract, hair loss, and so forth). Blood work with at least a complete blood cell count and a biochemistry panel should be obtained. After learning all the pertinent data, an individualized assessment and follow-up instructions are to be provided.

Management of Direct Contact with Chemotherapy or Chemotherapy Spills

The US Occupational Safety Health Administration categorizes chemotherapy spills as small or large using a threshold of 5 g or 5 mL of undiluted cytotoxic agent.[33] If direct contact with cytotoxic agent occurs, contaminated clothing should be removed immediately and discarded into a hazardous waste container. Affected skin should be washed immediately with mild, additive-free soap without dyes or perfumes that may interact with the cytotoxic agent. If the affected area is the eye, it should be flooded immediately with water or isotonic saline for 5 minutes. The staff member should then report the incident to the occupational health office.

A small spill should be blotted dry using absorbent pads and wiped up. The area should be washed three times with water and neutral soap. Then, the area can be cleaned in the routine manner. When clearing large spills special care should be taken to avoid creating aerosols. To clean up any kind of spill personnel should wear the protective barrier garments previously described (see **Table 3**), including a respirator mask for large spills.

Cleaning up the OR after HIPEC

Education about the meaning and risks of using chemotherapy in the OR needs to transcend to the cleaning personnel. Standard protective clothing described should be used. Special leak-proof bins should be used to discard all trash from the room. All bactericidal cleaning solutions should not be used to wash the contaminated area because they may react with the cytotoxic agents and do not inactivate them. Water with neutral soap is adequate to clean up the OR after HIPEC, performing this task three consecutive times. Seventy percent isopropilic alcohol is also safe and effective. Surgical instruments should be washed three times with water and pure soap before leaving the working area.

SUMMARY

HIPEC is one of the cornerstones in the curative-intent treatment of peritoneal surface malignancies. It is administered after complete cytoreductive surgery. Several methods of delivering HIPEC have been described but no significant differences in treatment outcomes, morbidity, or safety have been found among the methods. The ultimate choice is left to individual preference or institutional criteria.

Administration of HIPEC is safe for personnel working in the OR; chemotherapy exposure during the procedure is negligible provided universal precautions, individual protection measures, and environmental safety guidelines are followed. Exposure to potentially harmful electrosurgical smoke produced during cytoreductive surgery needs to be taken into consideration. Proper education of OR staff about the essentials of HIPEC and on the proper handling of chemotherapy is mandatory.

REFERENCES

1. Yan TD, Welch L, Black D, et al. A systematic review on the efficacy of cytoreductive surgery combined with perioperative intraperitoneal chemotherapy for diffuse malignancy peritoneal mesothelioma. Ann Oncol 2007;18:827–34.
2. Yan TD, Black D, Savady R, et al. A systematic review on the efficacy of cytoreductive surgery and perioperative intraperitoneal chemotherapy for pseudomyxoma peritonei. Ann Surg Oncol 2007;14:484–92.
3. Yan TD, Black D, Savady R, et al. Systematic review on the efficacy of cytoreductive surgery combined with perioperative intraperitoneal chemotherapy for peritoneal carcinomatosis from colorectal carcinoma. J Clin Oncol 2006;24:4011–9.
4. Glehen O, Gilly FN, Boutitie F, et al. Toward curative treatment of peritoneal carcinomatosis from nonovarian origin by cytoreductive surgery combined with perioperative intraperitoneal chemotherapy: a multi-institutional study of 1290 patients. Cancer 2010;116(24):5608–18.
5. Quenet F, Elias D. (principal investigators): Protocole Prodige 7. ACCORD 15/0608. EudraCT N°: 2006-006175–20. Essai de phase III évaluant la place de la chimiohyperthermie intrapéritonéale peropéraroire (CHIP) après résection maximale d'une carcinose péritonéale d'origine colorectale associée à une chimiothérapie sysstémique.
6. Elias D, Benizri E, Di Pietrantonio D, et al. Comparison of two kinds of intraperitoneal chemotherapy following complete cytoreductive surgery of colorectal peritoneal carcinomatosis. Ann Surg Oncol 2007;14:509–14.
7. Glehen O, Kwiatkowski F, Sugarbaker PH, et al. Cytoreductive surgery combined with perioperative intraperitoneal chemotherapy for the management of peritoneal carcinomatosis from colorectal cancer: a multi-institutional study. J Clin Oncol 2004;22:3284–92.
8. Cashin PH, Graf W, Nygren P, et al. Intraoperative hyperthermic versus postoperative normothermic intraperitoneal chemotherapy for colonic peritoneal carcinomatosis: a case-control study. Ann Oncol 2012;23:647–52.
9. González-Moreno S. Peritoneal surface oncology: a progress report. Eur J Surg Oncol 2006;32:593–6.
10. Sticca RP, Dach BW. Rationale for hyperthermia with intraoperative intraperitoneal chemotherapy agents. Surg Oncol Clin N Am 2003;12:689–701.
11. Sugarbaker PH. Technical handbook for the integration of cytoreductive surgery and perioperative intraperitoneal chemotherapy into the surgical management of gastrointestinal and gynecologic malignancy. 4th edition. Grand Rapids (MI): The Ludann Company; 2005. p. 52–6.
12. Fujimura T, Yonemura Y, Fujita H, et al. Chemo-hyperthermic peritoneal perfusion for peritoneal dissemination in various intra-abdominal malignancies. Int Surg 1999;84:60–6.
13. Yonemura Y, Ninomiya I, Kaji M, et al. Prophylaxis with intraoperative chemohyperthermia against peritoneal recurrence of serosal invasion-positive gastric cancer. World J Surg 1995;19:450–5.
14. Elias D, Antoun S, Goharin A, et al. Research on the best chemohyperthermia technique of treatment of peritoneal carcinomatosis after complete resection. Int J Surg Investig 2000;1:431–9.

15. Esquis P, Consolo D, Magnin G, et al. High intraabdominal pressure enhances the penetration and antitumor effect of intrapoeritoneal cisplatin on experimental peritoneal carcinomatosis. Ann Surg 2006;244:106–12.

16. Jacquet P, Stuart OA, Chang D, et al. Effects of intra-abdominal pressure on pharmacokinetics and tissue distribution of doxorubicin after intraperitoneal administration. Anticancer Drugs 1996;7:596–603.

17. Rat P, Benoit L, Cheynel N, et al. Intraperitoneal chemohypertehjrmia with "overflow" open abdomen. Ann Chir 2001;126:669–71.

18. Sugarbaker PH. An instrument to provide containment of intraoperative intraperitoneal chemoptherapy with optimized distribution. J Surg Oncol 2005;92:142–6.

19. Ortega-Deballon P, Facy O, Jambet S, et al. Which method to deliver hyperthermic intraperitoneal chemotherapy with oxaliplatin? An experimental comparison of open and closed techniques. Ann Surg Oncol 2010;17:1957–63.

20. Glehen O, Cotte E, Kusamura S, et al. Hyperthermic intraperitoneal chemotherapy: nomenclature and modalities of perfusion. J Surg Oncol 2008;98:242–6.

21. Sugarbaker PH, Clarke L. The approval process for hyperthermic intraoperative intraperitoneal chemotherapy. Eur J Surg Oncol 2006;32:637–43.

22. Ortega-Deballon P, Facy O, Magnin G, et al. Using a heating cable within the abdomen to make hyperthermic intraperitoneal chemotherapy easier: feasibility and safety study in a pig model. Eur J Surg Oncol 2010;36:324–8.

23. González-Bayón L, González-Moreno S, Ortega-Pérez G. Safety considerations for operating room personnel during hyperthermic intraoperative intraperitoneal chemotherapy perfusion. Eur J Surg Oncol 2006;32:612–24.

24. Näslund Andréasson S. Work environment in the operating room during cytoreductive surgery and hyperthermic intraperitoneal chemotherapy: factors influencing the choice of protective equipment. Digital Comprehensive Summaries of Uppsala Dissertations from the Faculty of Medicine 716. Uppsala (Sweden): Acta Universitatis Upsaliensis; 2011. p. 35–38.

25. Andréasson SN, Anundi H, Sahlberg B, et al. Peritonectomy with high voltage electrocautery generates higher levels of ultrafine smoke particles. Eur J Surg Oncol 2009;3:780–4.

26. Andréasson SN, Mahteme H, Sahlberg B, et al. Policyclic aromatic hydrocarbons in electrocautery smoke during peritonectomy procedures. In: Näslund Andréasson S, editor. Work environment in the operating room during cytoreductive surgery and hyperthermic intraperitoneal chemotherapy: factors influencing the choice of protective equipment. Digital Comprehensive Summaries of Uppsala Dissertations from the Faculty of Medicine 716. Uppsala (Sweden): Acta Universitatis Upsaliensis; 2011. p. 35–8.

27. NIOSH Hazard Controls. Control of smoke from laser/electrical surgical procedures. Publication number 96–128. US Department of Health and Human Services. Atlanta (GA): National Institute of Ocupational Safety and Health; 1996.

28. Ulmer BC. Air quality in the operating room. Surgical services management, vol. 3. Denver (CO): AORN; 1997.

29. Ross K, ECRI. Surgical smoke evacuators: a primer. Surgical services management, vol. 3. Denver (CO): AORN; 1997.

30. Stuart OA, Stephens AD, Welch L, et al. Safety monitoring of the coliseum technique for heated intraoperative intraperitoneal chemotherapy with mitomycin C. Ann Surg Oncol 2002;9(2):186–91.

31. Schmid K, Boettcher MI, Pelz JO, et al. Investigations on safety of hyperthermic intraoperative intraperitoneal chemotherapy (HIPEC) with mitomycin C. Eur J Surg Oncol 2006;32:1222–5.

32. Näslund Andréasson S, Anundi H, Thóren SB, et al. Is platinum present in the blood and urine from treatment givers during hyperthermic intraperitoneal chemotherapy? J Oncol 2010;2010:649–719.

33. Yodaiken RE, Bennett D. OSHA work practice guidelines for personnel dealing with cytotoxic (antineoplastic) drugs. Occupational Safety and Health Administration. Am J Hosp Pharm 1986;43:1193–204.

The Importance of the Learning Curve and Surveillance of Surgical Performance in Peritoneal Surface Malignancy Programs

Shigeki Kusamura, MD, PhD[a], Dario Baratti, MD[a],
Ionut Hutanu, MD[b], Piero Rossi, MD[c], Marcello Deraco, MD[a],*

KEYWORDS

- Cytoreductive surgery • Hyperthermic intraperitoneal chemotherapy
- Learning curve

KEY POINTS

- Cytoreductive surgery (CRS) and hyperthermic intraperitoneal chemotherapy (HIPEC) is a complex procedure with a very steep learning curve (LC).
- Sequential probability ratio test with risk adjustment was used to evaluate the LC of CRS and HIPEC in a single-center experience of peritoneal surface malignancies (PSM).
- Approximately 140 to 150 cases were necessary for the acquisition of competence in CRS and HIPEC with adequate radicality and acceptable safety. Eighty to 100 cases were necessary to assure short-term prognostic gains in rare PSMs.
- This study highlights how LC and the continuous monitoring of surgical performance is critical in evaluating the credibility of emerging and already established PSM centers in the world.

INTRODUCTION

The advent of the cytoreductive surgery (CRS) associated with hyperthermic intraperitoneal chemotherapy (HIPEC) in the early 1990s has dramatically changed the treatment of peritoneal surface malignancies (PSM). The combined treatment has been suggested as the standard of care for pseudomyxoma peritonei (PMP), peritoneal mesothelioma (PM), and peritoneal carcinomatosis arising from colorectal cancers.[1–6]

The authors declare that there is no funding or financial support to the present work.
The authors have no conflict of interest to disclose.
[a] Peritoneal Surface Malignancy Program, Department of Surgery, Fondazione IRCCS Istituto Nazionale dei Tumori, via Venezia 1, Milan 20133, Italy; [b] Department of Surgery, University of Medicine and Pharmacy 'Gr T Popa', Strada Universitătii 16, zip code 700115, Iasi, Romania; [c] Dipartimento di Chirurgia D'Urgenza, Senologica e dei Trapianti, Fondazione Policlinico Tor Vergata, Viale Oxford, 81 - zip code 00133, Roma, Italy
* Corresponding author.
E-mail address: marcello.deraco@istitutotumori.mi.it

The concept of proficiency in surgical procedures is multidisciplinary and encompasses a wide range of perioperative aspects. The expertise comprises variables related to indication of the treatment, surgical technique, management of HIPEC parameters, and short-term surgical and oncologic results.[7,8] The few studies published thus far on learning curve of CRS and HIPEC have reported a steep and long-lasting process until the acquisition of sufficient competence.[9–12]

Although originally developed for use in quality control studies in the realm of manufacturing,[13] the sequential probability ratio test (SPRT) has been largely used in medicine to monitor the safety of medical interventions such as interventional cardiology, cardiac surgery, emergency medical services, and other procedures[14–17] It offers an advantage by allowing formal hypothesis testing. By providing a graphic summary of changes in performance with time, SPRT can detect deteriorated or improved performance. Therefore, it is helpful to analyze the learning curve of surgical procedures.[18]

The authors recently conducted an analysis on learning using this statistic for the CRS and HIPEC in a series of 420 cases of PSM treated in the Istituto Nazionale dei Tumori (NCI), Milan, Italy.[19] One hundred forty-nine and 137 cases were necessary to assure acceptable reductions of the risk of severe morbidity and incomplete cytoreduction.

The present study attempted the following:

1. To reevaluate the learning curve of the same surgical team in CRS and HIPEC in an expanded case mix. As in the previous study, changes in short-term surgical outcomes in a case sequence composed of a variety of PSMs were reassessed. Evolution of short-term oncologic outcomes were evaluated separately in subsets of pseudomyxoma peritonei (PMP) and peritoneal mesotheliomas (PM).
2. To monitor the surgical performance of the same team in terms of G3-5 morbidity along the timeline after the acquisition of expertise (surveillance with audit intent).
3. To discuss the utility and implications of the present results for emerging PSM programs and already active ones.

PATIENTS AND METHODS

All patients were treated under an institutionally approved protocol and provided written informed consent. The eligibility requirements for treatment were as follows: histologically confirmed diagnosis of peritoneal surface malignancy judged resectable clinically and radiologically; age younger than 75 years; no distant metastasis; adequate renal, hematopoietic, and liver functions; and performance status according to Eastern Cooperative Oncology Group (ECOG) classification.

Data were extracted from a prospectively collected institutional database of the PSM program of the NCI in Milan. In total, 462 CRS and HIPEC procedures performed from August 1995 to February 2012 were included in the study.

CRS and HIPEC

The technique of CRS has been described elsewhere.[20,21] In brief, the goal of the surgical cytoreduction was to remove all visible tumor with a diameter greater than 2.5 mm by means of diaphragmatic, parietal anterior, and pelvic peritonectomy with greater and lesser omentectomy. Depending on disease involvement, multiorgan resections were performed, including removal of gallbladder, spleen, left/right or total colon, and uterus with annexes.

Peritoneal carcinomatosis was quantified according to the peritoneal cancer index (PCI). The mean PCI was 22 (range 0–39). Completeness of cytoreduction was classified as follows[22]: CC-0, no residual disease (RD); CC-1, RD of 0 to 2.5 mm; CC-2, RD of 2.5 mm to 2.5 cm; and CC-3, RD greater than 2.5 cm.[22] Incomplete cytoreduction was defined as RD greater than 2.5 mm (CC-2/3).

HIPEC was performed with a closed-abdomen technique using an extracorporeal device (Performer LRT; RAND, Medolla [MO], Italy), which maintained the intra-abdominal temperature at 42° to 43°C. Chemotherapy schedules were as follows: cisplatin (CDDP; 25 mg/m^2/L) and mitomycin C (MMC; 3.3 mg/m^2/L)[23,24] for colorectal cancer, gastric cancers, and pseudomyxoma peritonei; and CDDP (43 mg/L of perfusate) and doxorubicin (Dx; 15.25 mg/L of perfusate)[25] for ovarian cancer and peritoneal mesothelioma. Patients older than 70 years and those who had undergone previous chemotherapy received a 30% dose reduction of both drugs. The same surgical team guided by the same principal operator (D.M.) operated on all of the patients.

In the postoperative period, patients were assisted in an intensive care unit for at least 48 hours. In the successive in-hospital stay, patients were cared for by a multidisciplinary team comprising internists with a nutritional science specialization, anesthetists, rehabilitation professionals, and psychologists.

Study Parameters

Adverse events (morbidity, anastomotic leak, systemic toxicity) were graded according to the NCI CTCAE v3 criteria.[26] When more than 2 complications occurred during the same period in 1 patient, the complication was considered as more serious for analysis. Anastomotic leak was defined according to the criteria established elsewhere.[27] The procedure-related mortality (PRM) was defined as death occurring during the in-hospital stay after CRS and HIPEC.[28] G3-5 morbidity was defined as the combination of surgical and medical G3-5 morbidities, PRM, and G3-5 systemic toxicity. To assess surgical outcomes according to case sequence, they were divided into 6 subgroups of 70 for cases 1 to 420, while cases 421 to 462 were designated as another subgroup.

The outcomes of interest were rates of incomplete cytoreduction, G3-5 morbidity, and short-term oncologic failure. Potential confounders to the outcomes of interest were identified among the following clinicopathological parameters: age, sex, ECOG performance status, Charlson comorbidity index (combined condition and age-related score),[29] previous systemic chemotherapy, previous surgical score (PSS), body mass index (BMI), preoperative serum albumin, tumor histotype, PMP histologic subtype (disseminated peritoneal adenomucinosis [DPAM], peritoneal mucinous carcinomatosis [PMCA]), PM subtype (biphasic/sarcomatoid vs others), PCI, bowel anastomosis, number of peritonectomy procedures, operating time, CDDP dose for HIPEC, subgroups of case sequence, incomplete cytoreduction rate, and HIPEC drug schedule.

The risk modeling and elaboration of SPRT curves for oncologic outcomes were done separately for PMP and PM. Short-term oncologic failure was defined as emergence of recurrence and/or death within 1 year from the combined procedure for PMP patients and within 6 months for PM patients. Therefore, PMP cases with less than 1 year of follow-up and PM cases with less than 6 months of follow-up that did not present recurrence and/or death were excluded.

Statistical Analysis

One-way analysis of variance (ANOVA) and the χ^2 test were used to analyze changes of continuous and discrete variables, respectively, according to subgroups of case sequence.

The risk-adjusted SPRT plot was used to chart, across the case sequence, changes in the rates of incomplete cytoreduction, rates of G3-5 morbidity, and short-term oncologic failure. To elaborate the SPRT, 4 parameters were defined: estimated probabilities of outcomes of interest for each case, a prespecified odds ratio (OR) for the outcomes of interest, and type I and II error rates. Probability of type I and type II (α and β) error were both set at 0.05. From these, 2 control limits (h0 and h1) and the cumulative sum of log-likelihood ratio with risk adjustment were calculated according to equations outlined by Rogers and colleagues.[18]

The risk predictions for incomplete cytoreduction, G3-5 morbidity, and short-term oncologic failures were elaborated by multivariate analysis, using the logistic regression model. Clinical factors were selected as covariates when P values were less than .15 on univariate analysis. Using backward stepwise selection, independent factors were identified. The probability of event was calculated, which was adjusted with independent risk factors of incomplete cytoreduction, G3-5 morbidity, or short-term oncologic failures from the logistic regression model. Discrimination was measured by the area under the receiver-operating characteristic curve (AUC),[30] with values of 0.5 representing no discrimination and 1.0 representing perfect discrimination. Model fitness was assessed by the Hosmer-Lemeshow goodness-of-fit test,[31] with P values of greater than .05 indicating acceptable fit.

When creating the RA-SPRT curve, each case was plotted in sequence along the x-axis. When a success occurred (no G3-5 morbidity, optimal cytoreduction, or short-term oncologic success) a log-likelihood ratio with risk adjustment (s) was subtracted from the cumulative score. When a failure occurred, the constant 1 − s was added to the cumulative score. Thus, an ascending slope in the RA-SPRT line indicated deterioration of performance, whereas a descending slope indicated improvement of performance.

An unacceptable OR was set for increase in rates of incomplete cytoreduction and G3-5 morbidity, respectively, at 1.8 and 1.4, adopting the same boundary lines of the authors' previous experience of LC analysis.[19] In brief, these figures were obtained considering the highest and lowest rates of these outcomes available in the literature.[1,32,33] The upper and lower control limits were respectively defined as h1 (reject line) and h0 (accept line). OR was prespecified as 2 for short-term oncologic failure, for both PMP and PM.

If the RA-SPRT curve crossed the upper decision limit (h1) from below, this meant that the actual OR for outcome was equal to or higher than the prespecified OR with the probability of type I error of 0.05. If the line crossed the lower decision limit (h0 or accept line) from above, this indicated that the actual OR for the outcome being studied is less than the unacceptable OR with the probability of type II error of 0.05. When the line was between h0 and h1, no statistical inference could be made. Expertise was estimated to be achieved at point(s) in which the curve of RA-SPRT crossed the accept line (h0) for outcomes of interest. At the time of crossing to the lower boundary, the graph was reset to 0 to start the surveillance of surgical performance with audit intent.[16]

Once the expertise is acquired, the surveillance continues to monitor any eventual deterioration of the performance. The RA-SPRT curve could assume a positive slope in the case of enrollment of new surgeons in the surgical team, launch of new protocols using more toxic or more effective treatments, and the introduction of changes or innovations in surgical strategy based on new data obtained from other centers.

Evolution of predicted risk of incomplete cytoreduction and G3-5 morbidity along the case sequence was assessed with the moving-average (MA) method.[34] An MA order of 10 was used.

The applied statistical software was SPSS 18.0 (SPSS Inc, Chicago, IL), while the MA method and RA-SPRT model were calculated by Excel version 2003 (Microsoft Corporation, Redmond, WA). Statistical significance was set at $P<.05$.

RESULTS
Patients' Characteristics in the Entire Series

The mean age was 53.7 (SD ± 12.6). The male/female ratio was 172:290. Four hundred fifty-two (97.8%) cases had ECOG performance status of 0 or 1. The mean Charlson comorbidity index was 3.6 (±0.9). The mean BMI was 25.3 (±14.4) kg/m². The mean preoperative serum albumin level was 4.1 (±0.6) g/dL. Three hundred nineteen (69%) cases had a PSS of 0 or 1. Two hundred sixty-one cases (56.6%) had previous systemic chemotherapy. The histologic distribution was as follows: colon cancer 23 (5.0%), gastric cancer 12 (2.6%), ovarian cancer 56 (12.1%), PM 151 (32.7%), PMP 168 (36.4%), peritoneal sarcomatosis 34 (7.4%), and other tumors 18 (3.9%). The mean PCI was 18.1 (±9.9).

The mean number of peritonectomy procedures performed for each case was 8.0 (±4.4). The mean operating time was 557 (±164) minutes. The mean number of red cell units transfused intraoperatively was 2.8 (±3.5). Rate of incomplete cytoreduction was 10.2%. The HIPEC drug schedules were distributed as follows: 56.5% CDDP + Dx and 43.5% CDDP + MMC. The mean CDDP dose was 186 (±46) mg. The mean length of stay in the intensive care unit was 3 days (range 0–10) and the mean in-hospital stay was 23.7 (±15.3) days.

Rates of G3-5 morbidity, G3-5 hematologic toxicity, and PRM were 29.2%, 6.2%, and 2.4%, respectively. The most common G3-5 surgical complications were gastro-intestinal anastomotic leak/perforation (9.7%), infection (10.4%), and postoperative bleeding (3.2%).

The independent risk factors for the outcomes of interest (incomplete cytoreduction, G3-5 morbidity, short-term oncologic failures for PMP and PM) as well as goodness of fit and discriminant capacity of each risk modeling are outlined in **Table 1**. The MA of predicted risk of outcomes of interest along the case sequence are outlined in **Fig. 1**.

G3-5 Morbidity

After an initial phase of fluctuation the RA-SPRT curve for G3-5 morbidity assumed a negative slope from case 51 down to case 101 (**Fig. 2**A). The curve fluctuated again, before breaching the accept line (h0) at case 149. This point could be considered the cutoff at which the actual OR for G3-5 morbidity is less than the prespecified OR of 1.4 with a probability of type II error of 0.05. At no time did the G3-5 morbidity rate cross the unacceptable threshold (h1). The RA-SPRT at the breaking point was reset to 0 to restart the monitoring.

Incomplete Cytoreduction

The RA-SPRT curve for incomplete cytoreduction presented a positive slope (increase in the rates of CC-2/3) up to case 31 without breaching the upper boundary for unacceptable OR of incomplete cytoreduction (h1) (**Fig. 2**B). It then assumed a consistent negative slope and breached the lower boundary (h0) at case 140. This point could be considered the breaking point at which the actual OR for incomplete cytoreduction is less than the unacceptable OR of 1.8 with a probability of type II error of 0.05. The RA-SPRT at the breaking point was reset to 0 to restart the monitoring.

Short-Term Oncologic Outcomes

Regarding the rates of early oncologic results in PM patients, the surgical team experienced a consistent improvement in performance until case 101, where the accept line is crossed (**Fig. 2**C). The RA-SPRT curve assessing the performance of surgical

Table 1
Independent risk factors correlated with short-term surgical and oncologic outcomes in a case sequence with PSM patients

	Independent Risk Factors											
	Incomplete Cytoreduction			G3-5 Morbidity			Six-Month Recurrence/Death in 119 PM			One-Year Recurrence/Death in 136 PMP		
Dependent Variables	OR (adj)	95% CI	P	OR (adj)	95% CI	P	OR (adj)	95% CI	P	OR (adj)	95% CI	P
Age (>52 y)							11.09	1.37 90.12	.02			
Gender (male)										2.25	0.92–5.50	.08
ECOG PS (0 vs 1/2)	0.37	0.19–0.73	.04	0.52	0.31–0.87	.013						
Charlson comorbidity index (>4)												
Preoperative serum albumin <3.2 g/dL							6.36	1.21 33.51	.03			
BMI <20 kg/m²							4.54	1.19 17.30	.03			
PM histologic subtype	—	—		v			5.14	1.13 23.29	.03			
PMP histologic subtype	—	—		—			—	—	—	3.27	1.22–8.76	.02
PSS (0/1 vs 2/3)												
Previous sCT	2.16	1.12–4.19	.022									
PCI (>20)	4.13	2.04–8.38	<.001	2.44	1.57–3.80	<.001						
Anastomosis	0.38	0.19–0.76	.006							2.85	0.94–8.58	.06
Mean no. of peritonectomy procedures (>8)												

	Model 1 OR	95% CI	P	Model 2 OR	95% CI	P	Model 3	Model 4 OR	95% CI	P
CC	—	—	—	—	—	—	—	—	—	—
Ostomy	—	—	—	—	—	—	—	—	—	—
HIPEC drug schedule (CDDP + Dx vs CDDP+MMC)	—	—	—	1.72	1.10–2.69	.018	—	—	—	—
CDDP dose (>240 mg)	—	—	—	2.75	1.38–5.47	.004	—	—	—	—
Duration of the surgery (>570 min)										
Subgroups of case sequence[a]	0.77	0.65–0.92	.004	1.15	1.01–1.31	.032	—	—	—	—
G3-5 morbidity	—	—	—	—	—	—	—	2.43	1.01–5.86	.05
Expertise for CC and morbidity	—	—	—	—	—	—	—	0.16	0.04–0.62	.01
Model goodness of fit[b]	$\chi^2 = 5.69$; P = .68			$\chi^2 = 4.73$; P = .786			$\chi^2 = 2.78$; P = .427	$\chi^2 = 2.01$; P = .98		
Discriminant capacity (AUC)	0.78; 95% CI: 0.71–0.85			0.69; 95% CI: 0.63–0.74			0.81; 95% CI: 0.69–0.93	0.75; 95% CI: 0.66–0.85		

Abbreviations: adj, adjusted; AUC, area under the curve; BMI, body mass index; CC, completeness of cytoreduction; CDDP, cisplatin; CI, confidence interval; Dx, doxorubicin; MMC, mitomycin C; OR, odds ratio; PCI, peritoneal cancer index; PS, performance status; PSS, previous surgical score; sCT, systemic chemotherapy.

[a] Subgroups: 1–70; 71–140; 141–210; 211–280; 281–350; 351–420; 421–462.

[b] Hosmer-Lemeshow test.

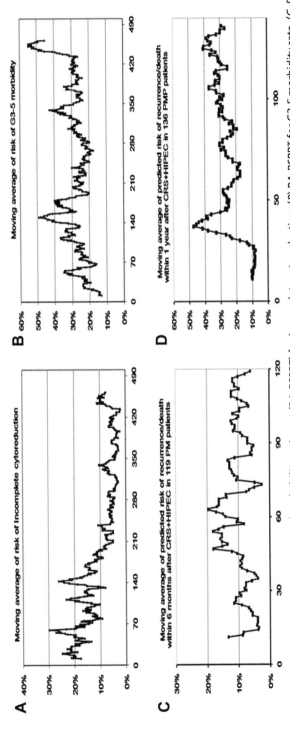

Fig. 1. (A) Risk-adjusted resetting sequential probability ratio test (RA-RSPRT) for incomplete cytoreduction. (B) RA-RSPRT for G3-5 morbidity rate. (C, D) RA-RSPRT for early recurrence/death in PMP and PM patients after CRS + HIPEC.

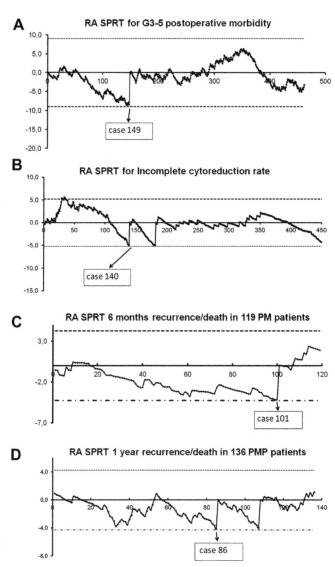

Fig. 2. (*A, B*) Moving average of predicted risk for incomplete cytoreduction and G3-5 morbidity in a case sequence of 462 peritoneal surface malignancies. RA-SPRT, risk-adjusted sequential probability ratio test; h0, lower boundary of control limit; h1, upper boundary of control limit. The x-axis represents operation number, not calendar time. The y-axis represents the cumulative summation of log-likelihood ratio. The lower boundaries were surpassed by the RA-RSPRT plots at 140th and 149th cases, respectively, for incomplete cytoreduction and G3-5 morbidities. Regarding oncologic outcome the proficiency was achieved after 86 PMP patients and after 101 PM patients. For RA-RSPRT, at the time of crossing to the lower boundary, the graph should be reset to 0. (*C, D*) Moving average of predicted risk of early recurrence/death in PMP and PM patients. RA-SPRT, risk-adjusted sequential probability ratio test; h0, lower boundary of control limit; h1, upper boundary of control limit. The x-axis represents operation number, not calendar time. The y-axis represents the cumulative summation of log-likelihood ratio. The lower boundaries were surpassed by the RA-RSPRT plots at 140th and 149th cases, respectively, for incomplete cytoreduction and G3-5 morbidities. Regarding oncologic outcome the proficiency was achieved after 86 PMP patients and after 101 PM patients. For RA-RSPRT, at the time of crossing to the lower boundary, the graph should be reset to 0. (*Data from* Grigg OA, Farewell VT, Spiegelhalter DJ. Use of risk-adjusted CUSUM and RSPRT charts for monitoring in medical contexts. Stat Methods Med Res 2003;12(2):147–70.)

team concerning rates of 1-year recurrence/death in PMP patients presented an initial fluctuation and then tended to gradually decrease with increasing experience until the 86th case, where the lower boundary, or accept line (h0), was surpassed. At that point actual OR for 1-year recurrence/death rate in PMP patients is less than 2 (**Fig. 2**D).

The clinicopathological variables, G3-5 morbidity, and rates of incomplete cytoreduction were analyzed regarding their distribution along the consecutive subgroups of the case sequence (**Table 2**).

Audit

The fifth (281st to 351st case) and seventh (421st to 462nd case) subgroups of patients presented a fairly higher level of morbidity with respect other periods of the program. G3-5 morbidity rates associated with these time points were 40% and 49%, respectively (see **Table 2**). Clusters of adverse events raised concerns regarding a possible deterioration in the surgical performance. Segments of RA-SPRT curve representative of these time periods revealed 2 peaks that did not surpass the upper boundary limit (reject line). This finding means that although patients operated on in these moments presented statistically significant higher morbidity rates with respect the rest of study period, the actual ORs pertaining to these time points were not sufficiently high to overcome the prespecified unacceptable limit. Therefore, no worsening of surgical performance was detected at any time point of the study period.

DISCUSSION

Different breaking points were obtained according to the outcomes considered. Those related to incomplete cytoreduction and G3-5 morbidity were located respectively at the 140th and 149th cases, confirming the results of the authors' previous study. Acceptable risks of short-term oncologic failures were achieved at the 86th and 101st cases, respectively, for PMP and PM patients.

Four studies have addressed the issue of the learning curve for CRS and HIPEC.[9–12] The methodology used in these works is not optimal in their approach to sequential data. All of them split arbitrarily the study population, according to period of time or according to the number of procedures performed. All of these studies demonstrated an inverse correlation between the outcomes of interest (morbidity rates, operating time, number of red cell units transfused, mortality rates, and in-hospital stay) and the proficiency of the surgical team. In other words, improvement in outcomes among almost all variables was observed as the surgical team became expert.

As none of these studies used a statistical process control tool such as SPRT, nor adjusted for differences in the risk profile of cases, it is impossible to infer whether such improvement in the outcomes was due to a progressive selection of less complex cases or to an actual improvement in surgical performance.

The estimated risk of an adverse outcome is expected to suffer a wide variation from case to case and does not depend exclusively on the expertise of the surgical team. Factors related to the characteristics of patients and tumors do contribute to the emergence of an adverse event. Therefore, an adjustment for prior risk is critical to ensure that unfavorable event rates that appear unusual are not erroneously attributed to technical aspects.

Each case from the case sequence is plotted on an x-axis and receives a score that is calculated by the RA-SPRT. The score depends on patient risk (estimated by the

Table 2
Distribution of demographic and clinical characteristics of 462 cases treated by CRS + HIPEC along the consecutive subgroups

Subgroups	1–70	71–140	141–210	211–280	281–350	351–420	421–462	P
Age (y)	50.2 ±11.3	53.0 ±11.9	53.0 ±12.5	53.2 ±13.5	54.6 ±12.2	56.4 ±13.8	56.6 ±12.5	.241[a]
Gender (male) (%)	35.7	37.1	28.6	30.0	42.9	47.1	40.5	.029[a]
ECOG PS (0 vs 1/2) (%)	88.6	97.1	95.7	98.6	91.4	97.1	100.0	<.001[a]
Charlson comorbidity index	3.2 ±0.5	3.4 ±0.6	3.5 ±0.7	3.6 ±0.8	3.7 ±1.0	3.9 ±0.9	3.8 ±1.4	<.001[b]
Preoperative serum albumin (g/dL)	3.7 ±0.5	4.1 ±0.5	4.0 ±0.5	4.3 ±0.5	4.4 ±0.6	4.3 ±0.6	4.2 ±0.5	0.065[b]
BMI (kg/m^2)	24.7 ±4.3	24.7 ±4.1	24.8 ±4.1	23.7 ±3.7	24.0 ±3.5	25.8 ±4.7	32.8 ±48.4	<.001[a]
Tumor histotype (PM & PMP vs other PSM) (%)	28.6	41.4	77.1	87.1	85.7	87.1	81.0	<.001[a]
PSS (2/3 vs 0/1) (%)	5.7	17.1	24.3	45.7	34.3	37.1	66.7	.051[a]
Previous systemic chemotherapy (%)	54.3	54.3	41.4	34.3	34.3	45.7	36.6	<.001[b]
PCI	15.3 ±6.4	19.8 ±8.3	21.3 ±10.4	17.1 ±10.8	21.6 ±12.1	16.0 ±9.2	14.2 ±7.9	.012[a]
Bowel anastomosis (%)	38.6	62.9	60.0	48.6	67.1	55.7	47.6	<.001[a]
Ostomies (%)	0.0	0.0	2.9	2.9	18.6	20.0	35.7	<.001[b]
Mean no. of peritonectomy procedures	3.0 ±3.7	6.4 ±4.7	8.0 ±3.9	8.7 ±3.3	10.8 ±3.3	10.1 ±3.1	9.4 ±2.8	<.001[a]
HIPEC drug schedule (CDDP + Dx vs CDDP + MMC) (%)	5.7	57.1	55.7	42.9	48.6	42.9	57.1	<.001[b]
HIPEC CDDP dose (mg)	234.8 ±38.3	198.5 ±51.0	202.3 ±39.5	178.0 ±31.3	179.0 ±38.2	147.0 ±20.1	146.4 ±23.1	<.001[b]
Operating time (min)	452.7 ±188.3	559.5 ±207.5	584.6 ±138.4	603.4 ±105.3	613.5 ±98.3	564.9 ±106.2	499.1 ±227.2	.001[b]
No. of red cell units transfused	1.2 ±2.0	3.4 ±5.6	3.2 ±3.6	2.3 ±2.9	2.9 ±2.8	3.2 ±2.5	3.8 ±3.3	<.001[b]
In-hospital stay (days)	30.0 ±20.4	23.4 ±16.3	19.6 ±9.5	20.9 ±14.9	23.7 ±13.2	20.9 ±8.1	32.5 ±20.8	<.001[b]
G3-5 morbidity (%)	22.9	24.3	31.4	28.6	40.0	15.7	50.0	.002[a]

Continuous variables are presented as mean ± SD.
Abbreviations: CDDP, cisplatin; Dx, doxorubicin; MMC, mitomycin-C; PCI, peritoneal cancer index; PM, peritoneal mesothelioma; PMP, pseudomyxoma peritonei; PS, performance status; PSS, previous surgical score.
[a] χ^2.
[b] ANOVA.

multivariate logistic regression method) and on the actual outcome (favorable or unfavorable). In practice there are 4 possible situations:

1. If a low-risk case happens to present an adverse outcome (G3-5 morbidity, incomplete cytoreduction, or early oncologic failure) the surgeon is penalized with a high positive score and the RA-SPRT curve ascends steeply.
2. If a low-risk case presents a favorable outcome (uneventful postoperative period, complete cytoreduction, or absence of early oncologic failure) the surgeon is granted a low negative score and the RA-SPRT curve descends mildly.
3. If a high-risk case presents an adverse event the surgeon is penalized with a low positive score (the curve ascends mildly).
4. If a high-risk case presents a favorable outcome the surgeon is granted a high negative score (the curve descends steeply).

The scores assigned to each case are sequentially summed and the accumulated values determine the finale feature of the RA-SPRT curve. If there is a continuous improvement the curve assumes a negative slope, and if there is a deterioration the curve assumes a positive slope.

Patient selection is critical in obtaining good surgical short-term and long-term oncologic results. Operability of cases in the present study was relatively stable throughout the case sequence. Good ECOG performance and nutritional status as well as low Charlson comorbidity indices were maintained along the case sequence (see **Table 2**). Smeenk and colleagues[11] conducted an analysis of the learning curve of 390 combined procedures and observed that the complexity of the cases decreased progressively along their cohort. These investigators concluded that this was a consequence of an improvement in patient selection, secondary to the learning process.

Different eligibility criteria for the combined procedure are applied for peritoneal carcinomatosis from colorectal cancer and rare malignancies such as PMP and PM. The former is characterized by a more restrictive case selection, so that only cases with limited peritoneal dissemination present better chances to benefit from the procedure. On the other hand, extensive peritoneal carcinomatosis (PCI >20) is not a reason to rule out PM and PMP from the combined procedure. These rare malignancies are characterized by narrow therapeutic windows, as they do not have potentially effective alternative treatments other than the CRS and HIPEC.

Table 2 is a sort of arbitrary splitting method applied to the study population. An apparent unexpected finding becomes evident. There were 2 critical time points at which increases in rates of morbidity were assessed: from the 281st to 350th case and from the 421st to 462nd case. Using a traditional frequentist statistical test (χ^2) there were significant higher percentages of severe adverse events in both periods with respect to the rest of the study period. One could hypothesize that once having overcome the learning curve, the surgical team is no longer expected to present increases in the adverse event rates.

A careful examination of evolution of patients' estimated risks in both periods reveals a concentration of complex cases (see **Fig. 2**B). High-risk cases tend to complicate even when operated on by proficient surgeons. A cluster of complications happening consecutively in high-risk cases is translated by a curve with a mild positive slope, which in the example here did not ascend sufficiently to breach the upper boundary or reject line. Therefore, the RA-SPRT did not signal deterioration in any performance. A similar phenomenon of expanded indication of a surgical procedure has been noted in previous studies that addressed the learning curve of other types of operation. Laparoscopic surgeons, once having gained proficiency, become more prone to approach complex cases, leading to an apparent increase in the morbidity.[35,36]

Only one study in the literature addressed the oncologic outcome as a parameter for evaluation of the learning curve. Smeenk and colleagues[11] divided the study group, comprising patients with PMP and peritoneal carcinomatosis from colorectal cancer, into 3 sequential subgroups, and observed that there were no significant differences among them in terms of prognosis. However, this approach, as pointed out by the investigators themselves, has a serious drawback, as determining the effect of the learning curve on survival is limited because of the differences in the length of follow-up periods. Patients treated in the first subgroup had a higher chance of presenting an adverse oncologic event with relative to those from the third subgroup, as the former require longer follow-up. Moreover, the methodology used by Smeenk and colleagues does not allow the definition of a breaking point for the learning curve.

To circumvent these limitations the authors adopted the following strategy. The assessment of the effects of oncologic outcomes on the learning curve required the adoption of a discrete surrogate marker of survival, that is, early oncologic failure. The substitution of a time-dependent outcome (oncologic adverse event) by a binary outcome (1 year and 6 months recurrence/death rates, respectively, to PMP and PM) allowed the application of RA-SPRT. Such a strategy was attempted because information about the occurrence of oncologic adverse events is reported at constant lags, according to the time schedule of the outpatient follow-up after the treatment (every 6 months in the first 2 years and once a year thereafter).[37]

The surgical team managed to overcome the learning curve regarding short-term oncologic results after 86 and 101 cases, respectively, for PMP and PM. These figures contrast with the breaking points for incomplete cytoreduction and G3-5 morbidity obtained from the analysis of the entire case sequence (140 and 149 cases, respectively). One could raise the following concern: why were fewer cases necessary to make evident a reduction in the OR for short-term oncologic failures for subsets of PM and PMP with respect to the number of cases necessary to assure proficiency in the adequate and safe cytoreduction?

In fact, the breaking points of the learning curve for early recurrence and death in PMP and PM should be interpreted cautiously, considering that the analysis was performed in the context of a high-volume center in the treatment of PSMs. During the study period, the surgeon performed several combined procedures not just for PM and PMP but also for other types of PSM. The experience acquired from peritonectomy performed for PSM, in general, improves the cytoreduction skill and facilitates better execution of CRS for PMP and PM, regardless of the fact that PMP and PM are usually characterized by more disseminated disease and consequently require more complex and challenging procedures.

By the time the breaking point for short-term oncologic failure for PMP was surpassed (86th case), the surgical team had already performed another 189 parallel procedures for the treatment of other types of PSMs. Similarly, when the 101st case of PM was performed, the surgical team had already accomplished another 242 parallel peritonectomies to treat PSM other than PM.

One possible criticism is that the analysis of the learning curve for single abnormalities is meaningless, as the combined procedure is the same for all histotypes, with only small variations. This concern is partially pertinent. From the various targets available to appraise the learning curve, the prognosis is the most critical, as it represents the synthetic end point that encompasses others such as case selection, disease biology and extension, the completeness of cytoreduction, and morbidity. Oncologic outcome depends not only on parameters related to the procedure but also on factors related to the patient.

An analysis of the surgical performance using RA-SPRT with early oncologic failure as end point is currently ongoing using the multicentric registry of PMP, the same cohort of 2298 PMP patients evaluated by Chua and colleagues.[38] This multi-institutional initiative could answer several questions. The application of RA-SPRT to evaluate the surgical performance of the main PSM centers in the world, in particular that of Pseudomyxoma Peritonei Centre located at Basingstoke and North Hampshire Hospital in the United Kingdom, would disclose the influence of parallel procedures in the surgical performance of single histology experiences.

One limitation of the present analysis is related to inherent imperfections of risk modeling. The noninclusion of numerous, likely unmeasured confounders in the risk-prediction models renders them not perfect enough to predict 100% of adverse outcomes. Some of the possible confounders are those pertaining to related disciplines that care for the perioperative aspects of the patients. The study period encompasses 15 years of experience, and changes in the perioperative anesthesiologic management (intraoperative interventions, postoperative analgesic techniques), perioperative nutritional support, and postoperative rehabilitation interventions were not included in the analysis.

Other nonassessed confounders are those related to the background of the surgical team. The experience of the surgical team accumulated before the first operation of the case sequence and the volume of the PSM program are aspects not included in the risk-prediction models. Before setting up the PSM program in Milan the principal surgeon (D.M.) had assisted in at least 40 procedures in a well-recognized European oncologic center (Gustave Roussy) in the early 1990s. Subsequently the principal surgeon (D.M.) attended an observer fellowship at Washington Hospital Center with Dr Paul Sugarbaker.

In the early phase of the Milan PSM program the operations started and continued to be performed without the presence of a more experienced surgeon in peritonectomy procedures, following a tentative and trial-and-error policy. Seven years were necessary to acquire proficiency, and the NCI of Milan gradually has become a high-volume referral center in the treatment of PSM, in particular of PM and PMP that correspond, nowadays, to at least 80% of the cases treated by CRS and HIPEC.

The NCI of Milan, after having overcome its own learning curve, has provided technical and scientific assistance to community-based hospitals in the northern part of Italy to set up other new PSM centers. One of these institutes was Bentivoglio Hospital, located 250 km from Milan. The first step of the tutorial consisted of visits to the NCI of Milan by members of the emerging center. The second step was the development of study protocols, the definition of a multidisciplinary team, and logistic troubleshooting. The third step was the selection of initial cases and performance of CRS and HIPEC at the emerging center with the assistance of the tutor. The expert (D.M.) supervised Bentivoglio's operations participating in the surgeries during the first 2 years. The visits of the tutor to the Bentivoglio center were maintained on a regular basis every 2 months thereafter. The tutorial system is under evaluation using RA-SPRT, and preliminary data suggest that it could represent a valuable means to reduce the length of a long and complex process of knowledge transfer.

González Bayón and colleagues[39] defined 12 clear-cut critical points to initiate a program in PSM nearly 10 years ago, in another special issue of the present journal dedicated to peritoneal carcinomatosis. These items highlighted fundamental aspects departing from logistic evaluation, creation of a multidisciplinary team, institutional commitment, and the importance of contextualizing the project within a clinical trial.

Since then a dramatic change has occurred in the scenario of locoregional treatment of PSM. The combined procedure has gathered an enormous popularity, and several new centers have emerged around the world. Despite the dissemination of the technique, there is still a wide gap between the demand and supply. In the United States or Germany only 1% to 3% of patients with colorectal peritoneal carcinomatosis amenable to CRS and HIPEC are having access to this treatment (González-Moreno S, 2011, personal communication).

At the time the González Bayón study was published, no data on the learning curve of the combined procedure were available. The learning process has proved to be steep in the present analysis. The acquisition of sufficient expertise to perform CRS and HIPEC safely and with an adequate radicality required nearly a decade. Moreover, to gather experience in 80 cases of PM and/or PMP is virtually unfeasible for most PSM centers in the world. In fact, in a recently published multi-institutional study on 2298 PMP cases, involving the 16 most prominent international PSM programs, only half of the centers have performed more than 100 procedures.[38] The emerging centers contributed only 8% of the entire cohort.

The need for new PSM centers is a consensual thought, given the worldwide estimated incidence of peritoneal carcinomatosis that is potentially treatable with the combined procedure. However, the process of expanding the access program must be considered cautiously, as differences in the level of complexity of the combined procedure according to the histotype range widely. Although the procedure apparently seems to be the same irrespective of the disease being treated, the approach to rare malignancies such as PM and PMP requires additional effort for the acquisition of expertise. Considering the breaking points reported in the present study, the required competence would be achievable for rare malignancies only if a large-scale referral mechanism was available.[40]

SUMMARY

The acquisition of proficiency in CRS and HIPEC requires a long-lasting training program. This article aims to evaluate the learning curve of CRS and HIPEC in treating PSMs.

CRS was performed using peritonectomy procedures, and HIPEC through the closed-abdomen technique used CDDP and MMC or CDDP and Dx. The RA-SPRT was used to assess the learning curve for a case sequence of 462 PSMs. The main outcomes were rates of incomplete cytoreduction and G3-5 morbidity (NCI CTCAE v3) and short-term oncologic results measured by the incidence of disease relapse and/or death within 1 year (for PMP) and within 6 months (for PM) from the treatment. Control limits were determined by setting the unacceptable OR for the outcomes being studied as well as type I and II error rates. Risk adjustment was performed by identifying the risk factors for the outcomes of interest using a logistic regression model.

Rates of G3-5 morbidity, G3-5 hematologic toxicity, and PRM were 29.2%, 6.2%, and 2.4%, respectively. The RA-SPRT curve crossed the lower control limit at the 140th and 149th case, respectively, for incomplete cytoreduction and G3-5 morbidity. Accordingly, the lower boundaries for acceptable short-term relapse rates were achieved at the 86th case of PMP and at the 101st case of PM. At those points the actual OR is lower than the prespecified OR for outcomes being studied.

CRS and HIPEC to treat PM and PMP has a steep learning curve that requires between 140 and 149 procedures to assure the performance of a safe procedure and acceptable rates of optimal RD. Favorable short-term oncologic results began to be observed after the 86th case of PMP and after the 101st case of PM.

REFERENCES

1. Elias D, Gilly F, Quenet F, et al, Association Française de Chirurgie. Pseudo-myxoma peritonei: a French multicentric study of 301 patients treated with cyto-reductive surgery and intraperitoneal chemotherapy. Eur J Surg Oncol 2010;36: 456–62.
2. Baratti D, Kusamura S, Nonaka D, et al. Pseudomyxoma peritonei: biological features are the dominant prognostic determinants after complete cytoreduction and hyperthermic intraperitoneal chemotherapy. Ann Surg 2009;249:243–9.
3. Yan TD, Deraco M, Baratti D, et al. Cytoreductive surgery and hyperthermic intra-peritoneal chemotherapy for malignant peritoneal mesothelioma: multi-institutional experience. J Clin Oncol 2009;27:6237–42.
4. Deraco M, Baratti D, Cabras AD, et al. Experience with peritoneal mesothelioma at the Milan National Cancer Institute. World J Gastrointest Oncol 2010;2:76–84.
5. Cao C, Yan TD, Black D, et al. A systematic review and meta-analysis of cytore-ductive surgery with perioperative intraperitoneal chemotherapy for peritoneal carcinomatosis of colorectal origin. Ann Surg Oncol 2009;16:2152–65 Review.
6. Esquivel J, Elias D, Baratti D, et al. Consensus statement on the loco regional treatment of colorectal cancer with peritoneal dissemination. J Surg Oncol 2008;98:263–7 Review.
7. Kusamura S, Younan R, Baratti D, et al. Cytoreductive surgery followed by intra-peritoneal hyperthermic perfusion: analysis of morbidity and mortality in 209 peri-toneal surface malignancies treated with closed abdomen technique. Cancer 2006;106:1144–53.
8. Deraco M, Baratti D, Kusamura S. Morbidity and quality of life following cytore-duction and HIPEC. Cancer Treat Res 2007;134:403–18 Review.
9. Yan TD, Links M, Fransi S, et al. Learning curve for cytoreductive surgery and perioperative intraperitoneal chemotherapy for peritoneal surface malignancy–a journey to becoming a Nationally Funded Peritonectomy Center. Ann Surg On-col 2007;14:2270–80.
10. Cavaliere F, Valle M, De Rosa B, et al. Peritonectomy and chemohyperthermia in the treatment of peritoneal carcinomatosis: learning curve. Suppl Tumori 2005; 4(3):S119–21 [in Italian].
11. Smeenk RM, Verwaal VJ, Zoetmulder FA. Learning curve of combined modality treatment in peritoneal surface disease. Br J Surg 2007;94:1408–14.
12. Mohamed F, Moran BJ. Morbidity and mortality with cytoreductive surgery and intraperitoneal chemotherapy: the importance of a learning curve. Cancer J 2009;15:196–9 Review.
13. Wald A. Sequential tests in industrial statistics. Ann Math Stat 1945;6:117–86.
14. Matheny ME, Ohno-Machado L, Resnic FS. Risk-adjusted sequential probability ratio test control chart methods for monitoring operator and institutional mortality rates in interventional cardiology. Am Heart J 2008;155(1):114–20.
15. Chen TT, Chung KP, Hu FC, et al. The use of statistical process control (risk-adjusted CUSUM, risk-adjusted RSPRT and CRAM with prediction limits) for monitoring the outcomes of out-of-hospital cardiac arrest patients rescued by the EMS system. J Eval Clin Pract 2011;17(1):71–7.
16. Grigg OA, Farewell VT, Spiegelhalter DJ. Use of risk-adjusted CUSUM and RSPRT charts for monitoring in medical contexts. Stat Methods Med Res 2003; 12(2):147–70.
17. Steiner SH, Cook RJ, Farewell VT. Risk-adjusted monitoring of binary surgical outcomes. Med Decis Making 2001;21:163–9.

18. Rogers CA, Reeves BC, Caputo M, et al. Control chart methods for monitoring cardiac surgical performance and their interpretation. J Thorac Cardiovasc Surg 2004;128(6):811–9.
19. Kusamura S, Baratti D, Deraco M. Multidimensional analysis of learning curve for cytoreductive surgery and hyperthermic intraperitoneal chemotherapy in peritoneal surface malignancies. Annals of Surgery 2011;255(2):348–56.
20. Sugarbaker PH. Peritonectomy procedures. Ann Surg 1995;221:29–42.
21. Deraco M, Baratti D, Kusamura S, et al. Surgical technique of parietal and visceral peritonectomy for peritoneal surface malignancies. J Surg Oncol 2009;100:321–8.
22. Jacquet P, Sugarbaker PH. Current methodologies for clinical assessment of patients with peritoneal carcinomatosis. J Exp Clin Cancer Res 1996;15:49–58.
23. Fujimoto S, Takahashi M, Kobayashi K, et al. Combined treatment of pelvic exenterative surgery and intra-operative pelvic hyperthermochemotherapy for locally advanced rectosigmoid cancer: report of a case. Surg Today 1993;23:1094–8.
24. Baratti D, Kusamura S, Nonaka D, et al. Pseudomyxoma peritonei: clinical pathological and biological prognostic factors in patients treated with cytoreductive surgery and hyperthermic intraperitoneal chemotherapy (HIPEC). Ann Surg Oncol 2008;15:526–34.
25. Rossi CR, Foletto M, Mocellin S, et al. Hyperthermic intraoperative intraperitoneal chemotherapy with cisplatin and doxorubicin in patients who undergo cytoreductive surgery for peritoneal carcinomatosis and sarcomatosis: phase I study. Cancer 2002;94:492–9.
26. Younan R, Kusamura S, Baratti D, et al. Morbidity, toxicity, and mortality classification systems in the local regional treatment of peritoneal surface malignancy. J Surg Oncol 2008;98:253–7 Review.
27. Younan R, Kusamura S, Baratti D, et al. Bowel complications in 203 cases of peritoneal surface malignancies treated with peritonectomy and closed-technique intraperitoneal hyperthermic perfusion. Ann Surg Oncol 2005;12:910–8.
28. Kusamura S, Baratti D, Younan R, et al. Impact of cytoreductive surgery and hyperthermic intraperitoneal chemotherapy on systemic toxicity. Ann Surg Oncol 2007;14:2550–8.
29. Charlson ME, Pompei P, Ales KL, et al. A new method of classifying prognostic comorbidity in longitudinal studies: development and validation. J Chronic Dis 1987;40(5):373–83.
30. Hanley JA, McNeil BJ. The meaning and use of the area under a receiver operating characteristic (ROC) curve. Radiology 1982;143:29–36.
31. Lemeshow S, Hosmer DW Jr. A review of goodness of fit statistics for use in the development of logistic regression models. Am J Epidemiol 1982;115:92–106.
32. Chua T, Yan TD, Saxena A, et al. Should the treatment of peritoneal carcinomatosis by cytoreductive surgery and hyperthermic intraperitoneal chemotherapy still be regarded as a highly morbid procedure? A systematic review of morbidity and mortality. Ann Surg 2009;249:900–7.
33. Glehen O, Gilly FN, Boutitie F, et al, French Surgical Association. Toward curative treatment of peritoneal carcinomatosis from nonovarian origin by cytoreductive surgery combined with perioperative intraperitoneal chemotherapy: a multi-institutional study of 1,290 patients. Cancer 2010;116:5608–18.
34. Park IJ, Choi GS, Lim KH, et al. Multidimensional analysis of the learning curve for laparoscopic resection in rectal cancer. J Gastrointest Surg 2009;13:275–81.
35. Son GM, Kim JG, Lee JC, et al. Multidimensional analysis of the learning curve for laparoscopic rectal cancer surgery. J Laparoendosc Adv Surg Tech A 2010; 20(7):609–17.

36. Schlachta CM, Mamazza J, Seshadri PA, et al. Defining a learning curve for laparoscopic colorectal resections. Dis Colon Rectum 2001;44:217–22.

37. Axelrod DA, Guidinger MK, Metzger RA, et al. Transplant center quality assessment using a continuously updatable, risk-adjusted technique (CUSUM). Am J Transplant 2006;6(2):313–23.

38. Chua TC, Moran BJ, Sugarbaker PH, et al. Early- and long-term outcome data of patients with pseudomyxoma peritonei from appendiceal origin treated by a strategy of cytoreductive surgery and hyperthermic intraperitoneal chemotherapy. J Clin Oncol 2012;30(20):2449–56.

39. González Bayón L, Sugarbaker PH, Gonzalez Moreno S, et al. Initiation of a program in peritoneal surface malignancy. Surg Oncol Clin N Am 2003;12(3): 741–53 Review.

40. Moran BJ. Establishment of a peritoneal malignancy treatment centre in the United Kingdom. Eur J Surg Oncol 2006;32(6):614–8.

Pharmacology of Perioperative Intraperitoneal and Intravenous Chemotherapy in Patients with Peritoneal Surface Malignancy

Kurt Van der Speeten, MD, PhD[a,b,*], O. Anthony Stuart, BS[c],
Paul H. Sugarbaker, MD, FRCS[c]

KEYWORDS

- Peritoneal metastases • Pharmacology • Intraperitoneal chemotherapy
- Intravenous chemotherapy

KEY POINTS

The main teaching points of this article are:

- To understand the pharmacologic principle of dose intensification, the main rationale for providing locoregional cancer chemotherapy.
- To provide an update on the pharmacologic data available concerning the cancer chemotherapy drugs used in locoregional cancer chemotherapy protocols.
- To identify current controversies regarding the use of intraperitoneal and intravenous cancer chemotherapy in patients with peritoneal carcinomatosis.

INTRODUCTION

Peritoneal surface malignancy (PSM) is a common secondary manifestation of digestive and gynecologic malignancies alike.[1–3] Less frequently, PSM originates from a primary peritoneal cancer such as mesothelioma.[4] Despite continuing advances in systemic chemotherapy, no long-term survival is reported in PSM patients with this treatment modality alone. By contrast, cytoreductive surgery (CRS) combined with perioperative intraperitoneal (IP) and intravenous (IV) chemotherapy has resulted in encouraging clinical results in both phase II and phase III trials.[5–13] Now that the proof of principle for these new treatment modalities has been demonstrated, the question

Conflict of interest: None.

[a] Department of Surgical Oncology, Ziekenhuis Oost-Limburg, Schiepse Bos 6, Genk 3600, Belgium; [b] Department of Medicine, Research Group Oncology, University of Hasselt, Hasselt, Belgium; [c] Department of Surgical Oncology, Washington Cancer Institute, Washington Hospital Center, Irving Street 106, NW, Suite 3900, Washington, DC 20010, USA
* Corresponding author. Department of Surgical Oncology, Ziekenhuis Oost-Limburg, Schiepse Bos 6, Genk 3600, Belgium.
E-mail address: kurt.vanderspeeten@zol.be

remains as to where further improvement is to be sought. Although further clinical trials are needed, an equally important role exists for pharmacologic research in this setting. A disturbing variety of perioperative chemotherapy protocols is used in PSM patients, based on often scant pharmacologic data. This article reviews the current pharmacologic data and offers guidance toward further improvement and standardization of these cancer chemotherapy regimens.

DOSE INTENSIFICATION

One of the main limiting factors governing dosimetry in systemic chemotherapy is hematological toxicity. In other words, the actual dose given IV is not so much the dose one wants to give based on cytotoxicity studies, but rather the dose tolerated by the patient's hematological reserve. By contrast, the dose intensification offered by the peritoneal membrane after IP administration gives a unique opportunity to expose the residual microscopic intraperitoneal tumor cells in PSM patients after CRS to very high doses of the cancer chemotherapy drug. This concept of dose intensification was first explored by Dedrick and colleagues.[14–18] In his landmark article of 1978 Dedrick concluded that the peritoneal permeability of several hydrophilic anticancer drugs may be considerably less than the plasma clearance of that same drug.[14] **Fig. 1** demonstrates his 2-compartment model. The transport over the membrane is modeled according to the equation:

$$\text{Rate of mass transfer} = PA\,(C_P - C_B)$$

where PA is permeability area (PA = effective contact area × permeability), C_P is concentration in peritoneal cavity, and C_B is concentration in the blood. Although the equation permits calculation of the pharmacokinetic advantage, the model does not tell anything about the specific penetration of the cancer chemotherapy drug

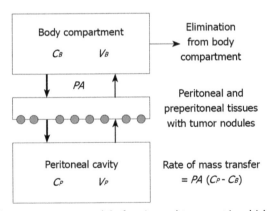

Fig. 1. Traditional 2-compartment model of peritoneal transport in which transfer of a drug from the peritoneal cavity to the blood occurs across the "peritoneal membrane." The permeability-area product (PA) governs this transfer, and can be calculated by measuring the rate of drug disappearance from the cavity and dividing by the overall concentration difference between the peritoneal cavity and the blood (or plasma). C_B = the free drug concentration in the blood (or plasma); V_B = volume of distribution of the drug in the body; C_P = the free drug concentration in the peritoneal fluid; V_P = volume of the peritoneal cavity. (*Modified from* Dedrick RL, Flessner MF. Pharmacokinetic problems in peritoneal drug administration: Tissue penetration and surface exposure. J Natl Cancer Inst 1997; 89(7):483; with permission.)

into the tissue or tumor nodule. Neither does it predict the value of the effective contact area. It simply describes the transfer between 2 compartments.

PERITONEAL MEMBRANE

The rationale of administering chemotherapeutic drugs into the peritoneal cavity is based on the relative transport barrier formed by the tissue surrounding the peritoneal space. The peritoneum is a complex 3-dimensional organ covering the abdominopelvic organs and the abdominal wall, and contains a potentially large space. The most elaborate description of the ultrastructure of the peritoneum in man was presented in 1941 by Baron.[19] The peritoneum consists of a monolayer of mesothelial cells supported by a basement membrane and 5 layers of connective tissue, which account for a total thickness of 90 μm. The connective-tissue layers include interstitial cells and a matrix of collagen, hyaluron, and proteoglycans. The cellular component consists of pericytes, parenchymal cells, and blood capillaries. This complex is often referred to as the peritoneal membrane, and the description is a working model derived from research on the peritoneum as a dialysis membrane. Contrary to intuitive thinking, the elimination of the mesothelial lining during peritonectomy procedures does not alter the pharmacokinetic properties of the peritoneum in the transport of chemotherapeutic agents from the peritoneal cavity to the plasma compartment. In a rodent model, Flessner and colleagues[20] demonstrated that neither removal of the stagnant fluid layer on the mesothelium nor removal of the mesothelial lining influences the mass transfer coefficient (MTC) over the barrier. There is indirect evidence supporting this hypothesis in humans in that the extent of the peritonectomy in peritoneal carcinomatosis (PC) patients does little to alter the intraperitoneal chemotherapy pharmacokinetics (PK) of mitomycin C or 5-fluorouracil.[21–23] Basic research indicates it is the blood capillary wall and the surrounding interstitial matrix that are the principal barriers for clearance of molecules from the abdominopelvic space, not the mesothelial lining.[24]

PHARMACOKINETICS VERSUS PHARMACODYNAMICS

PK describes what the body does to the drug whereas pharmacodynamics (PD) describes what the drug does to the body.

The basic way of depicting PK data is by a concentration × time graph. **Fig. 2** shows such a PK graph for IP doxorubicin during hyperthermic intraperitoneal perioperative

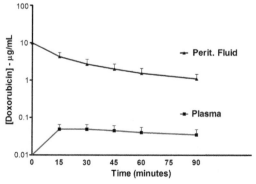

Fig. 2. Doxorubicin pharmacokinetics in 145 patients. Concentration-time graph of intraperitoneal doxorubicin during hyperthermic intraperitoneal perioperative chemotherapy in 145 patients.

chemotherapy (HIPEC).[24] The subsequent pharmacologic advantage is quantified by determining the area-under-the-curve (AUC) ratio of the peritoneal exposure over the intravenous exposure after IP administration. In this equation, AUC IP is responsible for efficacy and AUC IV is a measure of toxicity. Until recently all pharmacologic research regarding perioperative chemotherapy was PK research.

This PK strategy, however, leaves out all PD variables that are equally important for the final ability of the cancer chemotherapy drug to kill tumor cells. The basic way of depicting PD is by plotting a concentration × effect graph. However, this is not possible in vivo. The closest we can come is by adding the concentrations of the cancer chemotherapy drug inside the tumor nodule to the PK graph, as in **Fig. 3**.[25] The higher concentrations of the doxorubicin inside the tumor nodule when compared with the peritoneal levels are the result of irreversible binding at the level of the tumor cell membrane.

Box 1 summarizes all PK and PD variables involved in protocols for perioperative cancer chemotherapy. One could state that the PK variables influence the amount of drug showing up at the level of the tumor nodule and that the PD variables subsequently determine what goes on inside the tumor nodule. As such the tumor nodule should be considered the most appropriate end point in the pharmacologic exploration regarding these treatment strategies.

TIMING OF PERIOPERATIVE CANCER CHEMOTHERAPY IN RELATION TO TIMING OF CRS

In the clinical application of chemotherapy in PSM patients, intervention can occur at 4 points in the timeline. First, induction intraperitoneal and/or intravenous chemotherapy is suggested as an option for reducing dissemination to the extra-abdominal space, testing the tumor biology, and for reducing the extent of small PC nodules, and theoretically this approach, called neoadjuvant intraperitoneal and systemic chemotherapy (NIPS), may facilitate definitive CRS after initial exploratory laparoscopy or laparotomy.[26] Radiologic and clinical responses with NIPS have been reported by several groups.[26–28] However, although NIPS may reduce the tumor load to be addressed by CRS, it has several disadvantages. Adhesions from prior surgical interventions may interfere with adequate intraperitoneal drug distribution and, as complete responses are unusual, further cytoreduction chemotherapy is necessary if the approach is to be curative. NIPS is reported to add to morbidity and mortality of further surgical treatment, and extensive fibrosis, as a response to chemotherapy, may occur and render judgments concerning the extent of PC difficult or impossible to assess.[29]

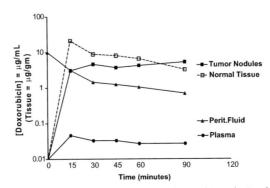

Fig. 3. Concentration-time graph of intraperitoneal doxorubicin during hyperthermic intraperitoneal perioperative chemotherapy.

Box 1
Pharmacokinetic and pharmacodynamic variables of perioperative cancer chemotherapy

Pharmacokinetic VR

- Dose
- Volume
- Duration
- Carrier solution
- Pressure
- Molecular weight

Pharmacodynamic VR

- Tumor nodule size
- Density
- Vascularity
- Interstitial fluid pressure
- Binding
- Temperature

HIPEC is the most widely explored modality that has shown consistent clinically improved outcomes in many phase II trials and several phase III trials.[5–13]

Early postoperative intraperitoneal chemotherapy (EPIC) has some conceptual advantages. It is administered after CRS at the time of minimal residual tumor burden, and intraperitoneal treatments initiated before wound healing occurs can minimize nonuniform drug distribution and eliminate residual cancer cell entrapment in postoperative fibrin deposits. The proper selection of chemotherapy agents based on pharmacologic principles suggests the use of cell-cycle–specific drugs such as 5-fluorouracil and the taxanes. Most EPIC regimens are administered postoperatively (day 1 to day 4/5) through both an inflow catheter and outflow drains inserted at the time of CRS, and can be applied with or without HIPEC.[30]

Several phase III trials of long-term combined intraperitoneal and systemic chemotherapy have demonstrated that intravenous plus intraperitoneal chemotherapy improves survival in patients with optimally debulked stage III ovarian cancer, compared with intravenous chemotherapy alone.[31–33] This approach may be used as chemotherapeutic bridging between incomplete initial surgery and definitive cytoreduction or second-look surgery. This type of chemotherapy is an adjuvant and not a perioperative use of chemotherapy.

Failure analysis for CRS plus perioperative chemotherapy indicates that recurrent cancer occurs most frequently within the abdominal and pelvic cavity.[34] Although systemic metastases occur, treatment failures rarely occur in liver, lungs, or other systemic sites. To optimize the treatment of patients with PC, the greatest benefit will probably result from a combination of the 4 treatment strategies.

AN UPDATE ON CANCER CHEMOTHERAPY DRUGS USED IN PROTOCOLS FOR PERIOPERATIVE CANCER CHEMOTHERAPY

Table 1 provides an overview of drugs commonly used in protocols for perioperative cancer chemotherapy, and their main pharmacologic characteristics.

Table 1
Molecular weight and area-under-the-curve ratios of intraperitoneal exposure to systemic exposure of chemotherapeutic agents used to treat peritoneal carcinomatosis

Drug	Molecular Weight (Da)	Area-Under-the-Curve Ratio
5-Fluorouracil	130.08	250
Carboplatin	371.25	10
Cisplatin	300.1	7.8
Docetaxel	861.9	552
Doxorubicin	579.99	230
Etoposide	588.58	65
Floxuridine	246.2	75
Gemcitabine	299.5	500
Irinotecan	677.19	No data available
Melphalan	305.2	93
Mitomycin C	334.3	23.5
Mitoxantrone	517.41	115–255
Oxaliplatin	397.3	16
Paclitaxel	853.9	1000
Pemetrexed	597.49	40.8

Mitomycin C

Mitomycin C is an alkylating antibiotic extracted from *Streptomyces* species, whose most important mechanism of action is through DNA cross-linking. Although mitomycin C is not regarded as a prodrug, it is not active against cancerous tissue as the unchanged molecule. The drug is modified as it enters the cell into an active state.[35] It is inactivated by microsomal enzymes in the liver and is metabolized in the spleen and kidneys. Jacquet and colleagues[22] reported a clear pharmacokinetic advantage after IP administration with an AUC IP/IV ratio of 23.5. Mitomycin C has been extensively studied in preclinical and clinical work, and is widely used for PC[36–39]; it is used for peritoneal carcinomatosis from colorectal cancer, appendiceal cancer, ovarian cancer, gastric cancer, and diffuse malignant peritoneal mesothelioma.[5,6,40–44] Barlogie and colleagues[36] suggested in vitro thermal enhancement of mitomycin C. A recent pharmacologic analysis of 145 HIPEC patients by the authors' group revealed that the largest proportion (62%) of the total drug administered remained in the body at 90 minutes.[45] Jacquet and colleagues[22] and Van Ruth and colleagues[46] presented similar data. The location and chemical state of this large amount of retained mitomycin C remains to be determined. It is possible that active drug remains in visceral surfaces, parietal peritoneum, and preperitoneal tissues. Unfortunately, a reliable assay of tissue mitomycin C concentrations does not exist; determination of the anatomic site and anticancer activity of this large proportion of the total mitomycin C administered has not been determined. Controversies still exist regarding the proper dosimetry of the chemotherapy solution. Some institutions use a single dose of mitomycin C, others a double dose, and still others a triple dose of the drug over a 90-minute time period.[46–48] A remarkable difference in drug dosimetry between different groups of investigators is reported. Van Ruth and colleagues[46] at the Dutch Cancer Institute reported a dose-finding study. Their data suggest that a dose of 35 mg/m² resulted in the highest peritoneal/plasma AUC ratio with acceptable toxicity. To maintain the concentration throughout the 90 minutes of perfusion time, the dose was divided into 3 fractions: 50% at the start, 25% after 30 minutes, and 25% at 60 minutes. The toxicity profile of mitomycin C, including anastomotic dehiscence and impaired wound healing, has been well characterized.[45,49–51]

Doxorubicin

Doxorubicin ($C_{27}H_{29}NO_{11}$) or hydroxyldaunorubicin (adriamycin) is an anthracycline antibiotic. Although traditionally categorized as a DNA-intercalating drug, the actual mechanism of action is a critical interaction of doxorubicin with the cell surface membrane as demonstrated by Tritton.[52] Lane and colleagues[53] reported on the temperature dependence of this phenomenon. Because of its wide in vitro and in vivo activity against a broad range of malignancies, its slow clearance from the peritoneal compartment owing to the high molecular weight of the hydrochloride salt (579.99 Da), its favorable AUC ratio of intraperitoneal to intravenous concentration times of 230, and the absence of risk for dose-limiting cardiotoxicity when used IP, doxorubicin was considered a potential beneficial agent for perioperative IP delivery. This notion was supported by both experimental and clinical PK data.[24,25,54–58] A moderate temperature enhancement has been postulated. Based on ex vivo experiments, Pilati and colleagues[59] suggested that this hyperthermic augmentation was based on increased drug uptake and sensitization of tumor cells (but not normal mucosal cells) to the cytotoxic effects of doxorubicin. More recently, PEGylated liposomal doxorubicin has generated interest for HIPEC application because of its favorable PK.[60] Doxorubicin-based HIPEC has been used in PSM from appendiceal, gastric, ovarian, and colon cancer, as well as in peritoneal mesothelioma.

Cisplatin

Cisplatin (cis-diamminedichloroplatinum-III, CDDP) causes apoptotic cell death by formation of DNA adducts.[61] It has been well studied in the setting of adjuvant normothermic postoperative IP chemotherapy for residual small-volume ovarian cancer after CRS. Three randomized trials showed a significant survival benefit.[31–33] In the setting of CRS and HIPEC, cisplatin has been used for intracavitary therapy for ovarian cancer, gastric cancer, desmoplastic small round cell tumor, and peritoneal mesothelioma. It is eliminated by renal excretion, and consequently the main concern with its use is renal toxicity. Urano and colleagues[62] showed an excellent in vitro and in vivo thermal augmentation of cisplatin. The penetration of cisplatin into tumor nodules was studied by several groups. Los and colleagues[63] for the first time described intratumoral distribution of cisplatin after IP administration and suggested that the advantage over IP versus IV administration was maximal in the first 1.5 mm. Van der Vaart and colleagues[64] investigated the cisplatin-induced DNA-adduct formation and were able to measure this 3 to 5 mm into the tumor tissue. Esquis and colleagues,[65] in an experimental model, reported an enhanced cisplatin penetration when cisplatin was administered with increased pressure.

Carboplatin

Carboplatin ((1,1-cyclobutanedicarboxylato)platinum(II)) is a platinum compound of higher molecular weight than cisplatin. Its main advantage is its decreased renal toxicity. As such it is currently explored in normothermic IP chemotherapy protocols in patients with advanced ovarian cancer.[66,67] Czejka and colleagues,[68] in a clinical study with normothermic carboplatin, reported a relative bioavailability (calculated as AUC values) that was at least 6 times higher in the IP fluid than in the serum for 48 hours. In 1991, Los and coworkers[69] compared carboplatin and cisplatin after IP administration in a rat model of PC. Their data demonstrated that despite a clear pharmacokinetic advantage of IP carboplatin over cisplatin; its capacity to penetrate into peritoneal cancer nodules and tumor cells is far lower than that of cisplatin. These data have limited its clinical application in the past. By contrast, a more recent direct comparison reveals a comparable or better drug penetration of IP carboplatin when compared with IP cisplatin given at equitoxic doses.[70] This finding has recently revived clinical interest in carboplatin for IP application.

Oxaliplatin

Oxaliplatin (oxalato-1,2-diaminocyclohexane-platinum(II)) is a third-generation platinum complex with a similar cytotoxic mechanism to that of cisplatin. In contrast to cisplatin, it has proven activity in colorectal and appendiceal malignancies.[71] Its clinical use in colorectal PSM patients was initiated by Elias and Sideris.[72,73] In a dose-escalation and pharmacokinetic study, they showed that 460 mg/m^2 of oxaliplatin in 2 L/m^2 of chemotherapy solution over 30 minutes was well tolerated.[72] The low AUC ratio is compensated by the rapid absorption of the drug into the tissue. In contrast to cisplatin and mitomycin, oxaliplatin is not stable in chloride-containing solutions,[74] thus necessitating a dextrose-based carrier that may result in serious electrolyte disturbances and hyperglycemia during the intracavitary therapy.[75] A recent murine pharmacokinetic study with oxaliplatin confirmed its substantial heath augmentation.[76] In a single-institution comparative study, Votanopoulos and colleagues[77] reported a higher hematologic toxicity with oxaliplatin-based HIPEC in comparison with mitomycin-based HIPEC. However, this was only statistically significant in the patients undergoing splenectomy as part of their CRS.

Taxanes

Paclitaxel and docetaxel are taxanes considered for IP chemotherapy. The taxanes stabilize the microtubule against depolymerization; thereby disrupting normal microtubule dynamics.[78] These agents exert cytotoxic activity against a broad range of tumors. Because of their high molecular weight, these molecules have a remarkable high AUC ratio of 853 and 861, respectively,[79] which translates into a clear pharmacokinetic advantage for intraperitoneal administration.[80] The data regarding possible thermal augmentation of taxanes are conflicting.[81–84] Taxanes have been used in a neoadjuvant intraperitoneal setting as well as intraoperatively and postoperatively. Their cell-cycle–specific mechanism of action makes them a particularly good candidate for repeat application such as in EPIC, NIPS, or normothermic adjuvant postoperative intraperitoneal chemotherapy.[26,31,32,85,86] Novel formulations of taxanes aiming at an increased bioavailability are under investigation.[87]

Pemetrexed

Pemetrexed is a multitargeted antifolate that belongs to the antimetabolites. It is an analogue of folic acid with cytotoxic activity against a variety of malignancies, especially mesothelioma, ovarian cancer, and colon cancer. Significant improvement in survival of patients with peritoneal and pleural mesothelioma after IV administration, and favorable PK, have generated interest in permetrexed's IP application.[88,89] Pemetrexed acts mainly as a thymidylate synthase inhibitor but is also unique in terms of cellular transport and lipid solubility.[90] Pestieau and colleagues[91] reported favorable IP PK with a 24-fold increase of peritoneal exposure after IP instillation when compared with IV administration. Pemetrexed is currently under investigation for the IP treatment of peritoneal mesothelioma and ovarian cancer.[92]

Gemcitabine

Gemcitabine (2′,2′-difluorodeoxycitidine) is a pyrimidine analogue with a wide range of in vitro cytotoxic activity, particularly against pancreatic cancer. Pestieau and colleagues[93] investigated the PK and tissue distribution of IP gemcitabine in a rat model. The AUC ratio (IP/IV) after IP administration was 26.8 ± 5.8, and as such was favorable for IP administration. Several investigators explored the use of normothermic IP gemcitabine in advanced cancer outside the setting of CRS.[94–96] Resected advanced pancreatic cancer with high risk of recurrence in the operative field is a potential indication for intraoperative IP administration of heated gemcitabine in an adjuvant setting.[97]

5-Fluorouracil

Since their introduction in 1957 by Heidelberger and colleagues,[98,99] the fluorinated pyrimidines have been successfully used for a wide variety of tumors, and are still an essential component of all successful chemotherapy regimens to treat gastrointestinal cancer. The thymidylate synthase inhibitor 5-fluorouracil binds covalently with the enzyme and prevents the formation of thymidine monophosphate, the DNA nucleoside precursor. The action of 5-fluorouracil is therefore cell-cycle specific. Moreover, 5-fluorouracil, via its metabolites 5-fluorouridine diphosphate and 5-fluorouridine triphosphate, is incorporated in RNA, resulting in a second cytotoxic pathway. Minor augmentation of 5-fluorouracil by mild hyperthermia is reported.[100,101] 5-Fluorouracil is not chemically compatible with other drugs in a mixed solution for infusion or instillation. These characteristics limit the use of 5-fluorouracil perioperatively to either EPIC or intraoperative IV 5-fluorouracil.

Ifosfamide

Ifosfamide is a prodrug that needs the cytochrome P450 system of liver or red blood cells to be activated to its active metabolite 4-hydroxyifosfamide. Consequently it requires IV administration rather than IP instillation for its cytotoxic activity. It is 1 of 4 drugs that show true heat synergy, with 5 to 10 times the duration of tumor control with 41.5°C heat in comparison with normal temperatures.[62] It may be an ideal systemic drug to increase the cytotoxicity of hyperthermic intraperitoneal perioperative chemotherapy. Pharmacokinetic data show the presence of ifosfamide and its active metabolite in peritoneal tumor nodules after continuous IV during bidirectional intraoperative chemotherapy.[102]

ONGOING CONTROVERSIES
Dosimetry of IP Chemotherapy

One of the main hurdles preventing a wider application of IP chemotherapy for PSM patients is the astonishing variety in the dosimetry available worldwide. These regimens are often based on few pharmacologic data. Standardization based on sound PK and PD data is the next leap to be taken. The current regimens can be divided into concentration-based protocols and body surface area (BSA)-based protocols. Most groups use a drug dose based on calculated BSA (mg/m^2) in analogy to systemic chemotherapy regimens. These regimens take BSA as a measure for the effective contact area (peritoneal surface area in the Dedrick formula). However, Rubin and colleagues[103] demonstrate that there is an imperfect correlation between actual peritoneal surface area and calculated BSA, and there may be sex differences in peritoneal surface areas, which in turn affect absorption characteristics. This phenomenon is also acknowledged in peritoneal dialysis literature. The female has a 10% larger peritoneal surface in proportion to body size than the male. There have been attempts to estimate the functional peritoneal surface area through applying stereologic methods to computed tomography (CT) scans and by extrapolating data from cadaver measurements and in animal models.[104–106]

By contrast, some groups use a totally different dosimetry regimen based on concentration. The total amount of cancer chemotherapy is mixed in a large volume of carrier solution (usually 6 L) that is placed in a reservoir. For example, Deraco and Rossi at the Milan Cancer Institute use doxorubicin, 15.25 mg/m^2/L and cisplatin, 43 mg/m^2/L in a total volume of 6 L. Glehen and Gilly from Lyon use mitomycin C, 0.5 mg/kg and cisplatin, 0.7 mg/kg in a total volume of 4 to 6 L.[107–110] From a pharmacologic point of view, the big advantage of a concentration-based system is that the residual tumor nodules after CRS are exposed to a constant diffusional force and, thus, cytotoxicity. Unfortunately the prize to be paid for a better prediction of the efficacy of the intraperitoneal chemotherapy is a high unpredictability of the levels of plasmatic cancer chemotherapy and, thus, toxicity. Indeed, according to the aforementioned Dedrick formula of transport over the peritoneal membrane, an increase in the volume of intraperitoneal chemotherapy solution will cause an increase in both diffusion surface and the amount of drug transferred from peritoneal space to plasma. For example, in 10 patients with renal insufficiency dialyzed with different volumes ranging from 0.5 up to 3 L, there is a linear increase in mass transfer.[111] PK data in PSM patients substantiate this hypothesis. **Fig. 4** demonstrates that in 10 PSM patients with a markedly contracted abdomen and small filling volume during HIPEC with mitomycin C, there is statistically significant less transfer of the drug over the peritoneal membrane.[112] Contrastingly, and clinically more important, is the situation in PSM patients with preoperative abdominal distention caused by ascites or mucus accumulation. Their significantly increased peritoneal surface area will result in higher plasmatic levels of the cancer chemotherapy drug, and thus increased risk or toxicity. The authors are currently pharmacologically investigating a CT-based correction on the dosimetry in this patient group.

Effect of Hyperthermia

Adding hyperthermia to protocols for perioperative cancer chemotherapy adds significantly to the logistic challenge of the procedure, and as such needs scientific validation. Adding hyperthermia to IP chemotherapy may increase the tumor response to cancer chemotherapy through several mechanisms. First, heat alone has a direct antitumor effect. Mild hyperthermia above 41°C induces selective cytotoxicity of malignant cells by several mechanisms: impaired DNA repair, protein denaturation, and inhibition of oxidative metabolism in the microenvironment of malignant cells. This process leads to increased acidity, lysosomal activation, and increased apoptotic cell death.[113–115] In this setting, thermal tolerance can be induced by upregulation of heat-shock proteins, which may limit the importance of a direct antitumor effect of heat.[116]

Second, applying mild hyperthermia augments the cytotoxic effects of some chemotherapeutic agents. Synergy between heat and cancer chemotherapy drugs may arise from multiple events such as heat damage to adenosine triphosphate–binding cassette transporters (drug accumulation), intracellular drug-detoxification pathways, and repair mechanisms of drug-induced DNA adducts.[117] Such augmented effects are postulated for doxorubicin,[59,118] platinum complexes,[36,62,119,120] mitomycin C,[36] melphalan,[120] and docetaxel, irinotecan, and gemcitabine.[121]

Third, hyperthermia may increase the penetration depth of the cancer chemotherapy solution into tissues and tumor nodules. Jacquet and colleagues[54] report

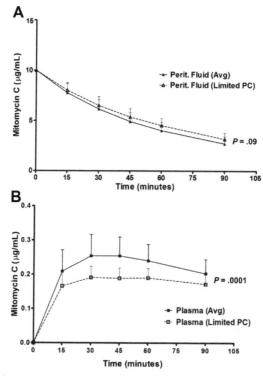

Fig. 4. Study of a limited peritoneal space (PC) and its effect on pharmacokinetics of mitomycin C during HIPEC. The peritoneal fluid (*A*) and plasma (*B*) area under the curve are plotted in 2 groups of patients. One subgroup of 10 patients was able to receive into the intraperitoneal space only 65% or less of the total volume of chemotherapy solution. The concentration of mitomycin C in this group was compared with the average of that in the 145 patients. With a limited peritoneal space there is less mitomycin C absorbed into the plasma (*P* = .0001).

that tissue penetration of doxorubicin is enhanced when the cancer chemotherapy solution is administered IP at 43°C. In addition, hyperthermia does not affect the pharmacokinetic advantages of IP doxorubicin, with low plasma and distant tissue levels. Leunig and colleagues[122] report a thermal dose-dependent decrease in interstitial fluid pressure in experimental solid tumors in an animal model after hyperthermia.

All these experimental data, however, were unable to establish a direct effect of hyperthermia on survival. Klaver and colleagues,[123] in a rat model of PSM, for the first time separated the intraoperative IP chemotherapy from the IP hyperthermia. Their study showed that the survival of the PSM rats after CRS was highly dependent on the presence of the chemotherapeutic agent in the perfusate but not on the hyperthermia. No similar human data are available at present.

Bidirectional (IP + IV) Intraoperative Chemotherapy

In 2002, Elias and colleagues[73] first reported the clinical use of intraoperative IV 5-fluorouracil and leucovorin in conjunction with oxaliplatin-based HIPEC. By combining intraoperative IV and intraoperative IP cancer chemotherapy, a bidirectional diffusion gradient is created through the intermediate tissue layer, which contains the cancer nodules as conceptualized in **Fig. 5**.[124] This approach offers opportunities for

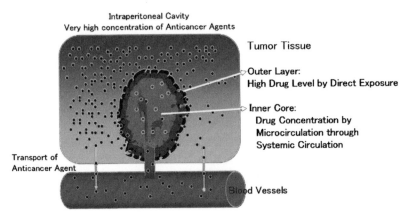

Fig. 5. Pharmacologic concept of bidirectional intravenous and intraperitoneal chemotherapy. (*Modified from* Fujiwara K. Three ongoing intraperitoneal chemotherapy trials in ovarian cancer. Int J Gynecol Cancer 2007;17(1):2; with permission.)

optimizing cancer chemotherapy delivery to the target peritoneal tumor nodules. **Fig. 6** demonstrates the concentrations of 5-fluorouracil in tumor nodules that were harvested during bidirectional (IP doxorubicin and mitomycin C plus rapid-infusion IV 5-fluorouracil) intraoperative chemotherapy treatment.[125] The rapid distribution of the 5-fluorouracil after IV administration affects all compartments similarly. The metabolism of the 5-fluorouracil, on the other hand, is mainly restricted to the plasma compartment by the liver. The high level of 5-fluorouracil persists within the peritoneal fluid because the drug can only leave the peritoneal space by back-diffusion through the peritoneal and subperitoneal tissues: the enzyme dihydropyrimidine dehydrogenase is not present in the artificial ascites fluid. These data show a clear pharmacokinetic advantage for the intraoperative IV administration of 5-fluorouracil. Although 5-fluorouracil is administered as a normothermic IV solution, it penetrates into the heated tumor nodules. Normothermically administered 5-fluorouracil becomes subject to augmentation of mild hyperthermia of the subperitoneal compartment. Therefore, heat targeting is achieved by modulating the timing of IV chemotherapy.

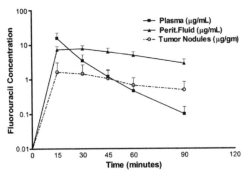

Fig. 6. 5-Fluorouracil concentrations in plasma, peritoneal fluid, and tumor nodules after intravenous administration during hyperthermic intraperitoneal chemotherapy procedure. (*From* Van der Speeten K, Stuart OA, Mahteme H, et al. Pharmacology of perioperative 5-fluorouracil. J Surg Oncol 2010;102(7):730–5; with permission.)

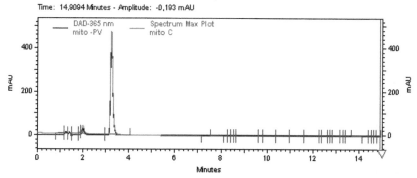

Fig. 7. Representative mitomycin C chromatogram in peritoneal fluid of a PSM patient during HIPEC at 75 minutes. Similar monospiked chromatograms were recovered from plasma, urine, and peritoneal fluid throughout HIPEC. The patient recurred at the peritoneal cavity 3 months after CRS and HIPEC.

Recently the authors were able to demonstrate a similar pharmacokinetic advantage and heat targeting of intraoperative IV ifosfamide (continuous infusion over 90 minutes).[102]

Individual Drug Sensitivity

The efficacy of perioperative cancer chemotherapy protocols is governed by both pharmacokinetic and nonpharmacokinetic variables. Ultimately, however, the individual drug sensitivity of a tumor to cancer chemotherapy may be equally important. There is evidence to support tumor-specific heterogeneous activity of cytotoxic drugs in cell cultures of different tumors.[126–128] Van der Speeten and colleagues[45] confirm the same heterogeneous cytotoxic response of cytotoxic drugs in PC samples in a variety of tumors, having recently identified PSM patients who did not metabolize mitomycin C during HIPEC after complete CRS. **Fig. 7** shows a representative high-pressure liquid chromatogram (HPLC) of a such a nonmetabolizer. Prospective clinical follow-up on these nonmetabolizers shows a risk for early recurrence. These preliminary data warrant close clinical follow-up for these patients. Based on these in vitro and clinical data, drug selection based on preoperative in vitro testing is a potential strategy for improving these protocols for perioperative cancer chemotherapy.

SUMMARY

The last 2 decades has witnessed the emergence of protocols for perioperative cancer chemotherapy in the treatment of PC patients, which has resulted in remarkable clinical successes in contrast to prior failures. Now that the concept has been proved, the time has come to further improve the treatment protocols. Assessment of further pharmacologic data on perioperative chemotherapy in PC patients should result in more standardization and a better clinical outcome.

REFERENCES

1. Jayne DG, Fook S, Loi C, et al. Peritoneal carcinomatosis from colorectal cancer. Br J Surg 2002;89(12):1545–50.

2. Chu DZ, Lang NP, Thompson C, et al. Peritoneal carcinomatosis in nongyneco-logic malignancy. A prospective study of prognostic factors. Cancer 1989;63(2): 364–7.
3. Sadeghi B, Arvieux C, Glehen O, et al. Peritoneal carcinomatosis from non-gynecologic malignancies: results of the EVOCAPE 1 multicentric prospective study. Cancer 2000;88(2):358–63.
4. Turner K, Varghese S, Alexander HR Jr. Current concepts in the evaluation and treatment of patients with diffuse malignant peritoneal mesothelioma. J Natl Compr Canc Netw 2012;10(1):49–57.
5. Verwaal VJ, Van Ruth S, De Bree E, et al. Randomized trial of cytoreduction and hyperthermic intraperitoneal chemotherapy versus systemic chemotherapy and palliative surgery in patients with peritoneal carcinomatosis of colorectal cancer. J Clin Oncol 2003;21(20):3737–43.
6. Verwaal VJ, Bruin S, Boot H, et al. 8-year follow-up of randomized trial: cytoreduction and hyperthermic intraperitoneal chemotherapy versus systemic chemotherapy in patients with peritoneal carcinomatosis of colorectal cancer. Ann Surg Oncol 2008;15(9):2426–32.
7. Glehen O, Mithieux F, Osinsky D, et al. Surgery combined with peritonectomy procedures and intraperitoneal chemohyperthermia in abdominal cancers with peritoneal carcinomatosis: a phase II study. J Clin Oncol 2003;21(5): 799–806.
8. Yan TD, Black D, Sugarbaker PH, et al. A systematic review and meta-analysis of the randomized controlled trials on adjuvant intraperitoneal chemotherapy for respectable gastric cancer. Ann Surg Oncol 2007;14(10):2702–13.
9. Bijelic L, Jonson A, Sugarbaker PH. Systematic review of cytoreductive surgery and heated intraoperative intraperitoneal chemotherapy for treatment of perito-neal carcinomatosis in primary and recurrent ovarian cancer. Ann Oncol 2007; 18(12):1943–50.
10. Yan TD, Welch L, Black D, et al. A systematic review of the efficacy of cytoreduc-tive surgery combined with perioperative intraperitoneal chemotherapy for diffuse malignancy peritoneal mesothelioma. Ann Oncol 2007;18(5):827–34.
11. Yan TD, Black D, Savady R, et al. A systematic review on the efficacy of cytore-ductive surgery and perioperative intraperitoneal chemotherapy for pseudo-myxoma peritonei. Ann Surg Oncol 2007;14(2):484–92.
12. Yan TD, Black D, Savady R, et al. Systematic review on the efficacy of cytore-ductive surgery combined with perioperative intraperitoneal chemotherapy for peritoneal carcinomatosis from colorectal carcinoma. J Clin Oncol 2006; 24(24):4011–9.
13. Elias D, Glehen O, Gilly F. Carcinose péritonéales d'origine digestive et primi-tive. Rapport du 110 éme congrès de l'AFC. Arnette: Wolters Kluwer France; 2008.
14. Dedrick RL, Myers CE, Bungay PM, et al. Pharmacokinetic rationale for perito-neal drug administration in the treatment of ovarian cancer. Cancer Treat Rep 1978;62(1):1–11.
15. Dedrick RL. Theoretical and experimental bases of intraperitoneal chemo-therapy. Semin Oncol 1985;12(3 Suppl 4):1–6.
16. Flessner MF, Fenstermacher JD, Dedrick RL, et al. A distributed model of peritoneal-plasma transport: tissue concentration gradients. Am J Physiol 1985;248(3):F425–35.
17. Flessner MF. The transport barrier in intraperitoneal therapy. Am J Physiol Renal Physiol 2005;288(3):433–42.

18. Flessner MF. Intraperitoneal drug therapy: physical and biological principles. Cancer Treat Res 2007;134:131–52.
19. Baron MA. Structure of the intestinal peritoneum in man. Am J Anat 1941;69: 439–97.
20. Flessner M, Henegar J, Bigler S, et al. Is the peritoneum a significant barrier in peritoneal dialysis? Perit Dial Int 2003;23(6):542–9.
21. de Lima Vazquez V, Stuart OA, Mohamed F, et al. Extent of parietal peritonectomy does not change intraperitoneal chemotherapy pharmacokinetics. Cancer Chemother Pharmacol 2003;52(2):108–12.
22. Jacquet P, Averbach A, Stephens AD, et al. Heated intraoperative intraperitoneal mitomycin C and early postoperative intraperitoneal 5-fluorouracil: pharmacokinetic studies. Oncology 1998;55(2):130–8.
23. Stelin G, Rippe B. A phenomenological interpretation of the variation in dialysate volume with dwell time in CAPD. Kidney Int 1990;38(3):456–72.
24. Sugarbaker PH, Van der Speeten K, Stuart OA, et al. Impact of surgical and clinical factors on the pharmacology of intraperitoneal doxorubicin in 145 patients with peritoneal carcinomatosis. Eur J Surg Oncol 2011;37(8):719–26.
25. Van der Speeten K, Stuart OA, Mahteme H, et al. A pharmacologic analysis of intraoperative intracavitary chemotherapy with doxorubicin. Cancer Chemother Pharmacol 2009;63(5):799–805.
26. Yonemura Y, Bandou E, Sawa T, et al. Neoadjuvant treatment of gastric cancer with peritoneal dissemination. Eur J Surg Oncol 2006;32(6):661–5.
27. Sugarbaker PH. Treatment of peritoneal carcinomatosis from colon or appendiceal cancer with induction intraperitoneal chemotherapy. Cancer Treat Res 1996;82:317–25.
28. Zylberberg B, Dormont D, Janklewicz S, et al. Response to neo-adjuvant intraperitoneal and intravenous immunochemotherapy followed by interval secondary cytoreduction in stage IIIC ovarian cancer. Eur J Gynaecol Oncol 2001;22(1):40–5.
29. Esquivel J, Vidal-Jove J, Steves MA, et al. Morbidity and mortality of cytoreductive surgery and intraperitoneal chemotherapy. Surgery 1993;113(6): 631–6.
30. Sugarbaker PH, Graves T, DeBruijn EA, et al. Early postoperative intraperitoneal chemotherapy as an adjuvant therapy to surgery for peritoneal carcinomatosis from gastrointestinal cancer: pharmacologic studies. Cancer Res 1990;50(18): 5790–4.
31. Armstrong DK, Bundy B, Wenzel L, et al. Intraperitoneal cisplatin and paclitaxel in ovarian cancer. N Engl J Med 2006;354(1):34–43.
32. Markman M, Bundy BN, Alberts DS, et al. Phase III trial of standard-dose intravenous cisplatin plus paclitaxel versus moderately high-dose carboplatin followed by intravenous paclitaxel and intraperitoneal cisplatin in small-volume stage III ovarian carcinoma: an intergroup study of the Gynecologic Oncology Group, Southwestern Oncology Group, and Eastern Cooperative Oncology Group. J Clin Oncol 2001;19(4):1001–7.
33. Alberts DS, Liu PY, Hannigan EV, et al. Intraperitoneal cisplatin plus intravenous cyclophosphamide versus intravenous cisplatin plus intravenous cyclophosphamide for stage III ovarian cancer. N Engl J Med 1996;335(26):1950–5.
34. Bijelic L, Yan TD, Sugarbaker PH. Failure analysis of recurrent disease following complete cytoreduction and perioperative intraperitoneal chemotherapy in patients with peritoneal carcinomatosis from colorectal cancer. Ann Surg Oncol 2007;14(8):2281–8.

35. Bachur NR, Gordon SL, Gee MV, et al. NADPH cytochrome P-450 reductase activation of quinine anticancer agents to free radicals. Proc Natl Acad Sci U S A 1979;2:954–7.

36. Barlogie B, Corry PM, Drewinko B. In vitro thermochemotherapy of human colon cancer cells with cis-dichlorodiammineplatinum(II) and mitomycin C. Cancer Res 1980;40(4):1165–8.

37. Link KH, Leder G, Pillasch J, et al. In vitro concentration response studies and in vitro phase II tests as the experimental basis for regional chemotherapeutic protocols. Semin Surg Oncol 1998;14(3):189–201.

38. Fujita T, Tamura T, Yamada H, et al. Pharmacokinetics of mitomycin C (MMC) after intraperitoneal administration of MMC-gelatin gel and its anti-tumor effects against sarcoma-180 bearing mice. J Drug Target 1997;4(5):289–96.

39. Gilly FN, Carry PY, Sayag AC, et al. Tolerance of intraperitoneal chemohyperthermia with mitomycin C: in vivo study in dogs. Int J Hyperthermia 1992;8(5):659–66.

40. Helm CW, Richard SD, Pan J, et al. Hyperthermic intraperitoneal chemotherapy in ovarian cancer: first report of the HYPER-O registry. Int J Gynecol Cancer 2010;20(1):61–9.

41. Sugarbaker PH. Epithelial appendiceal neoplasms. Cancer J 2009;15(3):25–235.

42. Murphy EM, Sexton R, Moran BJ. Early results of surgery in 123 patients with pseudomyxoma peritonei from perforated appendiceal neoplasm. Dis Colon Rectum 2007;50(1):37–42.

43. Scaringi S, Kianmanesh R, Sabate JM, et al. Advanced gastric cancer with or without peritoneal carcinomatosis treated with hyperthermic intraperitoneal chemotherapy: a single western center experience. Eur J Surg Oncol 2008; 34(11):1246–52.

44. Baratti D, Kusamura S, Cabras AD, et al. Diffuse malignant peritoneal mesothelioma: failure analysis following cytoreduction and hyperthermic intraperitoneal chemotherapy (HIPEC). Ann Surg Oncol 2009;16(2):463–72.

45. Van der Speeten K, Stuart OA, Chang D, et al. Changes induced by surgical and clinical factors in the pharmacology of intraperitoneal mitomycin C in 145 patients with peritoneal carcinomatosis. Eur J Surg Oncol 2011;37(8):719–26.

46. Van Ruth S, Verwaal VJ, Zoetmulder FAN. Pharmacokinetics of intraperitoneal mitomycin C. Surg Oncol Clin N Am 2003;12:771–80.

47. Sugarbaker PH. Successful management of microscopic residual disease in large bowel cancer. Cancer Chemother Pharmacol 1999;43(Suppl):S15–25.

48. Esquivel J. Technology of hyperthermic intraperitoneal chemotherapy in the United States, Europe, China, Japan, and Korea. Cancer J 2009;15:249–54.

49. Smeenk RM, Verwaal VJ, Zoetmulder FA. Toxicity and mortality of cytoreduction and intraoperative hyperthermic intraperitoneal chemotherapy in pseudomyxoma peritonei. A report of 103 procedures. Eur J Surg Oncol 2006;32(2):186–90.

50. Glehen O, Osinsky D, Cotte E, et al. Intraperitoneal chemohyperthermia using a closed abdominal procedure and cytoreductive surgery for the treatment of peritoneal carcinomatosis: morbidity and mortality analysis of 216 consecutive procedures. Ann Surg Oncol 2003;10(8):863–9.

51. Sugarbaker PH, Alderman R, Edwards G, et al. Prospective morbidity and mortality assessment of cytoreductive surgery plus perioperative intraperitoneal chemotherapy to treat peritoneal dissemination of appendiceal mucinous malignancy. Ann Surg Oncol 2006;13(5):635–44.

52. Tritton TR. Cell surface actions of adriamycin. Pharmacol Ther 1991;49(3): 293–309.
53. Lane P, Vichi P, Bain DL, et al. Temperature dependence studies of adriamycin uptake and cytotoxicity. Cancer Res 1987;47(15):4038–42.
54. Jacquet P, Averbach AM, Stuart OA, et al. Hyperthermic intraperitoneal doxorubicin: pharmacokinetics, metabolism and tissue distribution in a rat model. Cancer Chemother Pharmacol 1998;41(2):147–54.
55. Johansen PB. Doxorubicin pharmacokinetics after intravenous and intraperitoneal administration in the nude mouse. Cancer Chemother Pharmacol 1981; 5(4):267–70.
56. Ozols RF, Grotzinger KR, Fisher RI, et al. Kinetic characterization and response to chemotherapy in a transplantable murine ovarian cancer. Cancer Res 1979; 39(8):3202–8.
57. Ozols RF, Locker GY, Doroshow JH, et al. Pharmacokinetics and tissue penetration in murine ovarian cancer. Cancer Res 1979;39(8):3209–14.
58. Ozols RF, Young RC, Speyer JL, et al. Phase I and pharmacological studies of adriamycin administered intraperitoneally to patients with ovarian cancer. Cancer Res 1982;42(10):4265–9.
59. Pilati P, Mocellin S, Rossi CR, et al. Doxorubicin activity is enhanced by hyperthermia in a model of ex-vivo vascular perfusion of human colon carcinoma. World J Surg 2003;27(6):640–6.
60. Harrison LE, Bryan M, Pliner L, et al. Phase-I trial of pegylated liposomal doxorubicin with hyperthermic intraperitoneal chemotherapy in patients undergoing cytoreduction for advanced intra-abdominal malignancy. Ann Surg Oncol 2008;15(5):1407–13.
61. Cepeda V, Fuertes MA, Castilla J, et al. Biochemical mechanisms of cisplatin cytotoxicity. Anticancer Agents Med Chem 2007;7(1):3–18.
62. Urano M, Kuroda M, Nishimura Y. For the clinical application of thermochemotherapy given at mild temperatures. Int J Hyperthermia 1999;15(2): 79–107.
63. Los G, Mutsaers PH, Van der Vijgh WJ, et al. Direct diffusion of cis-diamminedichloroplatinum(II) in intraperitoneal rat tumors after intraperitoneal chemotherapy: a comparison with systemic chemotherapy. Cancer Res 1989; 49(12):3380–4.
64. Van der Vaart PJ, van der Vange N, Zoetmulder FA, et al. Intraperitoneal cisplatin with regional hyperthermia in advanced ovarian cancer: pharmacokinetics and cisplatin-DNA adduct formation in patients and ovarian cancer cell lines. Eur J Cancer 1998;34(1):148–54.
65. Esquis P, Consolo D, Magnin G, et al. High intraabdominal pressure enhances the penetration and antitumor effect of intraperitoneal cisplatin on experimental carcinomatosis. Ann Surg 2006;244(1):106–12.
66. Milczek T, Klasa-Mazurkiewicz D, Sznurkowski J, et al. Regimens with intraperitoneal cisplatin plus intravenous cyclophosphamide and intraperitoneal carboplatin plus intravenous cyclophosphamide are equally effective in second line intraperitoneal chemotherapy for advanced ovarian cancer. Adv Med Sci 2012;57(1):46–50.
67. Morgan MA, Sill MW, Fujiwara K, et al. A phase I study with an expanded cohort to assess the feasibility of intraperitoneal carboplatin and intravenous paclitaxel in untreated ovarian, fallopian tube, and primary peritoneal carcinoma: a Gynecologic Oncology Group study. Gynecol Oncol 2011;121(2): 264–8.

68. Czejka M, Jäger W, Schüller J, et al. Pharmacokinetics of carboplatin after intraperitoneal administration. Arch Pharm (Weinheim) 1991;324(3):183–4.

69. Los G, Verdegaal EM, Mutsaers PH, et al. Penetration of carboplatin and cisplatin into rat peritoneal tumor nodules after intraperitoneal chemotherapy. Cancer Chemother Pharmacol 1991;28(3):159–65.

70. Jandial DD, Messer K, Farshchi-Heydari S, et al. Tumor platinum concentration following intraperitoneal administration of cisplatin versus carboplatin in an ovarian cancer model. Gynecol Oncol 2009;115(3):362–6.

71. Stewart JH 4th, Shen P, Russell G, et al. A phase I trial of oxaliplatin for intraperitoneal hyperthermic chemoperfusion for the treatment of peritoneal surface dissemination from colorectal and appendiceal cancers. Ann Surg Oncol 2008;15(8):2137–45.

72. Elias DM, Sideris L. Pharmacokinetics of heated intraoperative intraperitoneal oxaliplatin after complete resection of peritoneal carcinomatosis. Surg Oncol Clin N Am 2003;12(3):755–69.

73. Elias D, Bonnay M, Puizillou JM, et al. Heated intraoperative intraperitoneal oxaliplatin after complete resection of peritoneal carcinomatosis: pharmacokinetic and tissue distribution. Ann Oncol 2002;13(2):267–72.

74. Jerremalm E, Hedeland M, Wallin I, et al. Oxaliplatin degradation in the presence of chloride: identification and cytotoxicity of the monochloro monooxalato complex. Pharm Res 2004;21(5):891–4.

75. De Somer F, Ceelen W, Delanghe J, et al. Severe hyponatremia, hyperglycemia and hyperlactatemia are associated with intraoperative hyperthermic intraperitoneal chemoperfusion with oxaliplatin. Perit Dial Int 2008;28(1):61–6.

76. Piché N, Leblond FA, Sideris L, et al. Rationale for heating oxaliplatin for the intraperitoneal treatment of peritoneal carcinomatosis: a study of the effect of heat on intraperitoneal oxaliplatin using a murine model. Ann Surg 2011; 254(1):138–44.

77. Votanopoulos K, Ihemelandu C, Shen P, et al. A comparison of hematological toxicity profiles after heated intraperitoneal chemotherapy with oxaliplatin and mitomycin C. J Surg Res 2012. [Epub ahead of print].

78. Ceelen WP, Pahlman L, Mahteme H. Pharmacodynamic aspects of intraperitoneal cytotoxic therapy. Cancer Treat Res 2007;134:195–214.

79. Sugarbaker PH, Mora JT, Carmignani P, et al. Update on chemotherapeutic agents utilized for perioperative intraperitoneal chemotherapy. Oncologist 2005;10(2):112–22.

80. Mohamed F, Sugarbaker PH. Intraperitoneal taxanes. Surg Oncol Clin N Am 2003;12(3):825–33.

81. Rietbroek RC, Katschinski DM, Reijers MH, et al. Lack of thermal enhancement for taxanes in vitro. Int J Hyperthermia 1997;13(5):525–33.

82. Schrump DS, Zhai SP, Nguyen DM, et al. Pharmacokinetics of paclitaxel administered by hyperthermic retrograde isolated lung perfusion techniques. J Thorac Cardiovasc Surg 2002;123(4):686–94.

83. Cividalli A, Cruciani G, Livdi E, et al. Hyperthermia enhances the response of paclitaxel and radiation in a mouse adenocarcinoma. Int J Radiat Oncol Biol Phys 1999;44(2):407–12.

84. Mohamed F, Stuart OA, Glehen O, et al. Docetaxel and hyperthermia: factors that modify thermal enhancement. J Surg Oncol 2004;88(1):14–20.

85. Fujiwara Y, Takiguchi S, Nakajima K, et al. Intraperitoneal docetaxel combined with S1 for advanced gastric cancer with peritoneal dissemination. J Surg Oncol 2012;105(1):38–42.

86. Kurita N, Shimeda M, Iwata T, et al. Intraperitoneal infusion of paclitaxel with S1 for peritoneal metastases of advanced gastric cancer: phase I study. J Med Invest 2011;58(1–2):134–9.

87. Bouquet W, Ceelen W, Adriaens E, et al. In vivo toxicity and bioavailability of Taxol and a paclitaxel-cyclodextrin formulation in a rat model during HIPEC. Ann Surg Oncol 2012;17(9):2510–7.

88. Janne PA, Wozniak AJ, Belani CP, et al. Open-label study of pemetrexed alone or in combination with cisplatin for the treatment of patients with peritoneal mesothelioma: outcomes of an expanded access program. Clin Lung Cancer 2005;7(1):40–6.

89. Vogelzang NJ, Rusthoven JJ, Symanowski J, et al. Phase III study of pemetrexed in combination with cisplatin versus cisplatin alone in patients with malignant pleural mesothelioma. J Clin Oncol 2003;21(14):2636–44.

90. Takimoto CH. Antifolates in clinical development. Sem Oncol 1997;24(Suppl 18): S18–40.

91. Pestieau SR, Stuart OA, Sugarbaker PH. Multi-targeted antifolate (MTA): pharmacokinetics of intraperitoneal administration in a rat model. Eur J Surg Oncol 2000;26(7):696–700.

92. Chambers SK, Chow HH, Janicek MF, et al. Phase I trial of intraperitoneal pemetrexed, cisplatin, and paclitaxel in optimally debulked ovarian cancer. Clin Cancer Res 2012;18(9):2668–78.

93. Pestieau SR, Stuart OA, Chang D, et al. Pharmacokinetics of intraperitoneal gemcitabine in a rat model. Tumori 1998;84(6):706–11.

94. Sabbatini P, Aghajanian C, Leitao M, et al. Intraperitoneal cisplatin with intraperitoneal gemcitabine in patients with epithelial ovarian cancer: results of a phase I/II trial. Clin Cancer Res 2004;10:2962–7.

95. Morgan RJ Jr, Synold TW, Bixin X, et al. Phase I trial of intraperitoneal gemcitabine in the treatment of advanced malignancies primarily confined to the peritoneal cavity. Clin Cancer Res 2007;13(4):1232–7.

96. Gamblin TC, Egorin MJ, Zuhowski EG, et al. Intraperitoneal gemcitabine pharmacokinetics: a pilot and pharmacokinetic study in patients with advanced adenocarcinoma of the pancreas. Cancer Chemother Pharmacol 2008;62(4): 647–53.

97. Sugarbaker PH, Stuart OA, Bijelic L. Intraperitoneal gemcitabine chemotherapy treatment for patients with resected pancreatic cancer: rationale and report of early data. Int J Surg Oncol 2011;2011:161862.

98. Heidelberger C, Chaudhuri NK, Danneberg P, et al. Fluorinated pyrimidines, a new class of tumour-inhibitory compounds. Nature 1957;179(4561):663–6.

99. Muggia FM. Heidelberger Symposium on the 50th anniversary of fluoropyrimidines. Mol Cancer Ther 2009;8(5):991.

100. Jacquet P, Averbach A, Stephens AD, et al. Heated intraoperative intraperitoneal mitomycin C and early postoperative 5-fluorouracil: pharmacokinetic studies. Oncology 1998;55(2):130–8.

101. Diasio RB, Lu Z. Dihydropyrimidine dehydrogenase activity and fluorouracil chemotherapy. J Clin Oncol 1994;12(11):2239–42.

102. Van der Speeten K, Stuart OA, Mahteme H, et al. Pharmacokinetic study of perioperative intravenous ifosfamide. Int J Surg Oncol 2011;2011:185092.

103. Rubin J, Clawson M, Planch A, et al. Measurements of peritoneal surface area in man and rat. Am J Med Sci 1988;295(5):453–8.

104. Chagnac A, Herskovitz P, Weinstein T, et al. The peritoneal membrane in peritoneal dialysis patients: estimation of its functional surface area by applying

stereologic methods to computerized tomograpphy scans. J Am Soc Nephrol 1999;10(2):342–6.

105. Albanese AM, Albanese EF, Mino JH, et al. Peritoneal surface area: measurement of 40 structures covered by peritoneum: correlation between total peritoneal surface area and the surface calculated by formulas. Surg Radiol Anat 2009;31(5):369–77.

106. Breton E, Choquet P, Bergua L, et al. In vivo peritoneal surface measurement in rats by micro-computed tomography (microCT). Perit Dial Int 2008;28(2):188–94.

107. Rossi CR, Deraco M, De Simone M, et al. Hyperthermic intraperitoneal intraoperative chemotherapy after cytoreductive surgery for the treatment of abdominal sarcomatosis: clinical outcome and prognostic factors in 60 consecutive patients. Cancer 2004;100(9):1943–50.

108. Baratti D, Kusamura S, Martinetti A, et al. Prognostic value of circulating tumor markers in patients with pseudomyxoma peritonei treated with cytoreductive surgery and hyperthermic intraperitoneal chemotherapy. Ann Surg Oncol 2007;14(8):2300–8.

109. Glehen O, Schreiber V, Cotte E, et al. Cytoreductive surgery and intraperitoneal chemohyperthermia for peritoneal carcinomatosis arising from gastric cancer. Arch Surg 2004;139(1):20–6.

110. Gilly FN, Carry PY, Sayag AC, et al. Regional chemotherapy (with mitomycin C) and intra-operative hyperthermia fro digestive cancers with peritoneal carcinomatosis. Hepatogastroenterology 1994;41(2):124–9.

111. Keshaviah P, Emerson PF, Vonesh EF, et al. Relationship between body size, fill volume, and mass transfer area coefficient in peritoneal dialysis. J Am Soc Nephrol 1994;4(10):1820–6.

112. Van der Speeten K, Stuart OA, Chang D, et al. Changes induced by surgical and clinical factors in the pharmacology of intraperitoneal mitomycin C in 145 patients with peritoneal carcinomatosis. Cancer Chemother Pharmacol 2011; 68(1):147–56.

113. Sticca RP, Dach BW. Rationale for hyperthermia with intraoperative intraperitoneal chemotherapy agents. Surg Oncol Clin N Am 2003;12(3):689–701.

114. Dahl O, Dalene R, Schem BC, et al. Status of clinical hyperthermia. Acta Oncol 1999;38(7):863–73.

115. Sugarbaker PH. Laboratory and clinical basis for hyperthermia as a component of intracavitary chemotherapy. Int J Hyperthermia 2007;23(5):431–42.

116. Lepock JR. How do cells respond to their thermal environment? Int J Hyperthermia 2005;21(8):681–7.

117. Kampinga HH. Cell biological effects of hyperthermia alone or combined with radiation or drugs: a short introduction to newcomers in the field. Int J Hyperthermia 2006;22(3):191–6.

118. Hahn GM, Braun J, Har-Kedar I. Thermochemotherapy: synergism between hyperthermia (42–43°) and adriamycin (or bleomycin) in mammalian cell inactivation. Proc Natl Acad Sci U S A 1975;72(3):937–40.

119. Kusumoto T, Holden SA, Teicher BA. Hyperthermia and platinum complexes: time between treatments and synergy in vitro and in vivo. Int J Hyperthermia 1995;11(4):575–86.

120. Urano M, Ling CC. Thermal enhancement of melphalan and oxaliplatin cytology in vitro. Int J Hyperthermia 2002;18(4):307–15.

121. Mohamed F, Marchettini P, Stuart OA, et al. Thermal enhancement of new chemotherapeutic agents at moderate hyperthermia. Ann Surg Oncol 2003; 10(4):463–8.

122. Leunig M, Goetz AE, Dellian M, et al. Interstitial fluid pressure in solid tumors following hyperthermia: possible correlation with therapeutic response. Cancer Res 1992;52(2):487–90.
123. Klaver YL, Hendriks T, Lomme RM, et al. Hyperthermia and intraperitoneal chemotherapy for the treatment of peritoneal carcinomatosis: an experimental study. Ann Surg 2011;254(1):125–30.
124. Fujiwara K, Armstrong D, Morgan M, et al. Principles and practice of intraperitoneal chemotherapy for ovarian cancer. Int J Gynecol Cancer 2007;17(1):1–20.
125. Van der Speeten K, Stuart OA, Mahteme H, et al. Pharmacology of perioperative 5-fluorouracil. J Surg Oncol 2010;102(7):730–5.
126. Nygren P, Fridborg H, Csoka K, et al. Detection of tumor-specific cytotoxic drug activity in vitro using the fluorometric microculture cytotoxicity assay and primary cultures of tumor cells from patients. Int J Cancer 1994;56(5):715–20.
127. Larsson R, Kristensen J, Sandberg, et al. Laboratory determination of chemotherapeutic drug resistance in tumor cells from patients with leukemia, using a fluorometric microculture cytotoxicity assay (FMCA). Int J Cancer 1992; 50(2):177–85.
128. Mahteme H, von Heideman A, Grundmark B, et al. Heterogeneous activity of cytotoxic drugs in patient samples of peritoneal carcinomatosis. Eur J Surg Oncol 2008;34(5):547–52.

Current Status and Future Directions in Appendiceal Cancer with Peritoneal Dissemination

Konstantinos I. Votanopoulos, MD, PhD, Perry Shen, MD,
John H. Stewart IV, MD, Edward A. Levine, MD*

KEYWORDS

- Appendiceal cancer • Peritoneal surface disease
- Hyperthermic intraperitoneal perfusion • Chemotherapy • Surgery

KEY POINTS

- The term "pseudomyxoma peritonei" should be used to describe a clinical sign and not a disease. It can be developed by a variety of mucin-producing primaries.
- Increased volume of peritoneal disease (PCI >18) is not a contraindication for cytoreduction in low-grade appendiceal primaries.
- Increased volume of disease is associated with decreased survival, even in cases of complete cytoreduction. Early diagnosis and treatment is crucial.
- Low-grade lesions, including DPAM, may present with positive lymph nodes. The prognosis of this group is decreased and similar to high-grade node-positive appendiceal primaries.

INTRODUCTION

Appendiceal cancer is a rare disease with an incidence in the reported literature that varies depending on the histologic types included in the classification of appendiceal malignancies. Historic evidence suggests that appendiceal primaries are diagnosed in approximately 1% of all appendectomy specimens.[1] In a Surveillance, Epidemiology and End-Results database retrospective analysis that excluded low-grade carcinoid tumors, the annual age-adjusted incidence of appendiceal primaries was 0.12 cases per 1,000,000 of population. Appendiceal adenocarcinoma represented 66.5% of these patients.[2] Extrapolating from the fact that the Surveillance, Epidemiology and End-Results program collects data from 14% of the US population, the annual incidence of appendiceal adenocarcinoma in the country should be around 300 to 400

Surgical Oncology Section, Department of General Surgery, Wake Forest University School of Medicine, Medical Center Boulevard, Winston-Salem, NC 27157, USA
* Corresponding author. Surgical Oncology Service, Department of General Surgery, Wake Forest University School of Medicine, Medical Center Boulevard, Winston-Salem, NC 27157.
E-mail address: elevine@wakehealth.edu

Surg Oncol Clin N Am 21 (2012) 599–609
http://dx.doi.org/10.1016/j.soc.2012.07.012
1055-3207/12/$ – see front matter © 2012 Elsevier Inc. All rights reserved.

cases, although estimates of up to 2000 cases annually in the United States have been made.

The rarity of the disease has unique implication in diagnosis, classification, terminology, and treatment of these patients. Therefore, several misconceptions are still prevalent among clinicians. First, because most pseudomyxoma peritonei (PMP) cases occur in association with appendiceal primaries the term "pseudomyxoma peritonei" has been used as a synonym to the variant of appendiceal-induced peritoneal surface disease (PSD) that was associated with excessive production of mucin. This is far from accurate given that the term is descriptive and can be applied to any primary (including ovarian, colon, or even pancreatic mucinous) cancer that has the ability to produce mucinous ascites.[3] For the same reason, a diagnosis of PMP lacks prognostic information. Therefore, the term "pseudomyxoma peritonei" is better used as a clinical sign rather than as a distinct disease. Second, not every PMP or appendiceal cancer is associated with long-term survival. Such factors as histologic grade, tumor biology of the primary lesion, age, functional status, and extent of disease at the time of diagnosis determine the prognosis of these patients. Third, not every appendiceal primary is associated with mucin production or ascites. Many patients present with solid peritoneal disease that has no phenotypic difference from any other gastrointestinal malignancy with peritoneal dissemination.

The early symptoms of appendiceal cancer are not disease specific, which in part explains why most of these patients are diagnosed incidentally during surgical exploration or late when peritoneal or systemic dissemination has already occurred. In patients with low-grade tumors, peritoneal dissemination begins with tumor-induced obstruction of the appendiceal lumen. The obstruction in the face of continued mucin production frequently leads to perforation and subsequent dissemination of mucous-producing epithelial cells throughout the peritoneal cavity. The pattern of spread is clearly related to the grade of disease. Low-grade mucin-producing lesions are associated with implantation and spread along the peritoneal surfaces with distant or lymphatic metastases in less than 10% of cases. Dissemination starts in the right lower quadrant of the abdomen, followed by the pelvis, right upper quadrant, then diffusely throughout the peritoneal spaces. This is distinguished from high-grade lesions, which have more substantial risks of systemic metastasis, resulting in poor prognosis. In addition, approximately 7% of low-grade lesions have lymph node involvement and another 16% dedifferentiate into higher-grade lesions during the course of the disease.[4,5]

The management of patients with PSD from appendiceal neoplasms is still a matter of intense debate. These patients have been traditionally treated with systemic chemotherapy or only debulking procedures.[3,6] Although low-grade appendiceal tumors treated with debulking procedures can provide some patients with prolonged survival, they are by nature unable to remove all microscopic disease and deal with tumor entrapment in surgical scars. Therefore, more than 90% of these patients inevitably develop local recurrence and death from bowel obstruction. To deal with the problem of postdebulking residual microscopic disease, a variety of "adjuvant" therapies have been evaluated. Intraperitoneal photodynamic therapy, radiation (with ^{32}P), and chemotherapy instillation have been tried and largely abandoned. In 1980, hyperthermic intraperitoneal chemotherapy (HIPEC) was described.[7] Sugarbaker and coworkers[8,9] published their early experience in combining cytoreduction with heated intraperitoneal chemotherapy. This combined approach has been more thoroughly evaluated to the point that in many centers, HIPEC is now considered a standard of care in the treatment of peritoneal dissemination from appendiceal cancer.

Systemic chemotherapy for PSD of low-grade appendiceal neoplasms is considered largely ineffective because of the inability of systemically delivered drugs to reach effective intraperitoneal concentrations and the slow kinetics of the malignant cells. Recently, a phase II study in advanced unresectable low-grade appendiceal primaries with concurrent mitomycin C and capecitabine showed a response in 38% of the patients in the form of either stabilization or radiologic reduction in the volume of disease.[10] For high-grade lesions it seems that systemic chemotherapy might improve progression-free survival with the overall survival benefit being derived from the ability to achieve a complete cytoreduction.[11] Chemotherapy with FOLFOX in the neoadjuvant setting for high-grade appendiceal mucinous lesions was related with progression of disease in 50% of patients who had surgical exploration. Tumor response was observed in 29% of the examined specimens.[12] In addition, groups have evaluated several alternative treatment modalities including photodynamic therapy[13] and external-beam radiation therapy.[3] None of these treatments have significantly altered the clinical course of these patients.

Our group's approach to peritoneal dissemination from appendiceal tumors has been optimal cytoreduction surgery (CRS) with the goal of removal of all gross disease if feasible. This typically entails peritoneal stripping (peritonectomy procedures) and multivisceral resection followed by HIPEC. Selected patients on recurrence undergo repeat exploration and perfusion as dictated by their performance status and symptoms.[14] This article focuses on the use of HIPEC for the treatment of peritoneal dissemination from appendiceal primary tumors. The first part details patient selection criteria used at the Wake Forest University School of Medicine and the use of preoperative imaging and endoscopic evaluation in the management of this cohort of patients. The second part focuses on clinical outcomes for patients undergoing HIPEC for peritoneal dissemination from appendiceal tumors. Finally, future challenges for the use of HIPEC for appendiceal primary tumors are explored.

PREOPERATIVE PATIENT EVALUATION
Patient Selection

Appropriate patient selection is of paramount importance in the management of patients with PSD. All patients presenting to our multidisciplinary clinic have a complete history and physical examination followed by computed tomography (CT) of the chest, abdomen, and pelvis (with oral and intravenous contrast) and tumor markers including CEA, CA19–9, and CA125. All patients undergo pathologic review of previous biopsy or resected tissue.

In general, we use the following eligibility criteria for any patient presenting with documented peritoneal surface malignancy:

1. Patients should be medically fit with an Eastern Cooperative Oncology Group (ECOG) performance status ≤2.
2. There is no extraabdominal disease.
3. The peritoneal disease is resectable.
4. The primary lesion has been resected or is resectable.
5. Parenchymal hepatic metastases if present must be easily resectable.
6. There is no bulky retroperitoneal disease.

In cases of appendiceal cancer specifically, our selection criteria are modified somewhat based on the grade of the appendiceal primary. For low-grade appendiceal cancer a cytoreduction is attempted regardless of the volume of disease. This is because we recognize that the specific tumor biology is typically indolent and even in cases of incomplete cytoreduction patients receive the benefit of symptomatic control and improved overall survival that can often be measured in years.[6] This is supported by a multi-institutional retrospective review of 2298 patients with PMP where low-grade patients with peritoneal carcinomatosis index (PCI) 31 to 30 had a 10-year survival of 68% when a complete cytoreduction was achieved.[15] The decision to proceed with heated intraperitoneal chemotherapy after incomplete cytoreduction depends on the volume of residual disease and the amount of ascites. In general, patients with voluminous liquid ascites are perfused because their symptoms are effectively controlled at least 75% of the time. In patients without symptomatic ascites but with excessive post-CRS residual disease the perfusion is aborted. In high-grade nonmucinous appendiceal primaries the PCI along with the specific distribution of the peritoneal disease is taken into consideration before proceeding with cytoreduction. Patients with imaging of disease not amenable to complete cytoreduction are not taken into the operating room. These patients are treated with systemic chemotherapy followed by restaging imaging to evaluate for resectability.

Preoperative Imaging

All patients have a contrast-enhanced CT of the thorax, abdomen, and pelvis or magnetic resonance imaging (MRI) within 50 days of the scheduled operation. We prefer CT for low-grade appendiceal malignancies to obtain a rough estimate of the distribution of disease and avoid surprises of possible extra-abdominal involvement. Even though MRI with gadolinium has increased sensitivity in identifying smaller peritoneal implants, we believe that this additional information would not change the clinical decision-making process for low-grade appendiceal patients. In addition, it increases the cost of the preoperative evaluation and patient discomfort.

The strength of the CT is its fundamental ability to detect anatomic details and differences in tissue density. Unfortunately, in peritoneal carcinomatosis one often encounters subcentimeter lesions spread in a carpet fashion. This is consistent with the Netherlands Cancer Institute, which compared intraoperative findings with CT findings and reported CT scan sensitivity between 25% and 37% with a negative predictive value that ranged between 47% and 51%. In the same study the sensitivity for lesions less than 1 cm was between 9% and 24%.[16] In a similar study the false negative rate for the CT to detect small bowel lesions was 60%.[17] Therefore, we explain to our patients that what we see in the preoperative imaging is rarely what we get in the operating room. There is also significant variability among radiologists in the interpretation of the extent of peritoneal carcinomatosis.[15] Therefore, it is imperative for the surgeon who treats PSD to develop expertise in the interpretation of abdominal imaging. Despite thorough preoperative imaging approximately 5% to 10% of patients are deemed not to be operative candidates on exploration.

Conversely, MRI with dilute oral barium and delayed enhanced intravenous gadolinium for mucinous appendiceal lesions when compared with intraoperative findings has been shown to be superior to CT scan in detecting peritoneal metastasis with a sensitivity of 82% to 89%.[18] We use either CT or MRI, but do not routinely obtain both.

Positron emission tomography (PET) imaging has been shown to have decreased sensitivity (10%) for low-volume disease in patients with peritoneal carcinomatosis.[19] The voluminous mucin and low cellular density combined with a low metabolic rate severely limits the use of PET imaging for appendiceal cancers. A retrospective analysis of 33 low- and high-grade appendiceal patients in our institution showed a PET sensitivity of 21% and 8%, respectively. Combing PET with CT increased the sensitivity to 30% and 41%, respectively, for low- and high-grade lesions. PET with or without CT has serious limitations in predicting the extent of carcinomatosis for appendiceal cancer and rarely changes the decision to operate or not on these patients.[20] Therefore, a PET-CT is rarely if ever obtained in our institution.

Colonoscopy for Appendiceal Tumors

We offer colonoscopy in patients with low-grade appendiceal primaries who have not had one in the previous 5 years. This is because we have found that 44% of patients with appendiceal primaries have synchronous colonic polyps. Given the potential of these patients for long survival, we prefer to address a potential need of an additional colonic resection at the same time as CRS-HIPEC. Colonoscopy itself for identification of appendiceal cancer is successful (diagnostic) less than 5% of the time, with most endoscopists finding only a smooth, submucosal cecal mass at the appendiceal orifice with or without free-flowing intraluminal mucin. For high-grade appendiceal tumors, a colonoscopic examination does not commonly alter the course of the disease and is requested in selected patients.[21]

All patients have preoperatively drawn CEA, CA125, and CA19–9. The likelihood of having increased tumor markers has been observed to be equivalent in low- and high-grade lesions. It has been shown that normal preoperative levels of all three are associated with increased likelihood to obtain a complete cytoreduction, probably functioning as a marker of low-volume disease. In addition, normal preoperative CA125 (in male and female patients) has been shown to be associated with prolonged overall survival.[22] Postoperatively, tumor markers are obtained in 3- to 6-month intervals. Levels are taken into consideration along with diagnostic imaging findings and the presence or not of symptoms in evaluating patients for possible recurrence. Patients with voluminous disease and normal preoperative levels rarely benefit from further testing for those markers after HIPEC. A decision to offer a repeat cytoreduction is never based exclusively on the laboratory tumor marker values.

CLINICAL OUTCOMES FOR APPENDICEAL TUMORS

Clinical outcomes of appendiceal peritoneal surface malignancies after optimal cytoreduction depend primarily on histology and the extent of peritoneal seeding at the time of diagnosis and comorbidities.[23,24] Appendiceal primaries can be grouped based on their ability to produce mucin. In general, mucin-producing primaries have a better biologic behavior than their non–mucin-producing counterparts and are clinically related with the development of PMP.

At Wake Forest University, we consider the term "pseudomyxoma" as a mixed basket containing pathologies with a wide spectrum of biologic behavior. Ronnett and Sugarbaker had classified patients with pseudomyxoma in three groups in terms of survival: (1) disseminated peritoneal adenomucinosis (DPAM) with 5- and 10-year survival of 75% and 68%; (2) mucinous carcinomatosis with intermediate or discordant features (peritoneal mucinous carcinomatosis [PMCA] I/D) with 5- and 10-year survival of 50% and 21%; and (3) PMCA with 5- and 10-year survival of 14% and 3%, respectively.[25] In our clinical experience, DPAM was prognostically indistinguishable from what Ronnett had defined as PMCA I/D. Therefore, we concluded that categorizing mucinous appendiceal primaries into low- and high-grade lesions is more predictive of overall survival and response to CRS-HIPEC.[26,27] DPAM and intermediated primaries also had similar outcomes in a recent review of 2298 patients with PMP ($P<.001$).[14] In the Wake Forest classification, low-grade mucinous carcinoma peritonei includes all cases formerly classified as DPAM, well-differentiated mucinous carcinomatosis, PMCA I/D, and well-differentiated variants of mucinous adenocarcinoma or low-grade appendiceal mucinous neoplasms.[26] High-grade mucinous carcinoma peritonei applies to cases histologically recognized as either moderately or poorly differentiated adenocarcinoma, PMCA, and cases with signet-ring cell component.

The 5-year survival for the low- and high-grade mucinous cohorts was 62.5% and 37.7%, respectively. Similarly, 5-year survival of 45% for the high-grade group has been recently reported for patients with PCI greater than 20 who had a complete cytoreduction. High-grade mucinous patients with PCI less than 20 who had a complete cytoreduction achieved a 5-year survival of 66%.[28] However, high-grade nonmucinous appendiceal primaries that include appendiceal adenocarcinoma, goblet cell, and carcinoid tumors derive significantly less benefit from a CRS-HIPEC procedure with a 3-year survival of approximately 15%.[29]

Recently, the efforts of our group have focused on correlating survival with the genetic signatures of appendiceal primaries, bypassing the pitfalls of histologic classifications. More specifically, it was demonstrated that patients with low-grade appendiceal primaries can be subdivided based on global gene expression analysis into low- and high-risk groups that correlates with survival. We have also shown that the genetic traces of appendiceal and colon cancer are different, questioning directly the use of colon cancer directed chemotherapy regimens in patients with appendiceal primaries.[30]

Patients who develop PMP from appendiceal primaries have been considered the best candidates for CRS-HIPEC with 5-year survival ranging between 60% and 97%.[24,26,31–34] The 15-year overall survival has been recently reported as 59%.[15] Several factors influence these outcomes. In our series of 110 patients (from 2006),[29] a complete CRS had superior outcomes compared with those who underwent incomplete CRS. The 5-year survival rate for patients with an R0/R1 resection was 70%, whereas 5-year survival for R2 resections was approximately 40%.[29] This finding confirms data from our institution and others that demonstrate a significant survival advantage for patients undergoing R0/R1 resection compared with those with R2 resections.[23,24,35]

The extent of disease, as described by the PCI at the time of CRS-HIPEC, seems to be a significant factor in overall survival even in cases where a complete cytoreduction was achieved. Elias and colleagues reported that in 206 patients with pseudomyxoma treated with complete cytoreduction the 5-year survival was 57% for patients with a PCI greater than 19 and 83% for patients with PCI less than 19 ($P = .004$).[23] These data underline the importance of early diagnosis and treatment. At the same time, increased PCI by itself should not function as an exclusion criterion for operative treatment, given that increased PCI is not incompatible with prolonged survival especially in low-grade lesions.[15]

The role of lymph nodes in the prognosis of metastatic disease has been debated. However, it is clear that low-grade lesions have a rate of nodal metastasis low enough to be able to avoid a right colectomy if the margins of the appendix are negative. However, in high-grade mucinous appendiceal neoplasm with peritoneal dissemination, nodal metastasis seems to be prognostic of decreased survival predominantly when a complete cytoreduction is not feasible. Nodal positivity in high-grade mucinous patients with R0 resection had a 5-year survival of 73%.[36] Low-grade mucinous lesions, without excluding DPAM, may also present with positive lymph nodes defining a separate group of patients that have a prognosis similar to node-positive high-grade primaries with a 5-year survival of 50% and 43%, respectively.[15,37]

Preoperative performance status is a significant prognosticator of survival. In general, we have used the ECOG performance status to evaluate patients with PSD. In our experience patients with HIPEC (from a variety of primary sites) with ECOG scores of 2 to 3 have significantly poorer overall survival (median survival,

9.5 months) than patients with ECOG scores of 0 or 1 (median survival, 21.7 months) ($P = .02$).[38] This is also true for appendiceal primaries where ECOG preoperative performance status significantly affects survival after CRS-HIPEC. For each stepwise increase in ECOG score, the risk of death is increased 8.8-fold. Patients with ECOG scores of 2 or 3 have a median survival of 20.4 months ($P = .0001$).[29] We no longer offer CRS-HIPEC to patients with performance status of 3 or worse.

Age is another variant that has to be taken into serious consideration when selecting operative candidates for CRS-HIPEC. We have found a clear correlation between age and outcome after CRS and HIPEC for appendiceal malignancies in the multivariate analysis. More specifically, for each 1 year of increase in age, the risk of death from appendiceal neoplasms increases by 4%.[39] Age older than 53 was also found to be an independent predictor of poor survival only on low-grade appendiceal neoplasms and not on high-grade lesions.[15] The reasons are unclear and age itself has not been found by other authors in major series to be significant in predicting survival.[23,24,35] We do not use age as an exclusion criteria for CRS-HIPEC, but rather as another factor to be considered before the procedure.

Prior debulking surgeries not followed by intraperitoneal chemotherapy have been shown to be associated with poorer progression-free survival and overall survival.[15] For the proponents of HIPEC, this is attributed to dissection-induced exposure of the retroperitoneum, which leads to implantation of malignant cells that eventually result in multilevel bowel obstruction and death. Although extensive prior surgery clearly makes CRS-HIPEC more difficult, is should not, in and of itself, exclude patients from the procedure.

For all patients who had a CRS-HIPEC for PSD, approximately 7% ultimately have a repeat cytoreduction to treat recurrent disease. For appendiceal primary cases, this number is slightly higher at 9.4%. Patients selected in our institution for repeat HIPEC are those who have maintained an ECOG 0 to 1 functional status; have adequate nutritional reserves (albumin >3 g/dL); had a low-grade tumor without nodal metastatic disease; and had an interval between the two procedures that was at least a year long. Incomplete (R2a,b) first cytoreduction is not an absolute contraindication to an attempted second cytoreduction because 20% of these patients achieve a complete R0/R1 repeat cytoreduction. We and others have reported that in appendiceal primaries the R status of resection of the repeat cytoreduction and not the first cytoreduction is the one that determines long-term survival ($P = .013$).[14,40] This is also true for the interval between the two CRS-HIPEC procedures ($P = .009$). This underscores the importance of proper patient selection and tumor biology in the outcomes of PSD. The observed morbidity and mortality of repeat CRS-HIPEC was 3.2% and 48.4%, respectively, which is similar with the first operation.

CRS-HIPEC procedures are demanding for the patient and the surgeon, require significant expertise, have a significant learning curve, and are associated with considerable morbidity and mortality. The currently reported mortality rate for CRS-HIPEC procedures applied in the treatment of appendiceal primaries is between 0% and 9% with an associated morbidity between 12% and 67%.[23,29,34,35,41-44] The importance of the volume of treated patients with PSD in survival has been demonstrated in a European multi-institutional review where survival was better in centers treating at least 10 patients with pseudomyxoma per year ($P = .004$).[23] No doubt the learning curve for a peritoneal surface malignancy center continues to evolve over a period of several years. Kusamura and coworkers[45] recently reported that 140 cases are necessary for a center to develop expertise in the treatment of PSD. We have found that outcomes improve after 125 cases.[46] There clearly is a substantial learning curve for these procedures in terms of patient selection and operative therapy. Although the precise length of that curve varies from surgeon to surgeon and center to center, it clearly shows substantial value to the patient treated at a center with extensive experience.

FUTURE DIRECTIONS

Several factors will determine the future directions of HIPEC in PSD from appendiceal malignancies. Currently, there is significant heterogeneity in intraperitoneal chemotherapy protocols among different institutions. Open and closed techniques, intraoperative and perioperative delivery of monotherapy or combination of different drugs (mitomycin, oxaliplatin, cisplatin, 5-fluorouracil, and irinotecan), varying perfusate temperatures, and durations of perfusion are currently used at active centers. In addition, multi-institutional reviews have failed to prove the superiority of one therapeutic protocol over the other. Although we have always been struck by the similarity of outcome data from the larger centers, a more uniform approach is called for.

Looking at the data through different lenses and comparing patients that have historically been treated with cytoreduction only, it seems that there is a trend in the progression-free survival in favor of the patients that received HIPEC. More specifically, the Mayo Clinic reported 50% recurrence rate at 2.5 years (most of them detected with physical examination),[3] whereas Memorial Sloan-Kettering had 91% recurrence rate at a median of 2 years for the patients who underwent a complete cytoreduction.[6] Elias and colleagues[23] have recently reported a 5-year disease-free survival of 56% in a multi-institutional European study of 301 patients. In the largest experience reported to date, a multi-institutional multivariate analysis of 2298 patients with a median survival of 16.3 years found that HIPEC was significant in predicting progression-free survival ($P = .03$) but not significant in predicting overall survival.[15] Even if progression-free survival is the only advantage to adding HIPEC to CRS, it is something we would continue to strongly recommend.

There is only one key question to answer before going forward. What is the exact role of heated intraperitoneal chemotherapy after cytoreduction? There is no debate on the value of the CRS. To date, there is no published prospective randomized trial comparing CRS with CRS/HIPEC (although several trials have been attempted). The premature closure of the ACOSOG Z6091 trial for colorectal cancer is indicative of the difficulties in execution of a similar project on an even more rare disease, such as PSD from appendiceal primaries. Currently, in France, the Prodige 7 trial is attempting to define the role of HIPEC post-CRS in PSD from colorectal cancer and has already accrued more than half of the required patients.[47] If HIPEC proves to be beneficial, then new directions in new drugs, delivery systems, and standardization of technique will flourish. If HIPEC proves not to be beneficial for colorectal cancer, then questions regarding its application in other primaries (eg, appendiceal) will immediately emerge. Regardless of what the role of HIPEC proves to be, it is almost certain that two things will not slow down. The first is the effort to compliment or replace histology with genetic signatures that will drastically improve selection of proper surgical candidates. The second is the development of centers of excellence for the treatment of PSD given the impressive current results of CRS-HIPEC in the treatment of patients otherwise considered only as hospice candidates.

REFERENCES

1. Collins DC. 71,000 human appendix specimens. A final report, summarizing forty years' study. Am J Proctol 1963;14:265–81.

2. McCusker ME, Cote TR, Clegg LX, et al. Primary malignant neoplasms of the appendix: a population-based study from the Surveillance, Epidemiology and End-Results program, 1973–1998. Cancer 2002;94(12):3307–12.

3. Gough DB, Donohue JH, Schutt AJ, et al. Pseudomyxoma peritonei. Long-term patient survival with an aggressive regional approach. Ann Surg 1994;219(2): 112–9.

4. Foster JM, Gupta PK, Carreau JH, et al. Right hemicolectomy is not routinely indicated in pseudomyxoma peritonei. Am Surg 2012;78(2):171–7.

5. Chua TC, Al-Zahrani A, Saxena A, et al. Secondary cytoreduction and perioperative intraperitoneal chemotherapy after initial debulking of pseudomyxoma peritonei: a study of timing and the impact of malignant dedifferentiation. J Am Coll Surg 2010;211(4):526–35.

6. Miner TJ, Shia J, Jaques DP, et al. Long-term survival following treatment of pseudomyxoma peritonei: an analysis of surgical therapy. Ann Surg 2005;241(2):300–8.

7. Spratt J, Adcock M, Miskovin M, et al. Clinical delivery system for intraperitoneal hyperthermic chemotherapy. Cancer Res 1980;40:256–60.

8. Sugarbaker PH, Landy D, Pascal R. Intraperitoneal chemotherapy for peritoneal carcinomatosis from colonic or appendiceal cystadenocarcinoma: rationale and results of treatment. Prog Clin Biol Res 1990;354B:141–70.

9. Sugarbaker PH, Kern K, Lack E. Malignant pseudomyxoma peritonei of colonic origin. Natural history and presentation of a curative approach to treatment. Dis Colon Rectum 1987;30(10):772–9.

10. Farquharson AL, Pranesh N, Witham G, et al. A phase II study evaluating the use of concurrent mitomycin C and capecitabine in patients with advanced unresectable pseudomyxoma peritonei. Br J Cancer 2008;99(4):591–6.

11. Lieu CH, Lambert LA, Wolff RA, et al. Systemic chemotherapy and surgical cytoreduction for poorly differentiated and signet ring cell adenocarcinomas of the appendix. Ann Oncol 2012;23(3):652–8.

12. Sugarbaker PH, Bijelic L, Chang D, et al. Neoadjuvant FOLFOX chemotherapy in 34 consecutive patients with mucinous peritoneal carcinomatosis of appendiceal origin. J Surg Oncol 2010;102(6):576–81.

13. Sindelar WF, DeLaney TF, Tochner Z, et al. Technique of photodynamic therapy for disseminated intraperitoneal malignant neoplasms. Phase I study. Arch Surg 1991;126(3):318–24.

14. Votanopoulos KI, Ihemelandu C, Shen P, et al. Outcomes of repeat cytoreductive surgery with hyperthermic intraperitoneal chemotherapy for the treatment of peritoneal surface malignancy. J Am Coll Surg 2012;215(3):412–7.

15. Chua TC, Moran BJ, Sugarbaker PH, et al. Early- and long-term outcome data of patients with pseudomyxoma peritonei from appendiceal origin treated by a strategy of cytoreductive surgery and hyperthermic intraperitoneal chemotherapy. J Clin Oncol 2012;30(20):2449–56.

16. de BE, Koops W, Kroger R, et al. Peritoneal carcinomatosis from colorectal or appendiceal origin: correlation of preoperative CT with intraoperative findings and evaluation of interobserver agreement. J Surg Oncol 2004;86(2):64–73.

17. Dromain C, Leboulleux S, Auperin A, et al. Staging of peritoneal carcinomatosis: enhanced CT vs. PET/CT. Abdom Imaging 2008;33(1):87–93.

18. Low RN, Barone RM, Gurney JM, et al. Mucinous appendiceal neoplasms: preoperative MR staging and classification compared with surgical and histopathologic findings. AJR Am J Roentgenol 2008;190(3):656–65.

19. Sobhani I, Tiret E, Lebtahi R, et al. Early detection of recurrence by 18FDG-PET in the follow-up of patients with colorectal cancer. Br J Cancer 2008;98(5):875–80.

20. Rohani P, Scotti SD, Shen P, et al. Use of FDG-PET imaging for patients with disseminated cancer of the appendix. Am Surg 2010;76(12):1338–44.

21. Trivedi AN, Levine EA, Mishra G. Adenocarcinoma of the appendix is rarely detected by colonoscopy. J Gastrointest Surg 2009;13(4):668–75.

22. Ross A, Sardi A, Nieroda C, et al. Clinical utility of elevated tumor markers in patients with disseminated appendiceal malignancies treated by cytoreductive surgery and HIPEC. Eur J Surg Oncol 2010;36(8):772–6.

23. Elias D, Gilly F, Quenet F, et al. Pseudomyxoma peritonei: a French multicentric study of 301 patients treated with cytoreductive surgery and intraperitoneal chemotherapy. Eur J Surg Oncol 2010;36(5):456–62.

24. Smeenk RM, Verwaal VJ, Antonini N, et al. Survival analysis of pseudomyxoma peritonei patients treated by cytoreductive surgery and hyperthermic intraperitoneal chemotherapy. Ann Surg 2007;245(1):104–9.

25. Ronnett BM, Zahn CM, Kurman RJ, et al. Disseminated peritoneal adenomucinosis and peritoneal mucinous carcinomatosis. A clinicopathologic analysis of 109 cases with emphasis on distinguishing pathologic features, site of origin, prognosis, and relationship to "pseudomyxoma peritonei." Am J Surg Pathol 1995; 19(12):1390–408.

26. Bradley RF, Stewart JH, Russell GB, et al. Pseudomyxoma peritonei of appendiceal origin: a clinicopathologic analysis of 101 patients uniformly treated at a single institution, with literature review. Am J Surg Pathol 2006;30(5):551–9.

27. Misdraji J, Yantiss RK, Graeme-Cook FM, et al. Appendiceal mucinous neoplasms: a clinicopathologic analysis of 107 cases. Am J Surg Pathol 2003; 27(8):1089–103.

28. El HH, Gushchin V, Francis J, et al. The role of cytoreductive surgery and heated intraperitoneal chemotherapy (CRS/HIPEC) in patients with high-grade appendiceal carcinoma and extensive peritoneal carcinomatosis. Ann Surg Oncol 2012; 19(1):110–4.

29. Stewart JH, Shen P, Russell GB, et al. Appendiceal neoplasms with peritoneal dissemination: outcomes after cytoreductive surgery and intraperitoneal hyperthermic chemotherapy. Ann Surg Oncol 2006;13(5):624–34.

30. Levine EA, Blazer DG III, Kim MK, et al. Gene expression profiling of peritoneal metastases from appendiceal and colon cancer demonstrates unique biologic signatures and predicts patient outcomes. J Am Coll Surg 2012;214(4): 599–606.

31. Sugarbaker PH, Chang D. Results of treatment of 385 patients with peritoneal surface spread of appendiceal malignancy. Ann Surg Oncol 1999;6(8): 727–31.

32. Elias D, Laurent S, Antoun S, et al. Pseudomyxoma peritonei treated with complete resection and immediate intraperitoneal chemotherapy. Gastroenterol Clin Biol 2003;27(4):407–12 [in French].

33. Deraco M, Baratti D, Inglese MG, et al. Peritonectomy and intraperitoneal hyperthermic perfusion (IPHP): a strategy that has confirmed its efficacy in patients with pseudomyxoma peritonei. Ann Surg Oncol 2004;11(4):393–8.

34. Yan TD, Links M, Xu ZY, et al. Cytoreductive surgery and perioperative intraperitoneal chemotherapy for pseudomyxoma peritonei from appendiceal mucinous neoplasms. Br J Surg 2006;93(10):1270–6.

35. Chua TC, Yan TD, Smigielski ME, et al. Long-term survival in patients with pseudomyxoma peritonei treated with cytoreductive surgery and perioperative intraperitoneal chemotherapy: 10 years of experience from a single institution. Ann Surg Oncol 2009;16(7):1903–11.

36. Halabi HE, Gushchin V, Francis J, et al. Prognostic significance of lymph node metastases in patients with high-grade appendiceal cancer. Ann Surg Oncol 2012;19(1):122–5.
37. Gonzalez-Moreno S, Brun E, Sugarbaker PH. Lymph node metastasis in epithelial malignancies of the appendix with peritoneal dissemination does not reduce survival in patients treated by cytoreductive surgery and perioperative intraperitoneal chemotherapy. Ann Surg Oncol 2005;12(1):72–80.
38. Shen P, Levine EA, Hall J, et al. Factors predicting survival after intraperitoneal hyperthermic chemotherapy with mitomycin C after cytoreductive surgery for patients with peritoneal carcinomatosis. Arch Surg 2003;138(1):26–33.
39. Stewart JH, Shen P, Levine EA. Patient selection for cytoreduction and hyperthermic intraperitoneal chemoperfusion. Cancer Treat Res 2007;134:215–29.
40. Esquivel J, Sugarbaker PH. Second-look surgery in patients with peritoneal dissemination from appendiceal malignancy: analysis of prognostic factors in 98 patients. Ann Surg 2001;234(2):198–205.
41. Elias D, Honore C, Ciuchendea R, et al. Peritoneal pseudomyxoma: results of a systematic policy of complete cytoreductive surgery and hyperthermic intraperitoneal chemotherapy. Br J Surg 2008;95(9):1164–71.
42. Loungnarath R, Causeret S, Bossard N, et al. Cytoreductive surgery with intraperitoneal chemohyperthermia for the treatment of pseudomyxoma peritonei: a prospective study. Dis Colon Rectum 2005;48(7):1372–9.
43. Sugarbaker PH, Alderman R, Edwards G, et al. Prospective morbidity and mortality assessment of cytoreductive surgery plus perioperative intraperitoneal chemotherapy to treat peritoneal dissemination of appendiceal mucinous malignancy. Ann Surg Oncol 2006;13(5):635–44.
44. Witkamp AJ, de BE, Kaag MM, et al. Extensive surgical cytoreduction and intraoperative hyperthermic intraperitoneal chemotherapy in patients with pseudomyxoma peritonei. Br J Surg 2001;88(3):458–63.
45. Kusamura S, Baratti D, Deraco M. Multidimensional analysis of learning curve for cytoreductive surgery and hyperthermic intraperitoneal chemotherapy in peritoneal surface malignancies. Ann Surg 2011;255(2):348–56.
46. Levine EA, Stewart JH, Russell GB, et al. Cytoreductive surgery and intraperitoneal hyperthermic chemotherapy for peritoneal surface malignancy: experience with 501 procedures. J Am Coll Surg 2007;204:943–55.
47. Elias D. Is intraperitoneal chemotherapy after cytoreductive surgery efficient? Knowing whether it is or not appears secondary! Ann Surg Oncol 2011;19(1):5–6.

Current Status and Future Directions in the Treatment of Peritoneal Dissemination from Colorectal Carcinoma

Dominique Elias, MD, PhD[a],*, François Quenet, MD[b], Diane Goéré, MD[a]

KEYWORDS

- Colon • Rectum • Peritoneal carcinomatosis • Cytoreductive surgery
- Intraperitoneal chemohyperthermia

KEY POINTS

- Peritoneal carcinomatosis (PC) carries a worse prognosis than the usual other sites of colorectal metastases.
- If incomplete resection of PC affords no benefit to patients, complete resection of PC is beneficial in selected patients.
- The combination of complete cytoreductive surgery to treat the visible PC and hyperthermic intraperitoneal chemotherapy (HIPEC) to treat the nonvisible PC is on the verge of becoming the gold-standard treatment when feasible.
- The prognostic impact of a complete resection is high, but that of HIPEC per se is more hypothetical (there is an ongoing trial on this topic).
- The presence of a few resectable liver metastases associated with PC is not a contraindication to surgery plus HIPEC.

Peritoneal dissemination, or carcinomatosis, from colorectal carcinoma is a form of disease progression that can affect 30% to 40% of patients.[1,2] Studies of the natural history of the disease show that peritoneal carcinomatosis (PC) is uniformly fatal, with a median survival not exceeding 6 months[3] in the past. At present, it continues to be uniformly fatal but with median survival approaching 20 months under chemotherapy.[4,5] Ten years ago, the discovery of PC by definition signified that palliative therapy and surgery was only attempted to provide comfort care. Recent data have taught us that new strategies can greatly increase median survival and can lead to cure in selected

The authors have nothing to disclose.
[a] Department of General Oncologic Surgery, Institut Gustave Roussy, Rue Camille Desmoulins, Villejuif 94805, France; [b] Département de Chirurgie, Centre anticancéreux Val d'Aurelle, 208 Rue des Apothicaires, Montpellier 34298, France
* Corresponding author.
E-mail address: elias@igr.fr

patients. A therapeutic package combining cytoreductive surgery to treat the visible peritoneal disease and hyperthermic intraperitoneal chemotherapy (HIPEC) to treat the remaining nonvisible peritoneal disease has been developed, which allows the surgical team to achieve cure in selected patients. The aim of this article is to review the different treatments of colorectal PC and to specify the indications for these respective options.

A REMINDER OF THE NATURAL HISTORY OF COLORECTAL PC

Of patients with metastatic disease at presentation, 5% to 7% exhibit synchronous PC, only one-third have isolated PC, and the disease is technically resectable in only some of these cases of isolated PC.[3,6,7] Virtually half of the patients suffering from PC also have liver metastases.[7] Metachronous PC is far more frequent, occurring during cancer progression. However, it is more complex to analyze because it is detected at different stages of the primary cancer and is frequently associated with distant metastases. Some cases of PC are isolated, moderately extended, and accessible to complete cytoreduction.

PC TREATED WITH CHEMOTHERAPY ALONE: CURRENT RESULTS

The results of systemic chemotherapy are modest. In 2003, the Amsterdam group published the first randomized trial on HIPEC.[8] It concerned 105 patients with colorectal PC treated between 1988 and 2001, without other metastases and with a good general status, and no signs of diffuse PC. Among them, 51 were randomized to the non-HIPEC group and received systemic chemotherapy. Their median survival was 12.6 months, twice as short ($P = .03$) as that observed in the HIPEC group.

Among patients with metastases, the presence of PC as a metastatic site worsens the prognosis: the analysis of the 2095 patients with metastases treated in the North American N9741 and N9841 trials, which compared chemotherapy with FOLFOX (leucovorin/5-fluorouracil/oxaliplatin) or FOLFIRI (leucovorin/5-fluorouracil/irinotecan), showed that median survival was 12.7 months for the 364 patients with PC versus 17.6 months for the 1731 patients without PC ($P<.001$).[4] The 5-year survival rate was 4.1% in the first group and 6% in the second group.

In 2012, the adjunction of targeted molecules such as bevacizumab or cetuximab prolonged median survival by 3 to 6 months. Thus, in the 1401 patients in the randomized study reported by Saltz and colleagues,[5] the median survival of patients receiving FOLFOX + bevacizumab was 21.3 months, compared with 19.9 months ($P = .07$) in the patients who received FOLFOX alone (**Fig. 1**).

Data are emerging on the effectiveness of modern chemotherapy in patients with isolated PC. Klaver and colleagues[9] recently showed in a population-based survival study of 904 patients with primary colorectal cancer who presented specifically with synchronous PC between 1995 and 2008 that PC was the only site of metastasis in 398 patients, and median overall survival was 19 months when patients received targeted therapy such as bevacizumab or cetuximab. This group achieved a higher survival rate than patients presenting with PC plus other metastases, for whom median overall survival was 14 months.

In conclusion, the presence of PC worsens the prognosis of patients with metastases, and currently the median survival of patients with PC is close to 22 months.

PC TREATED WITH SURGERY ALONE: RESULTS

Two situations are possible: either PC is completely resectable or it is not. A clear and wildly accepted definition of resectable PC does not exist. However, one may

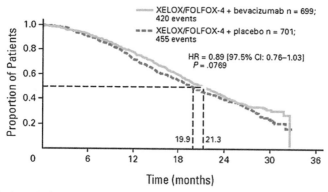

Fig. 1. Global survival curves of 1401 metastatic patients treated with intravenous FOLFOX with or without bevacizumab. (*From* Saltz LB, Clarke S, Diaz-Rubio E, et al. Bevacizumab in combination with oxaliplatin-based chemotherapy as first-line therapy in metastatic colorectal cancer: a randomized phase III study. J Clin Oncol 2008;26(12):2013–9; with permission.)

postulate that when the patient has a relatively good general status and when the extension of PC is limited, resection is technically possible.

When Complete Resection of PC is Not Possible, What are the Results of Incomplete (R2) Resection, and is This Option Beneficial?

In the French study[10] that included 523 patients with colorectal PC operated on between 1990 and 2007 in 23 centers, 84 patients (16%) were not amenable to complete resection of PC, and their median survival was less than 9 months, that is, exactly similar to that obtained with systemic chemotherapy alone during the same period. Recently, the Amsterdam group reported on a series of 43 patients with unresectable PC mainly defined based on the extent of the PC in 6 of the 7 areas of the abdomen, or on involvement of the small bowel.[11] Median survival for the whole group was 6.3 months, but was 9.3 months for the patients who received chemotherapy. Similar results were reported by the Erlangen group: median survival was 8 months (5-year survival: 3%) for the 94 patients who underwent an incomplete (R2) resection of PC, but 15 months (5-year survival: 6%) for the 17 who presented with PC alone.[6]

In conclusion, an incomplete resection of PC does not afford any benefit.

When Complete Resection Alone of PC is Feasible, is it Beneficial?

When one compares the 20 patients who underwent a complete resection of limited PC with the 96 patients who did not undergo a curative resection, as reported by a Japanese group, the 2-year survival rate was 65% in the first group versus 27% in the second (P = .004).[7] However, it was clear that only patients presenting very limited PC adjacent to the primary were included in the first group.

The Erlangen group recently reported the results of 31 selected patients who underwent complete (R0/R1) resection of their PC that was synchronous with the primary, who were operated on before 2006 (the date they began to use HIPEC).[6] Clearly this option was selected for patients with limited PC and in good general condition. Survival results were unexpectedly good, with a median survival of 25 months and a 5-year survival of 22%. These results were better than those obtained during the same period (before 2006) with systemic chemotherapy (18 months), but probably lower than those obtained with complete resection plus HIPEC. Indeed, the 5-year

Table 1
Median survivals (in days) of 5 groups of 10 rats with a PC treated without cytoreductive surgery but with different types of intraperitoneal treatments

Treatment	37°C	41.5°C	42.5°C	Mito 37°C	Mitomycin C + 41.5°C
Median (d)	16	19	51	19	103

Data from Koga S, Hamazoe R, Maeta M, et al. Treatment of implanted peritoneal cancer in rats by continuous hyperthermic peritoneal perfusion in combination with an anticancer drug. Cancer Res 1984;44:1840–2.

survival rate after complete surgery plus HIPEC was 48% for patients with minimal peritoneal extension (peritoneal index lower than 10) in the French study that included the learning curves of the 23 participating centers,[10] and 60% for the patients treated by 2 experienced teams reported by Quenet and colleagues.[12]

In conclusion, complete resection of resectable PC is beneficial to patients. The next point will be to prove that it is beneficial to add HIPEC.

PC TREATED WITH SURGERY PLUS HIPEC: CURRENT RESULTS
Rationale Behind the Use of HIPEC

This combined treatment associates cytoreductive surgery with HIPEC. The aim of HIPEC is to kill any residual microscopic disease in only one session. A very high concentration of chemotherapy is used together with the effect of hyperthermia. Cultured cancer cells begin to die at 42°C and are totally eradicated at 45°C,[13] explaining why 1°, more or less, is so important in the peritoneal cavity during HIPEC. To change the mean temperature of 43°C in the abdomen during HIPEC to a mean of 42°C divides the efficacy of hyperthermia by 2. Finally, 42° is the minimal temperature required, and a mean temperature of 43° to 44°C is adequate during HIPEC. It is also very important to obtain a high and homogeneous temperature throughout the abdominal cavity. An open procedure is therefore theoretically more efficient than a closed procedure.[14]

Several experimental trials in animals demonstrated the efficacy of this combination, 2 of which[15,16] are reported in **Tables 1** and **2**. **Table 1** shows results reported by Koga and colleagues[15] in rats, published as early as 1984, proving the superiority of HIPEC over chemotherapy alone and hyperthermia alone. **Table 2** shows similar results published by Pelz and colleagues[16] in 2006.

Table 2
Results on a PC (implanted 10 days before) of different treatments (4 groups of 6 rats; IP chemotherapy was made with mitomycin C)

Treatment	Laparotomy Alone	Hyperthermia 41°C	IP Chemotherapy Alone	HIPEC
Weight of tumor (g)	16.4	5.9	5.7	1.8
No. of implants	68	21	16	4

Data from Pelz J, Doerfer J, Dimmler A, et al. Histological response of peritoneal carcinomatosis after hyperthermic intraperitoneal chemoperfusion in experimental investigations. BMC Cancer 2006;2:162–9.

Moreover, experimental data show that chemotherapy penetrates only 1 mm in depth during HIPEC,[17] which signifies that HIPEC is only able to cure inframillimetric residual tumor deposits.

Clinical results in humans confirm these experimental data. There is no benefit to using HIPEC after incomplete cytoreductive surgery. Median survival of patients in whom resection is incomplete equates to that obtained with systemic chemotherapy alone, as clearly shown in the French registry[10]: when cytoreductive surgery was not complete, median survival was between 6 and 18 months **(Fig. 2)**, that is, not superior to that obtained with systemic chemotherapy alone.

In conclusion, there is a strong rationale for concluding that HIPEC is superior to intraperitoneal (IP) chemotherapy alone and to IP hyperthermia alone, but that it is logical to use it exclusively after complete cytoreductive surgery, leaving only undetectable tumor deposits no greater than 1 mm in diameter.

What Proof Do We Have of the Efficacy of This Combined Treatment in 2012?

A randomized study was published in 2003 concerning 105 patients with PC who were eligible for HIPEC and treated between 1998 and 2001.[8] Patients were randomly allocated to conventional treatment with chemotherapy alone versus cytoreductive surgery plus HIPEC. Median survival was 2-fold higher ($P = .03$) in the experimental group **(Fig. 3)**, although complete cytoreductive surgery could only be achieved in 38% of the patients, meaning that almost two-thirds of these patients were not truly good candidates for this combined treatment.

Another comparative study was not randomized, but compared similar patients,[18] all of whom underwent a laparotomy and had completely resectable PC. Forty-eight patients were treated with HIPEC in 1 experienced center, and 48 were treated in 5

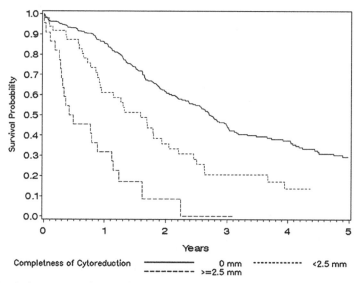

Fig. 2. Survival rates according to the completeness of the resection of the peritoneal carcinomatosis in the 523 patients of the French registry. (*From* Elias D, Gilly F, Boutitie F, et al. Peritoneal colorectal carcinomatosis treated with surgery and perioperative intraperitoneal chemotherapy: retrospective analysis of 523 patients from a multicentric French study. J Clin Oncol 2010;28(1):63–8; with permission.)

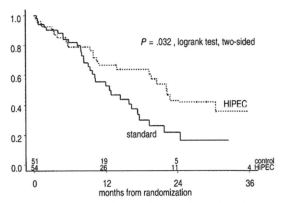

Fig. 3. Global survival rates in a randomized trial comparing cytoreductive surgery plus HIPEC with standard systemic chemotherapy alone (105 patients). (*From* Verwaal VJ, van Ruth S, de Bree E, et al. Randomized trial of cytoreduction and hyperthermic intraperitoneal chemotherapy versus systemic chemotherapy and palliative surgery in patients with peritoneal carcinomatosis of colorectal cancer. J Clin Oncol 2003;21(20):3737–43; with permission.)

other centers not using HIPEC at the time. The second group received 2.3 lines of different types of systemic chemotherapy. After a minimal follow-up of 63 months, overall 5-year survival was 51% for patients who had received HIPEC and 13% for patients in the no-HIPEC group ($P<.05$) (**Fig. 4**).

On considering the results of the largest series in the French registry,[10] they are the worst that could be obtained with HIPEC because they include the learning curves of 23 centers. Among the 523 patients with colorectal cancer and PC treated with HIPEC between 1990 and 2007, only 84% had undergone complete cytoreductive surgery,

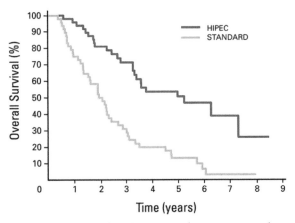

Fig. 4. Comparison of survival rates of similar operated patients treated even with complete cytoreductive surgery plus HIPEC or even with systemic chemotherapy alone (2 groups of 48 patients). (*From* Elias D, Lefèvre J, Chevalier J, et al. Complete cytoreductive surgery plus intraperitoneal chemohyperthermia with oxaliplatin for peritoneal carcinomatosis of colorectal origin. J Clin Oncol 2009;27(5):681–5; with permission.)

a prerequisite for the proper use of HIPEC. Yet the median survival of those patients was 33 months and 27% were alive at 5 years. Furthermore, it must be underlined that mortality was exclusively postoperative. Mortality and grade-3 to grade-4 morbidity were respectively only 3% and 30% at 1 month.

Far better were the results obtained prospectively by 2 experienced centers between 1998 and 2007 using intraperitoneal oxaliplatin at 43°C over 30 minutes: 5-year survival of the 143 patients was 42%, with median survival attaining 41 months (**Fig. 5**).[12] Finally, definitive cure of PC with HIPEC is possible. The authors recently followed up their patients who had no recurrence more than 5 years after their last treatment. Among 107 patients treated between 1995 and 2005, 16% were definitely cured, and the learning curve was included in the period concerned.[19]

In conclusion, it appears that the results obtained with HIPEC used to treat PC are the same as those obtained with hepatectomy used to treat liver metastases: both treatment options gave rise to an overall 5-year survival rate approximating 45%.[20] Hepatectomy, when feasible, is a standard treatment that has not been corroborated by a randomized study. HIPEC, on the other hand, has comparable results and more scientific data, and therefore could also be considered as the standard treatment of PC.

CURRENT INDICATIONS FOR HIPEC

The indications for HIPEC are based on absolute and relative contraindications. An absolute contraindication for complete cytoreductive surgery (CCRS) plus HIPEC is a poor general status, the presence of extraperitoneal metastases, and a huge and diffuse PC. Relative contraindications are a subocclusive syndrome caused by more than 1 digestive stenosis, peritoneal disease progressing under chemotherapy, and the presence of more than 3 resectable liver metastases (liver metastases are not contraindicated provided there are fewer than 4 and if they are easily resectable).[21]

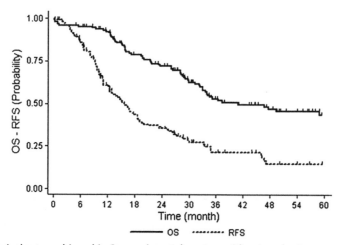

Fig. 5. Survival rates achieved in 2 experimental centers with cytoreductive surgery plus HIPEC in 146 patients with colorectal PC. (*From* Quenet F, Goéré D, Mehta SS, et al. Results of two bi-institutional prospective studies using intraperitoneal oxaliplatin with or without irinotecan during HIPEC after cytoreductive surgery for colorectal carcinomatosis. Ann Surg 2011;254(2):294–301; with permission.)

Response to systemic chemotherapy (decreasing or stabilizing the cancer) is usually considered a prerequisite before attempting to perform CCRS plus HIPEC. However, PC could eventually be a particular form of metastasis with a different natural history from that of liver or lung metastases, and may also have a different response to systemic chemotherapy. A recent study of 90 patients with PC treated with neoadjuvant systemic chemotherapy reported median survival duration of more than 30 months with 5-year survival reaching just over 20% in the group of patients who developed progressive disease under adjuvant systemic chemotherapy.[22] These results were not significantly different from those of the whole population. Progression under neoadjuvant systemic chemotherapy should not currently constitute an absolute contraindication for a curative procedure combining cytoreductive surgery plus HIPEC if complete cytoreduction can be achieved. Such results will have to be confirmed in further studies.

The extent of PC has a major prognostic impact, and there is a threshold beyond which complete surgery and HIPEC are not beneficial to the patient. The exact extent of PC is measured with the peritoneal cancer index (PCI),[23] which can only be determined at laparotomy (and not at laparoscopy). The authors recently reported that there was no difference in scores among surgeons in the assessment of the PCI, signifying that this score is a reliable tool for accurately evaluating PC. However, the PCI score increased by 2 points when it was determined at the beginning of surgery and at the end of surgery.[24] This finding means that if one takes into consideration the PCI to indicate or contraindicate cytoreductive surgery at the beginning of surgery, 2 points must be added to obtain the true definitive score. The important point to consider is that there is no 5-year survival when the PCI is greater than 20.[10,12,22] In the French registry that tracks patients treated before 2007, the median survival of patients with a PCI greater than 20 was close to 18 months, that is, similar to that obtained with systemic chemotherapy alone (**Fig. 6**).[10]

The authors recently compared similar patients who presented with colorectal PC except for the presence of synchronous resectable liver metastases.[25] Disease was completely resected in all patients, and they received HIPEC between 1993 and

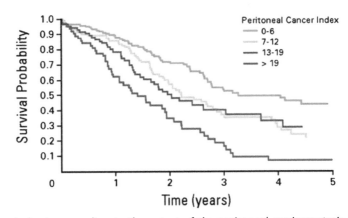

Fig. 6. Survival rates according to the extent of the peritoneal carcinomatosis (measured with the PCI), in the French registry (N = 523 patients). (*From* Elias D, Gilly F, Boutitie F, et al. Peritoneal colorectal carcinomatosis treated with surgery and perioperative intraperitoneal chemotherapy: retrospective analysis of 523 patients from a multicentric French study. J Clin Oncol 2010;28(1):63–8; with permission.)

2009. The median follow-up duration was 36 months. Thus, 61 patients with PC alone were compared with 37 patients with PC + liver metastases. At 3 years, the overall survival rates were 66% and 40%, respectively (P = .04), and the disease-free survival rates were 27% and 6%, respectively (P = .001). When the PCI was less than 12, median survival was 76 months in the PC-alone group and 40 months in the PC + liver metastases group (with 1–3 liver metastases). However, when the PCI was greater than 12 or when the number of liver metastases was greater than 3, median survival decreased to 27 months. Finally, the presence of liver metastases synchronous with PC decreases survival. However, when the extent of peritoneal disease is limited and when the number of liver metastases is not greater than 3, complete resection of both types of disease results in interesting prolonged survival.

In conclusion, a PCI greater than 20 is currently a contraindication for surgery and HIPEC, given that a postsurgical PCI score of 20 corresponds to a presurgical PCI score of 18.

FUTURE DIRECTIONS

The HIPEC procedure will have to be gradually standardized in the future in terms of the drugs, their concentration, the temperature of the infusate, and the duration and the use of the open or closed procedures. In theory, a randomized trial would be required for each modified parameter, but 100 or so different combinations would need to be tested. It is clear that multiple trials will not be conducted. It will therefore be up to the leaders in the HIPEC field to propose procedures based on known experimental data and to create a cocktail they think will ensure the maximum chances of success. At present there are two main different tendencies: one based on the use of mitomycin C over a long duration (60–90 minutes) at a low temperature (41°C), and one based on the use of oxaliplatin over only 30 minutes, but with a higher temperature (43°C) and preceded by a systemic injection of 5-fluorouracil plus leucovorin.

What is more urgently needed is an appraisal of the true efficacy of HIPEC alone in eradicating the residual nonvisible disease after CCRS, applying the usual HIPEC procedure. This approach is currently ongoing in a randomized multicentric French trial (Prodige 7) comparing HIPEC with no HIPEC after CCRS. Any type of systemic chemotherapy can be used before and after CCRS (**Fig. 7**). In January 2012, 150 of the 280 patients were already randomized. HIPEC is delivered with oxaliplatin (460 mg/m²), in 2 L/m² of dextrose 5%, over 30 minutes, at a minimal temperature of 42°C, and is

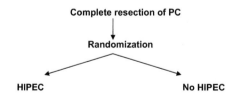

Fig. 7. Design of the ongoing French trial Prodige 7, concerning patients presenting a patent macroscopic colorectal PC.

preceded by an intravenous injection of leucovorin (20 mg/m^2) with 5-fluorouracil (400 mg/m^2).

One of the great promises of HIPEC lies in its use as prophylactic or its use very early during the development of PC in patients presenting a high risk of developing it. All of the series concerning the treatment of established macroscopic PC concluded that survival results are far better when peritoneal disease is less bulky.[14,17,18] In addition, postoperative morbidity and mortality are significantly lower when the peritoneal index is lower, because surgery is less extensive.[10,23] These 2 points are strong arguments in favor of operating on patients with the lowest peritoneal index. However, currently early PC is not detectable clinically, biologically, or with imaging. Early PC is only detectable by a second-look laparotomy. Second-look laparoscopy is not recommended because it does not allow the surgeon to "reexpose" all the dissection planes of the first surgical procedure, and because palpation cannot be used. The aim of this second-look procedure is to detect the early emergence of PC and to treat it with cytoreductive surgery plus HIPEC. As this is a rather aggressive and expensive treatment, it should be proposed exclusively to patients considered to be at high risk of developing PC after resection of the primary. A major proportion of the at-risk population was defined by Elias and colleagues[26]: (1) patients exhibiting a few nodules of synchronous PC that were completely resected with the primary tumor, (2) patients with ovarian metastasis, and (3) patients with a perforated primary tumor (spontaneous or iatrogenic). A second-look operation performed 1 year after the first surgical procedure and 6 months after the end of systemic adjuvant chemotherapy, in asymptomatic patients with a completely negative workup, was able to detect macroscopic PC in respectively 63%, 75%, and 33% of these subgroups. Patients with macroscopic PC were treated with cytoreductive surgery plus HIPEC. No mortality was observed, morbidity was low, and the survival rate was promising (2-year disease-free survival exceeding 50%). Patients without macroscopic PC were treated prophylactically with or without HIPEC.

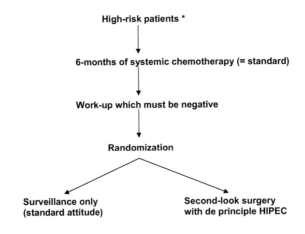

Fig. 8. Design of the ongoing French trial Prodige 15 (Prophylochip), concerning patients presenting a high risk of developing a colorectal PC.

The subgroup receiving HIPEC developed far fewer peritoneal recurrences than those who had not received HIPEC (17% vs 43%, respectively).

Based on this preliminary study, a multicentric randomized trial (Prodige 15) was designed, which began in France in 2011. All high-risk patients (see the aforestated definition) receive the standard adjuvant systemic chemotherapy with FOLFOX over 6 months. Afterward, a complete workup is performed. If it is negative, patients are randomized between simple surveillance (control group) and a second-look laparotomy with systematic HIPEC (**Fig. 8**). The main evaluation criterion will be the rate of peritoneal recurrences at 3 years. To date, the risk of developing PC has not been clearly established for patients with a pT4 lesion of the colon, with an occlusive tumor, or with positive peritoneal cytology.

SUMMARY

During the last years the frequency of complete resection of PC, mainly when limited, has increased. Resection increases survival and, at present, its association with HIPEC enables definite cure of patients. Like the increased use of hepatectomy for colorectal liver metastases observed 20 years ago, complete surgery plus HIPEC is also becoming the standard treatment for colorectal PC, with similar results in terms of survival. The real impact of HIPEC alone is currently being investigated in a randomized trial. This approach will probably be more useful for the treatment of PC at a very early stage when it can only be detected through second-look surgery proposed to well-defined high-risk patients. This aspect is also currently being investigated in a randomized trial.

ACKNOWLEDGMENTS

The authors thank Ms Lorna Saint-Ange for editing.

REFERENCES

1. Chu DZ, Lang NP, Thompson C, et al. Peritoneal carcinomatosis in nongynecologic malignancy. A prospective study of prognostic factors. Cancer 1989;63: 364–7.
2. Sadeghi B, Arvieux C, Glehen O, et al. Peritoneal carcinomatosis from non-gynecologic malignancies: results of the EVOCAPE 1 multicentric prospective study. Cancer 2000;88:358–63.
3. Jayne DG, Fook S, Loi C, et al. Peritoneal carcinomatosis from colorectal cancer. Br J Surg 2002;89:1545–50.
4. Franko J, Hhi Q, Goldman C, et al. Treatment of colorectal peritoneal carcinomatosis with systemic chemotherapy: a pooled analysis of NCCTG's phase III trials N9741 and N9841. J Clin Oncol 2011;29(Suppl) [abstract: 3571].
5. Saltz L, Clarke S, Diaz-Rubio E, et al. Bevacizumab in combination with oxaliplatin-based chemotherapy as first-line therapy in metastatic colorectal cancer: a randomized phase III study. J Clin Oncol 2008;26:1013–9.
6. Mulsow J, Merkel S, Agaimy A, et al. Outcomes following surgery for colorectal cancer with synchronous peritoneal metastases. Br J Surg 2011;98: 1785–91.
7. Kobayashi K, Enomoto M, Higushi T, et al. Validation and clinical use of the Japanese classification of colorectal metastases: benefit of surgical cytoreduction even without intraperitoneal chemotherapy. Dig Surg 2010;27:473–80.

8. Verwaal VJ, van Ruth S, de Bree E, et al. Randomized trial of cytoreduction and hyperthermic intraperitoneal chemotherapy versus systemic chemotherapy and palliative surgery in patients with peritoneal carcinomatosis of colorectal cancer. J Clin Oncol 2003;21:3737–43.

9. Klaver YL, Lemmens VE, Creemers GJ, et al. Population-based survival of patients with peritoneal carcinomatosis from colorectal origin in the era of increasing use of palliative chemotherapy. Ann Oncol 2011;22:2250–6.

10. Elias D, Gilly F, Boutitie F, et al. Peritoneal colorectal carcinomatosis treated with surgery and perioperative intraperitoneal chemotherapy: retrospective analysis of 523 patients from a multicentric French study. J Clin Oncol 2010;28:63–8.

11. Hompes D, Boot H, Van Tinteren H, et al. Unresectable peritoneal carcinomatosis from colorectal cancer: a single center experience. J Surg Oncol 2011;104: 269–73.

12. Quenet F, Goéré D, Mehta SS, et al. Results of two bi-institutional prospective studies using intraperitoneal oxaliplatin with or without irinotecan during HIPEC after cytoreductive surgery for colorectal carcinomatosis. Ann Surg 2011;254: 294–301.

13. Armour EZP, McEachern D, Wang G, et al. Sensitivity of human cells to mild hyperthermia. Cancer Res 1993;53:2740–4.

14. Elias D, Antoun S, Goharin A, et al. Research on the best chemohyperthermia technique for treatment of peritoneal carcinomatosis after complete resection. Int J Surg Investig 2000;1:431–9.

15. Koga S, Hamazoe R, Maeta M, et al. Treatment of implanted peritoneal cancer in rats by continuous hyperthermic peritoneal perfusion in combination with an anticancer drug. Cancer Res 1984;44:1840–2.

16. Pelz J, Doerfer J, Dimmler A, et al. Histological response of peritoneal carcinomatosis after hyperthermic intraperitoneal chemoperfusion in experimental investigations. BMC Cancer 2006;2:162–9.

17. van de Vaart P, van der Vange N, Zoetmulder F, et al. Intraperitoneal cisplatin with regional hyperthermia in advanced ovarian cancer: pharmacokinetics and cisplatin-DNA adduct formation in patients and ovarian cancer cell lines. Eur J Cancer 1998;34:148–54.

18. Elias D, Lefèvre J, Chevalier J, et al. Complete cytoreductive surgery plus intraperitoneal chemohyperthermia with oxaliplatin for peritoneal carcinomatosis of colorectal origin. J Clin Oncol 2009;27:681–5.

19. Goéré D, Tzanis D, Gava V, et al. Can patients with colorectal peritoneal carcinomatosis be cured after cytoreduction and intraperitoneal chemotherapy? Ann Surg, in press.

20. Elias D. Peritoneal carcinomatosis or liver metastases from colorectal cancer: similar standards for a curative surgery? Ann Surg Oncol 2004;11:122–3.

21. Elias D, Benizri E, Pocard M, et al. Treatment of synchronous peritoneal carcinomatosis and liver metastases from colorectal cancer. Eur J Surg Oncol 2006;32: 632–6.

22. Passot G, Vaudoyer D, Cotte E, et al. Ann Surg 2010;256:125–9.

23. da Silva RG, Sugarbaker PH. Analysis of prognostic factors in seventy patients having a complete cytoreduction plus perioperative intraperitoneal chemotherapy for carcinomatosis from colorectal cancer. J Am Coll Surg 2006;203: 878–86.

24. Elias D, Soudka A, Fayard F, et al. Variation in the Peritoneal Cancer Index scores between surgeons and according to when they are determined (before or after cytoreductive surgery). Eur J Surg Oncol 2012;38(6):503–8.

25. Maggiori L, Goéré D, Tzanis D, et al. Should patients with peritoneal carcinomatosis of colorectal origin with synchronous liver metastases be treated with a curative intent? A case control study. Ann Surg 2012, in press.
26. Elias D, Goere D, Di Pietrantonio D, et al. Results of systematic second-look surgery in patients at high risk of developing colorectal peritoneal carcinomatosis. Ann Surg 2008;247:445–50.

Current Status and Future Directions in Gastric Cancer with Peritoneal Dissemination

Gabriel Glockzin, MD[a], Pompiliu Piso, MD[b],*

KEYWORDS

- Peritoneal carcinomatosis • Gastric cancer • Treatment • Cytoreductive surgery
- HIPEC

KEY POINTS

- Combined cytoreductive surgery and hyperthermic intraperitoneal chemotherapy (HIPEC) might be an additional therapeutic option for highly selected patients with peritoneal carcinomatosis arising from gastric cancer.
- Complete macroscopic cytoreduction (CC-0/1) is a precondition for a possible survival benefit.
- Consistent preoperative patient selection including laparoscopy is crucial to obtain complete macroscopic cytoreduction.
- Further prospective randomized trials are needed to assess the roles of cytoreductive surgery and HIPEC as an inherent part of an interdisciplinary treatment concept for patients with advanced gastric cancer and to standardize HIPEC protocols.

INTRODUCTION

Although the incidence of gastric cancer decreased during the past years, it is still the fourth most common newly diagnosed cancer worldwide and the second leading cause of cancer-related death.[1] Peritoneal metastasis is a common sign of advanced tumor stage, tumor progression, or disease recurrence in patients with gastric cancer. It might be already present in 5% to 20% of patients undergoing gastric resection in curative intent.[2] In a retrospective analysis of 1172 patients with gastric cancer after R0 resection, the peritoneal recurrence rate was 29%. In this study, the median time from recurrence at any location to death was 6 months.[3] Sasako and colleagues[4] demonstrated the peritoneum to be the most frequent first site of recurrence (38.1%)

[a] Department of Surgery, University Medical Center Regensburg, Franz Josef Strauss Allee 11, 93053 Regensburg, Germany; [b] Department of Surgery, St. John of God Hospital Regensburg, Pruefeninger Street 86, 93049 Regensburg, Germany
* Corresponding author.
E-mail address: Pompiliu.Piso@klinik.uni-regensburg.de

Surg Oncol Clin N Am 21 (2012) 625–633
http://dx.doi.org/10.1016/j.soc.2012.07.002
1055-3207/12/$ – see front matter © 2012 Elsevier Inc. All rights reserved.

during a 5-year follow-up period after curative resection of gastric cancer. This tumor manifestation is mostly associated with poor prognosis. The multicentric prospective evolution of peritoneal carcinomatosis (EVOCAPE) 1 study reported a mean and a median overall survival for the natural course of the disease of 6.5 and 3.1 months, respectively. The mean age of the 125 included patients was 60.5 years (range 21–96 years). Most of the patients showed advanced T stage of the primary tumor (55 pT3, 62 pT4), 73 patients were diagnosed with synchronous peritoneal carcinomatosis (58.4%), and 19 patients had additional liver metastases (15.2%).[5] Despite the significant improvement in survival of patients with advanced gastric cancer during the past 20 years with the use of palliative systemic polychemotherapy, the results remain unsatisfactory.[6–9] Considering that patients with inoperable and/or locally advanced gastric cancer with or without distant and peritoneal metastases have been included, clinical trials with modern systemic chemotherapy show median survival rates ranging from 9 to 14 months.[10–12] Data for patients in the appropriate clinical condition with peritoneal metastasis only are not available. However, combined cytoreductive surgery (CRS) and hyperthermic intraperitoneal chemotherapy (HIPEC) as an inherent part of an interdisciplinary treatment concept might be a promising additional treatment option for a highly selected part of patients with limited peritoneal carcinomatosis arising from gastric cancer.

PATHOPHYSIOLOGY

In contrast to hematologic or lymphatic metastasis, peritoneal carcinomatosis is mostly caused by continuous tumor growth or tumor cell dissemination. Ikeguchi and colleagues[2] could demonstrate a strong correlation between the area of serosal invasion and the number of detectable free abdominal tumor cells. The first step in the development of peritoneal metastasis is the detachment of single tumor cells from the primary carcinoma. Based on fast tumor growth, lack of lymphatic drainage, and other mechanisms, these cells reach the abdominal cavity and are disseminated with the peritoneal fluid. Direct cell-to-cell contact via adhesion molecules such as intracellular adhesion molecule 1 and CD44 leads to binding to mesothelial cells with consecutive induction of apoptosis and breaking of their intercellular junctions. By reaching the extracellular matrix, the tumor cells bind integrins and cause degradation, leading to an invasion of submesothelial cell layers. Moreover, free tumor cells can directly bind to specific structures of the extracellular matrix or the greater omentum and cause tumor infiltration.[13]

CLINICAL PRESENTATION

In most cases, peritoneal carcinomatosis is oligosymptomatic or asymptomatic during a long period and therefore often initially diagnosed intraoperatively. The development of malignant ascites might be the first specific sign of progressive peritoneal tumor dissemination. Moreover, patients with peritoneal carcinomatosis may develop abdominal pain, stenosis of canalicular structures, and paralytic or mechanic ileus. These complications may be accompanied by general symptoms of malignant diseases such as deterioration of general condition, weight loss, and fever (**Box 1**).

THERAPEUTIC OPTIONS AND SURGICAL TECHNIQUE

It is beyond question that the treatment of patients with advanced or recurrent gastric cancer is the domain of palliative systemic chemotherapy. Wagner and colleagues[7] showed in a meta-analysis of several randomized clinical trials that compared

---

Box 1
Clinical signs of peritoneal carcinomatosis

- Malignant ascites
- Intestinal obstruction
- Palpable abdominal masses
- General symptoms of malignant diseases

---

chemotherapy with best supportive care a significant overall survival benefit in favor of systemic chemotherapy and combined chemotherapy, respectively. Two prospective randomized trials using epirubin, cisplatin, fluorouracil (ECF) demonstrated a median survival of 8.9 and 9.4 months, respectively.[10,14] Comparable results with a median survival of 9.2 months were achieved in a randomized controlled trial using docetaxel, cisplatin, fluorouracil (DCF).[11] Cunningham and colleagues[15] reported a median survival of 11.2 months in a group of patients treated with EOX (epirubin, oxaliplatin, capecitabine [xeloda]) in the prospective randomized multicentric Phase III study comparing capecitabine with fluorouracil and oxaliplatin with cisplatin in patients with advanced oesophagogastric cancer (REAL-2) trial. The addition of the anti-HER2 monoclonal antibody trastuzumab to a chemotherapeutic regimen consisting of cisplatin and 5-fluorouracil or capecitabine led to an improved overall median survival of 13.8 months in patients with *HER2*-positive advanced gastric cancer.[12] Nevertheless, the oncologic outcome of the subgroup of patients with peritoneal carcinomatosis is not reported in these trials and might be expected to be worse. Thus, additional treatment options are required to improve the oncologic outcome of this subset of patients.

The goal of the combined treatment concept consisting of CRS and HIPEC is to remove all visible tumor masses from the abdominal cavity as a precondition for peritoneal perfusion with highly concentrated chemotherapy to locally treat residual microscopic tumor cells. Hyperthermia may have additional antitumoral effects and enhances the penetration ability of the intraperitoneally administered cytostatic agents.[16,17] The surgical technique has been described in detail by Sugarbaker[18] in 1995. Although the principle of HIPEC is based on continuous peritoneal perfusion using inflow and outflow drainages and a heat-exchanger/pump system, the treatment protocol is not standardized. Thus, multiple different cytostatic agents are used for HIPEC and administered in open, semiopen, or closed abdomen technique. Intraperitoneal temperature is 40° to 42°C, and perfusion time ranges from 30 to 120 minutes.[19] A meta-analysis summarizing the results of 13 randomized trials evaluating adjuvant intraperitoneal chemotherapy (IPC) in 1648 patients (873 patients with and 775 patients without IPC) indicates an overall survival advantage for patients with IPC after curative gastric resection.[20] Moreover, Kuramoto and colleagues[21] could demonstrate in a prospective randomized trial comparing extensive intraperitoneal lavage and IPC with IPC and surgery only a significant 5-year survival benefit in favor of prophylactic extensive intraoperative peritoneal lavage and IPC after curative resection of gastric cancer. These data support the efficacy of HIPEC in patients with advanced gastric cancer.

DIAGNOSTIC PROCEDURES

Preoperative gastroscopy including endosonography should be performed in all patients with advanced gastric cancer to determine the resectability of the primary tumor and local lymph node status. Moreover, computed tomography (CT) scanning

---

Box 2
Preoperative diagnostics

Mandatory diagnostic procedures

- Gastroscopy including endosonography
- CT
- Sonography

Recommended diagnostic procedures

- Diagnostic laparoscopy

Additional diagnostic procedures

- Contrast-enhanced sonography
- Magnetic resonance imaging
- PET or PET/CT

---

of the thorax and abdomen with intravenous and intraluminal contrast media is mandatory to exclude distant metastasis and to determine the extent of peritoneal tumor dissemination. Liver metastasis should be assessed with additional ultrasonography.

In patients qualifying for CRS and HIPEC, a staging laparoscopy before cytoreduction is recommended to assess the extent of peritoneal tumor dissemination and to exclude disseminated small-nodule carcinomatosis of the small bowel. Additional diagnostics such as contrast-enhanced sonography, magnetic resonance imaging, and/or positron-emission tomography (PET)/CT may be helpful in case of unclear findings and should be performed if applicable (**Box 2**).

Diagnosis and Patient Selection

Several studies demonstrate that complete macroscopic resection (CC-0/1) is crucial for the improvement of survival after CRS and HIPEC in patients with peritoneal carcinomatosis arising from gastric cancer.[22,23] Thus, the achievability of CC-0/1 resection should be assessed with preoperative diagnostics as described. Moreover, survival was influenced by the intraoperative Peritoneal Cancer Index (PCI) showing

---

Box 3
Preoperative diagnostics

Selection criteria

- PCI <12
- Complete macroscopic cytoreduction probable
- No evidence of distant organ metastasis
- Eastern Cooperative Oncology Group performance status ≤1
- Limited clinical relevant comorbidities

Exclusion criteria (STOP signs)

- Disseminated small bowel infiltration
- Ureteral stenosis
- Bilary tract stenosis/cholestasis

Table 1
Median and overall survival after CRS and HIPEC

Author, Year	n	Median Survival, mo	Survival Rate, %
Fujimoto et al,[27] 1997	48	16	31 (5 y)
Loggie et al,[28] 2000	17	10	0 (1 y)
Hall et al,[29] 2004	34	11	21 (5 y) CC-0/1
Glehen et al,[30] 2004	49	10	29 (5 y) CC-0/1
Yonemura et al,[31] 2005	107	11.5	27 (5 y) CC-0/1
Cheong et al,[33] 2007 (EPIC)	154	11	32 (5 y) CC-0/1
Yang et al,[34] 2010	21	43.4 (CC-0) 9.4 (CC-1)	43 (2 y) CC-0/1
Glehen et al,[22,35] 2010	159	9 (CC-0/1: 15)	23 (5 y) CC-0/1
Yang et al,[23] 2011	34	11	15 (2 y)

Abbreviation: EPIC, early postoperative intraperitoneal chemotherapy.

a significant survival benefit for patients with a PCI of less than 12.[22] The PCI (Washington Cancer Center Washington, DC, USA) allows the assessment of the extent of peritoneal surface malignancy.[24,25] The numerical score ranging from 0 to 39 combines lesion size and tumor localization in 13 abdominopelvic regions (regions 0–12). Esquivel and Chua[26] showed that preoperative CT mostly underestimates the extent of peritoneal tumor dissemination. In particular, the involvement of small bowel that is common in patients with advanced gastric cancer is not sufficiently detected with CT. Thus, additional staging laparoscopy is recommended to assess the PCI before CRS and HIPEC and to allow for consistent preoperative patient selection. The main selection criteria are summarized in **Box 3**. Moreover, individual patient motivation, operative risk, and the expected postoperative quality of life should be taken into account. All patients's cases should be discussed in an interdisciplinary tumor board before the institution of CRS and HIPEC.

CLINICAL OUTCOMES IN THE LITERATURE

Several case series could demonstrate overall median survival rates between 9 and 16 months.[22,27–31] In a prospective randomized phase III clinical trial with 68 patients with peritoneal carcinomatosis arising from gastric cancer that compared CRS and HIPEC to CRS only, Yang and colleagues[23] could demonstrate median survival rates of 11 and 6.5 months, respectively. After complete macroscopic cytoreduction (CC-0/1),

Table 2
Morbidity and mortality after CRS and HIPEC

Author, Year	n	Overall Morbidity Rate, %	Mortality Rate, %
Glehen et al,[30] 2004	49	27	4
Yonemura et al,[31] 2005	107	21.5	7
Cheong et al,[33] 2007	154	22.7	2.6
Shen et al,[36] 2009	43	43	4
Yang et al,[34] 2010	21	14.3	10.7
Glehen et al,[22] 2010	159	n.r.	6.5

Table 3 Safety of gastric resections			
Author, Year	No. of Gastric Resections	Overall Leakage Rate, %	Leakage Rate After GE, %
Sugarbaker,[38] 2002	45	Not reported	0
Glehen et al,[30] 2004	39	5.1	0
Kusamura et al,[39] 2006	29	11	0
Levine et al,[40] 2007	60	Not reported	Not reported
Piso et al,[37] 2009	37	8.5	0

Abbreviation: GE, gastric resection.

median survival increased to 13.5 months in the CRS plus HIPEC group. Synchronous peritoneal carcinomatosis and additional systemic chemotherapy were positive prognostic factors. Gill and colleagues summarized the data of 1 prospective controlled study, 3 retrospective case series, and 6 prospective case series, for a total number of patients of 445. In this recent systematic review, the median survival after CC-0/1 resection was 15 months (range 9.5–43.4 months).[32] Overall median survival and 1- to 5-year survival rates are summarized in **Table 1**. Despite minimal improvement of the median survival with the use of CRS and HIPEC, the percentage of long-term survivors is up to 30% higher.

COMPLICATIONS AND CONCERNS

Postoperative complications after CRS and HIPEC consist of surgery-related morbidity and chemotherapy-associated toxicity. Although the classification of perioperative morbidity and toxicity is not standardized, the overall morbidity rates range from 14% to 43% (**Table 2**). In the systematic review published by Gill and colleagues, overall morbidity and mortality rates were 21.5% and 4.8%, respectively.

Piso and colleagues[37] showed that there is no increased leakage rate if gastric resection is performed during CRS and HIPEC. The leakage rates after gastric resection in patients with peritoneal carcinomatosis of different origins are summarized in **Table 3**.

In conclusion, published data show that CRS and HIPEC can be performed with low mortality and acceptable morbidity rates in patients with peritoneal carcinomatosis arising from gastric cancer. Nevertheless, the significant operative risk has to be considered during the patient selection process for the combined treatment concept.

SUMMARY

Although a substantial survival benefit after CRS and HIPEC could be demonstrated for patients with peritoneal carcinomatosis arising from other tumor entities such as colorectal cancer, the efficacy of the combined treatment concept in patients with gastric cancer remains controversial. Published data show that survival can be improved in a highly selected subgroup of patients with peritoneal carcinomatosis of arising from gastric cancer. However, complete macroscopic cytoreduction seems to be crucial for positive results. Further randomized clinical trials comparing CRS and HIPEC to modern systemic chemotherapy are needed to determine the role of CRS and HIPEC as part of an interdisciplinary treatment strategy. Moreover, the results of ongoing clinical trials using new intraperitoneal drugs, drug combinations, or intraperitoneal antibodies such as catumaxumab may help to optimize the intraperitoneal treatment and lead to further improvement of oncologic outcome.

REFERENCES

1. Jemal A, Bray F, Center MM, et al. Global cancer statistics. CA Cancer J Clin 2011;61:69–90.
2. Ikeguchi M, Oka A, Tsujitani S, et al. Relationship between area of serosal invasion and intraperitoneal free cancer cells in patients with gastric cancer. Anticancer Res 1994;14:2131–4.
3. D'Angelica M, Gonen M, Brennan MF, et al. Patterns of initial recurrence in completely resected gastric adenocarcinoma. Ann Surg 2004;240:808–16.
4. Sasako M, Sano T, Yamamoto S, et al. D2 lymphadenectomy alone or with para-aortic nodal dissection for gastric cancer. N Engl J Med 2008;359:453–62.
5. Sadeghi B, Arvieux C, Glehen O, et al. Peritoneal carcinomatosis from non-gynecologic malignancies: results of the EVOCAPE 1 multicentric prospective study. Cancer 2000;88:358–63.
6. Glimelius B, Ekstrom K, Hoffman K, et al. Randomized comparison between chemotherapy plus best supportive care with best supportive care in advanced gastric cancer. Ann Oncol 1997;8:163–8.
7. Wagner AD, Grothe W, Haerting J, et al. Chemotherapy in advanced gastric cancer: a systematic review and meta-analysis based on aggregate data. J Clin Oncol 2006;24:2903–9.
8. Pyrhonen S, Kuitunen T, Nyandoto P, et al. Randomised comparison of fluorouracil, epidoxorubicin and methotrexate (FEMTX) plus supportive care with supportive care alone in patients with non-resectable gastric cancer. Br J Cancer 1995;71:587–91.
9. Murad AM, Santiago FF, Petroianu A, et al. Modified therapy with 5-fluorouracil, doxorubicin, and methotrexate in advanced gastric cancer. Cancer 1993;72:37–41.
10. Webb A, Cunningham D, Scarffe JH, et al. Randomized trial comparing epirubicin, cisplatin, and fluorouracil versus fluorouracil, doxorubicin, and methotrexate in advanced esophagogastric cancer. J Clin Oncol 1997;15:261–7.
11. Ajani JA, Moiseyenko VM, Tjulandin S, et al. Clinical benefit with docetaxel plus fluorouracil and cisplatin compared with cisplatin and fluorouracil in a phase III trial of advanced gastric or gastroesophageal cancer adenocarcinoma: the V-325 Study Group. J Clin Oncol 2007;25:3205–9.
12. Bang YJ, Van Cutsem E, Feyereislova A, et al. Trastuzumab in combination with chemotherapy versus chemotherapy alone for treatment of HER2-positive advanced gastric or gastro-oesophageal junction cancer (ToGA): a phase 3, open-label, randomised controlled trial. Lancet 2010;376:687–97.
13. Ceelen WP, Bracke ME. Peritoneal minimal residual disease in colorectal cancer: mechanisms, prevention, and treatment. Lancet Oncol 2009;10:72–9.
14. Ross P, Nicolson M, Cunningham D, et al. Prospective randomized trial comparing mitomycin, cisplatin, and protracted venous-infusion fluorouracil (PVI 5-FU) with epirubicin, cisplatin, and PVI 5-FU in advanced esophagogastric cancer. J Clin Oncol 2002;20:1996–2004.
15. Cunningham D, Starling N, Rao S, et al. Capecitabine and oxaliplatin for advanced esophagogastric cancer. N Engl J Med 2008;358:36–46.
16. Glockzin G, Schlitt HJ, Piso P. Peritoneal carcinomatosis: patient selection, perioperative complications and quality of life related to cytoreductive surgery and hyperthermic intraperitoneal chemotherapy. World J Surg Oncol 2009;7:5.

17. Ceelen WP, Flessner MF. Intraperitoneal therapy for peritoneal tumors: biophysics and clinical evidence. Nat Rev Clin Oncol 2010;7:108–15.

18. Sugarbaker PH. Peritonectomy procedures. Ann Surg 1995;221:29–42.

19. Gonzalez-Moreno S, Gonzalez-Bayon LA, Ortega-Perez G. Hyperthermic intraperitoneal chemotherapy: rationale and technique. World J Gastrointest Oncol 2010;2:68–75.

20. Yan TD, Black D, Sugarbaker PH, et al. A systematic review and meta-analysis of the randomized controlled trials on adjuvant intraperitoneal chemotherapy for resectable gastric cancer. Ann Surg Oncol 2007;14:2702–13.

21. Kuramoto M, Shimada S, Ikeshima S, et al. Extensive intraoperative peritoneal lavage as a standard prophylactic strategy for peritoneal recurrence in patients with gastric carcinoma. Ann Surg 2009;250:242–6.

22. Glehen O, Gilly FN, Arvieux C, et al. Peritoneal carcinomatosis from gastric cancer: a multi-institutional study of 159 patients treated by cytoreductive surgery combined with perioperative intraperitoneal chemotherapy. Ann Surg Oncol 2010;17:2370–7.

23. Yang XJ, Huang CQ, Suo T, et al. Cytoreductive surgery and hyperthermic intraperitoneal chemotherapy improves survival of patients with peritoneal carcinomatosis from gastric cancer: final results of a phase III randomized clinical trial. Ann Surg Oncol 2011;18:1575–81.

24. Jacquet P, Sugarbaker PH. Clinical research methodologies in diagnosis and staging of patients with peritoneal carcinomatosis. Cancer Treat Res 1996;82:359–74.

25. Glehen O, Gilly FN. Quantitative prognostic indicators of peritoneal surface malignancy: carcinomatosis, sarcomatosis, and peritoneal mesothelioma. Surg Oncol Clin N Am 2003;12:649–71.

26. Esquivel J, Chua TC. CT versus intraoperative peritoneal cancer index in colorectal cancer peritoneal carcinomatosis: importance of the difference between statistical significance and clinical relevance. Ann Surg Oncol 2009;16(9):2662–3.

27. Fujimoto S, Takahashi M, Mutou T, et al. Improved mortality rate of gastric carcinoma patients with peritoneal carcinomatosis treated with intraperitoneal hyperthermic chemoperfusion combined with surgery. Cancer 1997;79:884–91.

28. Loggie BW, Fleming RA, McQuellon RP, et al. Cytoreductive surgery with intraperitoneal hyperthermic chemotherapy for disseminated peritoneal cancer of gastrointestinal origin. Am Surg 2000;66:561–8.

29. Hall JJ, Loggie BW, Shen P, et al. Cytoreductive surgery with intraperitoneal hyperthermic chemotherapy for advanced gastric cancer. J Gastrointest Surg 2004;8:454–63.

30. Glehen O, Schreiber V, Cotte E, et al. Cytoreductive surgery and intraperitoneal chemohyperthermia for peritoneal carcinomatosis arising from gastric cancer. Arch Surg 2004;139:20–6.

31. Yonemura Y, Kawamura T, Bandou E, et al. Treatment of peritoneal dissemination from gastric cancer by peritonectomy and chemohyperthermic peritoneal perfusion. Br J Surg 2005;92:370–5.

32. Gill RS, Al-Adra DP, Nagendran J, et al. Treatment of gastric cancer with peritoneal carcinomatosis by cytoreductive surgery and HIPEC: a systematic review of survival, mortality, and morbidity. J Surg Oncol 2011;104:692–8.

33. Cheong JH, Shen JY, Song CS, et al. Early postoperative intraperitoneal chemotherapy following cytoreductive surgery in patients with very advanced gastric cancer. Ann Surg Oncol 2007;14:61–8.

34. Yang XJ, Li Y, Yonemura Y. Cytoreductive surgery plus hyperthermic intraperitoneal chemotherapy to treat gastric cancer with ascites and/or peritoneal carcinomatosis: results from a Chinese center. J Surg Oncol 2010;101:457–64.
35. Glehen O, Gilly FN, Boutitie F, et al. Toward curative treatment of peritoneal carcinomatosis from nonovarian origin by cytoreductive surgery combined with perioperative intraperitoneal chemotherapy: a multi-institutional study of 1290 patients. Cancer 2010;116:5608–18.
36. Shen P, Stewart JH 4th, Levine EA. Cytoreductive surgery and intraperitoneal hyperthermic chemotherapy for peritoneal surface malignancy: non-colorectal indications. Curr Probl Cancer 2009;33:168–93.
37. Piso P, Slowik P, Popp F, et al. Safety of gastric resections during cytoreductive surgery and hyperthermic intraperitoneal chemotherapy for peritoneal carcinomatosis. Ann Surg Oncol 2009;16:2188–94.
38. Sugarbaker PH. Cytoreduction including total gastrectomy for pseudomyxoma peritonei. Br J Surg 2002;89:208–12.
39. Kusamura S, Younan R, Baratti D, et al. Cytoreductive surgery followed by intraperitoneal hyperthermic perfusion: analysis of morbidity and mortality in 209 peritoneal surface malignancies treated with closed abdomen technique. Cancer 2006;106:1144–53.
40. Levine EA, Stewart JH 4th, Russell GB, et al. Cytoreductive surgery and intraperitoneal hyperthermic chemotherapy for peritoneal surface malignancy: experience with 501 procedures. J Am Coll Surg 2007;204:943–53 [discussion: 53–5].

Peritoneal Mesothelioma
Current Status and Future Directions

Terence C. Chua, MBBS (UNSW), MRCS (Ed)[a,b,*],
Chanel H. Chong, MBBS (UNSW)[a], David L. Morris, MD, PhD[a,b]

KEYWORDS

- Peritoneal mesothelioma • Pemetrexed • Cytoreductive surgery
- Hyperthermic intraperitoneal chemotherapy

KEY POINTS

- Peritoneal mesothelioma remains a rare primary disease of the peritoneum where survival advantage may be achieved through cytoreductive surgery and hyperthermic intraperitoneal chemotherapy over systemic treatment alone.
- Recognition of the histopathologic subtype of a malignant peritoneal mesothelioma is essential in treatment planning.
- Future diagnostic and treatment outcomes should be mapped and staged against the new staging criteria for future validation.

INTRODUCTION

Peritoneal mesothelioma is a rare and fatal cancer. Studies indicate an incidence that is demonstrating a rising trend and a global 15-year cumulative mortality rate of 213,200 cases.[1,2] Malignant mesothelioma affects the pleura, peritoneum, pericardium, and tunica vaginalis with each site-specific cancer surprisingly showing some epidemiologic differences.[3] Disease affecting the pleura accounts for 70% and peritoneum accounts for 30% of all mesothelioma. Instead of the male predominance and approximate mean age of mortality at 70 years seen in the other types of mesothelioma, peritoneal mesothelioma is more commonly seen in females and occurs earlier in life with a younger mean age at mortality of 66 years.[4,5] This disease is mostly seen in higher income countries because of the historical use of asbestos and the

Financial disclosures: None declared.
Conflict of interests: None declared.
[a] Hepatobiliary and Surgical Oncology Unit, Department of Surgery, University of New South Wales, St George Hospital, Sydney, NSW 2217, Australia; [b] St George Clinical School, University of New South Wales, NSW 2032, Australia
* Corresponding author. Department of Surgery, University of New South Wales, St George Hospital, Sydney, NSW 2217, Australia.
E-mail address: terence.chua@unsw.edu.au

Surg Oncol Clin N Am 21 (2012) 635–643
http://dx.doi.org/10.1016/j.soc.2012.07.010
1055-3207/12/$ – see front matter © 2012 Elsevier Inc. All rights reserved.

availability of expertise and technology that allow identification of this disease.[4] This article focuses on peritoneal mesothelioma and describes the current knowledge and recent clinical research findings in this disease entity.

PATHOPHYSIOLOGY

Asbestos is recognized as an etiologic factor in the formation of mesothelioma. Risk increases throughout life after asbestos exposure despite removal of the offending agent.[4] The evolution of mesothelial cells into cancer has been widely studied and several hypotheses have been put forward. It is theorized that the asbestos is inhaled, expectorated, and subsequently swallowed. Its favorable physical characteristics allow the mineral to penetrate the bowel lumen and enter into the lymphatics and splanchnic circulation.[6] The foreign body reaction triggered by asbestos fibers results in a series of host inflammatory response. In a study of immortalized human pleural mesothelial cells, ferritin heavy chain present within asbestos leads to production of reactive oxygen species and reactive nitrogen species. The phagocytotic process by alveolar macrophages also results in the production of these proinflammatory cytokines.[7,8] Overall, these processes lead to disruption of the genetic makeup of the mesothelial cells.[8] Direct disruption of the normal mitotic activity by asbestos fibers has also been recognized to cause aneuploidy and other abnormal chromosomal arrangements. This carcinogenic process occurs with incessant activation of kinases and early expression of the proto-oncogene (FOS or JUN or activated protein 1 family members) in mesothelial cells that confers the neoplastic mesothelial cell a persistent proliferating capacity.[5] Results from clinical studies have indicated that patients with malignant mesothelioma are observed to have higher levels of interleukin-10, a cytokine that drives further production of transforming growth factor-β. Interleukin-10 and transforming growth factor-β are postulated to play a role in asbestos-related carcinogenesis.[9,10] In some cases, whereby there is an absence of asbestos exposure, the role of other etiologic agents, such as the simian vacuolating virus (SV 40), has been implicated to contribute to the formation of the malignancy but the role of this oncogenic virus remains a postulate because there are conflicting studies that seem to suggest otherwise.[11]

CLINICAL PRESENTATION AND EXAMINATION

Patients typically present with an account of prolonged symptoms including complaints of abdominal pain (33%), increase in abdominal girth (31%), or both (10%). Other findings also include new onset of hernia, weight loss, dyspnea, fever, or night sweats and further history may reveal the absence of menstruation or complaints of infertility.[12,13] Attempts to classify the presenting complaints into three groups, namely classical (73%), surgical (16%), and medical (11%), are described in **Table 1**.[14,15] Although it is useful to have a clinical structure in approaching this malignancy, it may not be applicable at all times because some cases may not necessarily have the entire constellation of symptoms or fit into any of the three groups. At times, rarer instances of peritoneal mesothelioma may present with the development of subcutaneous swelling, oral gingivitis, or paraneoplastic syndrome.[16–18]

DIAGNOSTIC INVESTIGATIONS

The entire diagnostic work-up to arrive at a confirmatory diagnosis of peritoneal mesothelioma is lengthy and involves a series of serologic, imaging, and histopathologic tests. This is comprised of common blood tests including full blood count; erythrocyte

Table 1
Classification of symptoms

Classical	Medical	Surgical
Abdominal pain	Abdominal pain	Hernia
Ascites	Weight loss	Ileus
Abdominal mass	Fever	Abdominal perforation
	Diarrhea	
	Vomiting	
	Asthenia	
	Anorexia	

sedimentation rate; C-reactive protein; and tumor markers (CEA, CA199, CA125, and mesothelin). Tumor markers CA-125 and mesothelin are known to be elevated in peritoneal mesothelioma but are not entirely specific because these proteins are also observed to be elevated in other malignancies, such as ovarian cancer, and infective processes, such as tuberculosis.[19–22] CA-125 has a sensitivity of 53.3% and is more useful in supporting a diagnosis and for disease monitoring during the follow-up period.[19] Mesothelin, which is detected in pleural and peritoneal effusions, may be a valuable diagnostic marker because its serum level is shown to progressively increase in patients with a history of asbestos exposure who were later diagnosed with the mesothelioma.[23,24] Creaney and colleagues[25] adopted a logistic regression model combining the two index markers, CA-125 and mesothelin, and examined its sensitivity for detecting mesothelioma but found that using both biomarkers did not improve the sensitivity of mesothelioma diagnosis over a single biomarker alone. Other tumor markers, including CA 15.3, have been reported to have a baseline diagnostic sensitivity of 48.5%, whereas CEA and CA 19.9 have not been found to be helpful.[19] Recent studies have discovered a redox-active protein known as the "serum thioredoxin-1" and tenascin-X in effusions, which may act as diagnostic markers; however, this remains experimental and further research is required.[26,27] Hence, tumor markers have only a supportive role in arriving at the diagnosis and do not have sufficient sensitivity and specificity that is required of a diagnostic tool.

CT scan may detect overt peritoneal lesions by demonstrating well-defined masses, omental thickening, and modularity present within the mesentery.[28–30] Yan and colleagues[31] examined the CT scans of a series of 33 patients with peritoneal mesothelioma and described the presence of pleural abnormalities in 8 (24%) of 33 patients, 91% of patients having involvement of the greater omentum, 97% of patients having vesico, rectal, or uterine pouches, and 66% of patients having ascites. This predominant central abdominal and pelvic disease burden observed may seem to be a characteristic pattern in the presentation of this disease. Park and colleagues[32] used the terminology of "dry" and "wet" as descriptors of the CT features of peritoneal mesothelioma, with the dry appearance consisting of peritoneal-based lesions and the wet appearance consisting of ascites, irregular or nodular thickening of the peritoneum, and an omental mass that may scallop or directly invade adjacent abdominal viscera. After these imaging findings, it is important to exclude the presence of any intestinal primaries as cause of these peritoneal lesions. Commonly, an esophagogastroduodenoscopy and colonoscopy are required. After this, the diagnosis of peritoneal lesions arising from mesothelioma and not an intestinal primary is confirmed through a histologic assessment of biopsies obtained during laparoscopy. Macroscopically, peritoneal mesothelioma appear as multiple whitish nodules that may coalesce to form plaques or masses or layers out evenly to cover the peritoneal surface partially or completely. The diagnostic laparoscopy procedure could also provide an opportunity to evaluate the peritoneal disease burden and assess the potential for cytoreduction. Laterza and colleagues[33] reported 33 patients with peritoneal mesothelioma who underwent diagnostic laparoscopy and judged 30 patients to be amendable to complete cytoreduction, for which 29 patients eventually underwent cytoreduction with complete cytoreduction attained.

Histopathologic examination of pathologic specimens for the diagnosis of mesothelioma requires hematoxylin and eosin stain, which typically reveals an epithelioid type (79%) or sarcomatoid and biphasic type (12%).[34] Epithelioid mesothelioma has a prominent papilla-tubular structure and this must be differentiated from an adenocarcinoma of other origins. Sarcomatoid mesothelioma depicts proliferation of spindle cells and must be differentiated from sarcoma of the abdominal wall or retroperitoneum. Biphasic mesothelioma consists of dedifferentiated cells comprising epithelioid and sarcomatoid variant in varying proportions. A rare form of low malignant potential mesothelioma, multicystic variant, is also recognized and accounts for approximately 6.4% of all mesothelioma.[35,36] Immunohistochemical stains are then used to confirm the diagnosis after histomorphologic assessment with mesothelial cell markers including calretinin, WT1, thrombomodulin, mesothelin, and D2-40. These are tested against a panel of marks that are expressed in other malignancies to serve as a negative predictor to support the diagnosis (ie, CEA, CD15, Ber-EP4, MOC-31, ER). For sarcomatoid tumors, cytokeratins (AE1/AE3 or CAM5.2) are highly specific and are useful in arriving at a diagnosis.[37]

STAGING OF PERITONEAL MESOTHELIOMA

The peritoneal disease burden of mesothelioma is typically assessed systematically using Sugarbaker's peritoneal cancer index (PCI). The PCI is comprised of a score ranging between 0 and 3 assessed based on lesion size and computed in total out of a score ranging from 1 to 39 by a summation of specific scores from 13 abdomino-pelvic regions.[38] The Peritoneal Surface Oncology Group International (PSOGI) has collaborated to combine their experiences of managing patients with peritoneal mesothelioma to enroll patients collectively into a multi-institutional registry database to formulate a clinicopathologic staging system through prognostic parameters identified from patients treated uniformly with cytoreductive surgery (CRS) and hyperthermic intraperitoneal chemotherapy (HIPEC) at eight international institutions. The staging system adopts the common nomenclature of the tumor-node-metastasis (TNM) system comprised of tumor burden (T) assessed by the PCI subgrouped into four categories: T1 being PCI 1–10, T2 being PCI 11–20, T3 being PCI 21–30, and T4 being PCI 30–39. Abdominal nodal disease commonly affected by peritoneal mesothelioma includes the iliac chain, para-aortic, celiac axis, mesenteric, and the portocaval lymph nodes; any involvement of nodes is classified as N1. The M element refers to the presence or absence of extra-abdominal metastases. Formal stage-wise classification was done in a reverse fashion after analysis of the prognostic impact of the PCI, lymph node, and metastasis status before arriving at four clinical stages (**Table 2**). Patients with T1N0M0 were designated as stage I; T2–3N0M0 as stage II; and stage III was comprised of patients with T4, N1, or M1 disease. From the complete clinicopathologic data of the 294 patients that formed the cohort used to derive this staging system, stratification of stage-based survival was achieved with 5-year survival associated with stage I, II, and III disease being 87%, 53%, and 29%, respectively. This proposed TNM staging system is being evaluated in further prospective studies and it is hoped it will be formally endorsed by the American Joint Committee on Cancer.[39]

Table 2
Proposed TNM staging for DMPM with corresponding survival rates

Stage	Tumor	Node	Metastasis	Survival Rates (%)
I	T1	N0	M0	87
II	T2–3	N0	M0	53
III	T4	N0–1	M0–1	29
	T1–4	N1	M0–1	
	T1–4	N0–1	M1	

Abbreviations: DMPM, diffuse malignant peritoneal mesothelioma; M0, nil metastasis; M1, metastatic disease; N0, nil lymph node; N1, positive lymph node involvement; T1, PCI 1–10; T2, PCI 11–20; T3, PCI 21–30; T4, PCI 30–39.

THERAPEUTIC OPTIONS

A variety of chemotherapeutic drugs have been reported to be effective and used in peritoneal mesothelioma, with the most commonly used agents being cisplatin, gemcitabine, doxorubicin, and pemetrexed. Historical data from the Dana-Farber Cancer Institute and Brigham and Women's Hospital's experience of 180 patients with mesothelioma showed 37 patients with peritoneal mesothelioma reported a median survival of 15 months after a variety of palliative chemotherapy treatments.[40] In a randomized trial by the Cancer and Leukemia Group B comparing cisplatin and mitomycin versus cisplatin and doxorubicin for patients with pleural or peritoneal mesothelioma, this 79-patient trial reported an overall response rate of 26% with a median time to treatment failure of 3.6 months and 4.8 months, and 7.7 months and 8.8 months in the cisplatin-mitomycin and cisplatin-doxorubicin groups, respectively.[41] More recent data seem to indicate that inclusion of pemetrexed as a combination with cisplatin or carboplatin may improve efficacy and outcome. In the Expanded Access Program where 109 patients with peritoneal mesothelioma were treated with pemetrexed or pemetrexed combination chemotherapy, response rates for the platinum-based (cisplatin/carboplatin) combination with pemetrexed seemed to achieve superior results over pemetrexed alone with response rates of 24.1% versus 12.5% and 1-year survival of 57.4% and 41.5%, respectively.[42] Pemetrexed in combination with gemcitabine was demonstrated to have a synergistic effect in preclinical models and was recently evaluated in a phase II trial comprising 20 patients with peritoneal mesothelioma to evaluate its clinical efficacy and safety. This combination regimen achieved a response rate of 15% with median time to disease progression and overall survival of 10.4 months and 26.8 months, respectively. However, there was a high incidence of grade 3/4 neutropenia (60%).[43] There are isolated reports of the role of whole-abdominal radiation; however, this treatment has not been adequately studied naturally because of the potentially high morbidity. Nonetheless, a study on surgery and intraperitoneal chemotherapy with whole-abdominal radiation was reported to achieve improved disease-free survival.[44]

Because peritoneal mesothelioma seems to be confined within the peritoneal surfaces of the abdominal cavity before metastasizing to lymph nodes and extraabdominal regions later in the disease history, a proof of concept to treat this disease with intraperitoneal chemotherapy to allow direct targeting of disease by Markman and Kelsen[45] was conducted, treating 19 patients with intraperitoneal cisplatin and mitomycin. In this study, the treatment was well tolerated with control of ascites achieved in 47% of patients. Among the 19 patients, the median survival was 9 months; however, four patients with minimal volume peritoneal disease were reported to survive more than 3 years. This suggests that if peritoneal tumor

Table 3 Expected postcytoreduction outcomes of peritoneal mesothelioma by histopathologic subtype based on the multi-institutional registry	
Histologic Subtype	**Median Survival (Months)**
Multicystic	>54
Epithelioid	63
Mixed/sarcomatoid	16

cytoreduction could be achieved, intraperitoneal chemotherapy may serve as an adjunct to achieve peritoneal disease control and prolong the disease-free survival.

CRS for peritoneal tumors was introduced by Sugarbaker,[46] who described six peritonectomy procedures that allow removal of all peritoneal lining of the abdominopelvic cavity. It is important in peritoneal mesothelioma that complete peritonectomy be performed even for peritoneal surfaces that are uninvolved by tumor.[47] In a case-control study by Baratti and colleagues[48] comparing complete peritonectomy versus selective peritonectomy, 5-year survival was 63.9% and 40%, respectively, without any difference in morbidity and reoperation rates. Nodal sampling and its impact on outcome has been shown to be important in peritoneal mesothelioma. From the experience of the Milan group, Baratti and colleagues[49] identified in a multivariate analysis after controlling of other prognostic variables that negative lymph nodes were independent predictors of improved survival. In their study, negative nodes compared with positive or nonassessed nodes were associated with increased survival and hence the need for careful nodal sampling when performing cytoreduction for peritoneal mesothelioma. Although node positivity ultimately bears a poorer outcome and is unlikely to be modified through extended lymphadenectomy, an approach to standardized lymph node sampling would assist in disease staging (see **Table 2**).[39]

HIPEC has been commonly used as an intraoperative adjunct to cytoreduction. It may be administered using either an open or closed abdomen technique. For peritoneal mesothelioma, the drugs commonly used include cisplatin alone or cisplatin with doxorubicin. The abdominal cavity is perfused with the chemotherapy solution at a temperature of 40°C to 43°C. From the PSOGI registry of 405 patients treated uniformly with CRS and HIPEC, an overall median survival of 53 months, 3- and 5-year survival rates of 60% and 47% were achieved, respectively. Epithelioid tumor subtype, absence of lymph node metastasis, an optimal cytoreduction (CCR0/1), and using HIPEC were independently associated with an improved outcome.[34] Multicystic peritoneal mesothelioma, a variant of epithelioid mesothelioma, was also studied as a subgroup analysis from the PSOGI registry. There were 26 patients (6.4%) identified from the registry with multicystic tumors with a large preponderance of females having this histologic variant (20 women and 6 men). After cytoreduction and a median follow-up of 54 (range, 5–129) months, all patients treated are alive and free of disease. Clearly, this represents a distinct subtype with favorable disease biology where long-term survival may be achieved through complete eradication of the cystic peritoneal lesions (**Table 3**).[35]

SUMMARY

Peritoneal mesothelioma is a rare malignancy. Pemetrexed in combination with platinum-based chemotherapy seems to be the most effective treatment in patients whose disease is not amendable to surgery. Because of its rarity, it is unlikely that large-scale trials to obtain level one evidence of treatment efficacies will be a reality. Data based on large retrospective studies seem to be the most reliable to date.

PSOGI's multi-institutional registry study reporting the survival outcomes of 405 patients uniformly treated with CRS and HIPEC is the largest study reporting the best survival outcome in this disease. The newly proposed peritoneal mesothelioma staging system should be included in future clinical research of this disease. Ongoing translational research to identify specific molecular alterations and genetic signatures that are predictive of outcome may represent an ideal strategy to personalized peritoneal mesothelioma treatment to improve outcomes of patients with this disease.

REFERENCES

1. AIHW. Australian cancer incidence and mortality (ACIM) workbooks. Canberra (Australia): AIHW; 2011.
2. Park EK, Takahashi K, Hoshuyama T, et al. Global magnitude of reported and unreported mesothelioma. Environ Health Perspect 2011;119(4):514–8.
3. Gemba K, Fujimoto N, Kato K, et al. National survey of malignant mesothelioma and asbestos exposure in Japan. Cancer Sci 2012;103(3):483–90.
4. Delgermaa V, Takahashi K, Park E-K, et al. Global mesothelioma deaths reported to the World Health Organization between 1994 and 2008. Bull World Health Organ 2011;89(10):716–724C.
5. Robinson BW, Musk AW, Lake RA. Malignant mesothelioma. Lancet 2005; 366(9483):397–408.
6. Jeong YJ, Kim S, Kwak SW, et al. Neoplastic and non-neoplastic conditions of serosal membrane origin: CT findings. Radiographics 2008;28(3):801–18.
7. Kamp DW, Weitzman SA. The molecular basis of asbestos induced lung injury. Thorax 1999;54(7):638–52.
8. Matsuzaki H, Maeda M, Lee S, et al. Asbestos-induced cellular and molecular alteration of immunocompetent cells and their relationship with chronic inflammation and carcinogenesis. J Biomed Biotechnol 2012;2012:492608.
9. Murakami S, Nishimura Y, Maeda M, et al. Cytokine alteration and speculated immunological pathophysiology in silicosis and asbestos-related diseases. Environ Health Prev Med 2009;14(4):216–22.
10. Maeda M, Nishimura Y, Kumagai N, et al. Dysregulation of the immune system caused by silica and asbestos. J Biomed Biotechnol 2010;7(4):268–78.
11. Manfredi JJ, Dong J, Liu W-j, et al. Evidence against a role for sv40 in human mesothelioma. Cancer Res 2005;65(7):2602–9.
12. Sugarbaker PH, Acherman YIZ, Gonzalez-Moreno S, et al. Diagnosis and treatment of peritoneal mesothelioma: the Washington Cancer Institute experience. Semin Oncol 2002;29(1):51–61.
13. Uzüm N, Ozçay N, Ataoğlu O. Benign multicystic peritoneal mesothelioma. Turk J Gastroenterol 2009;20(2):138–41.
14. Manzini VDP. Malignant peritoneal mesothelioma. Tumori 2005;91(1):1–5.
15. Manzini VD, Recchia L, Cafferata M, et al. Malignant peritoneal mesothelioma: a multicenter study on 81 cases. Ann Oncol 2010;21(2):348–53.
16. Pappa L, Machera M, Tsanou E, et al. Subcutaneous metastasis of peritoneal mesothelioma diagnosed by fine-needle aspiration. Pathol Oncol Res 2006; 12(4):247–50.
17. Moser S, Beer M, Damerau G, et al. A case report of metastasis of malignant mesothelioma to the oral gingiva. Head Neck Oncol 2011;3:21.
18. Kimura N, Ogasawara T, Asonuma S, et al. Granulocyte-colony stimulating factor- and interleukin 6-producing diffuse deciduoid peritoneal mesothelioma. Mod Pathol 2004;18(3):446–50.

19. Baratti D, Kusamura S, Martinetti A, et al. Circulating CA125 in patients with peritoneal mesothelioma treated with cytoreductive surgery and intraperitoneal hyperthermic perfusion. Ann Surg Oncol 2007;14(2):500–8.

20. Hassan R, Remaley AT, Sampson ML, et al. Detection and quantitation of serum mesothelin, a tumor marker for patients with mesothelioma and ovarian cancer. Clin Cancer Res 2006;12(2):447–53.

21. Canney PA, Moore M, Wilkinson PM, et al. Ovarian cancer antigen CA 125: a prospective clinical assessment of its role as a tumour marker. Br J Cancer 1984;50(6):765–9.

22. Huang W-C, Tseng C-W, Chang K-M, et al. Usefulness of tumor marker CA-125 serum levels for the follow-up of therapeutic responses in tuberculosis patients with and without serositis. Jpn J Infect Dis 2011;64(5):367–72.

23. Creaney J, Yeoman D, Naumoff LK, et al. Soluble mesothelin in effusions: a useful tool for the diagnosis of malignant mesothelioma. Thorax 2007;62(7):569–76.

24. Creaney J, Olsen NJ, Brims F, et al. Serum mesothelin for early detection of asbestos-induced cancer malignant mesothelioma. Cancer Epidemiol Biomarkers Prev 2010;19(9):2238–46.

25. Creaney J, Bruggen Iv, Hof M, et al. Combined CA125 and mesothelin levels for the diagnosis of malignant mesothelioma. Chest 2007;132(4):1239–46.

26. Tabata C, Terada T, Tabata R, et al. Serum thioredoxin-1 as a diagnostic marker for malignant peritoneal mesothelioma. J Clin Gastroenterol 2012. [Epub ahead of print].

27. Yuan Y, Nymoen DA, Stavnes HT, et al. Tenascin-X is a novel diagnostic marker of malignant mesothelioma. Am J Surg Pathol 2009;33(11):1673–82. http://dx.doi.org/10.1097/PAS.0b013e3181b6bde3.

28. Ros PR, Yuschok TJ, Buck JL, et al. Peritoneal mesothelioma. Acta Radiol 1991;32(5):355–8.

29. Chen LY, Huang L-X, Wang J, et al. Malignant peritoneal mesothelioma presenting with persistent high fever. J Zhejiang Univ Sci B 2011;12(5):381–4.

30. Whitley N, Brenner D, Antman K, et al. CT of peritoneal mesothelioma: analysis of eight cases. AJR Am J Roentgenol 1982;138(3):531–5.

31. Yan TD, Haveric N, Carmignani CP, et al. Computed tomographic characterization of malignant peritoneal mesothelioma. Tumori 2005;91(5):394–400.

32. Park JY, Kim KW, Kwon H-J, et al. Peritoneal mesotheliomas: clinicopathologic features, CT findings, and differential diagnosis. Am J Roentgenol 2008;191(3):814–25.

33. Laterza B, Kusamura S, Baratti D, et al. Role of explorative laparoscopy to evaluate optimal candidates for cytoreductive surgery and hyperthermic intraperitoneal chemotherapy (HIPEC) in patients with peritoneal mesothelioma. In Vivo 2009;23(1):187–90.

34. Yan TD, Deraco M, Baratti D, et al. Cytoreductive surgery and hyperthermic intraperitoneal chemotherapy for malignant peritoneal mesothelioma: multi-institutional experience. J Clin Oncol 2009;27(36):6237–42.

35. Chua TC, Yan TD, Deraco M, et al. Multi-institutional experience of diffuse intraabdominal multicystic peritoneal mesothelioma. Br J Surg 2011;98(1):60–4.

36. Baratti D, Kusamura S, Sironi A, et al. Multicystic peritoneal mesothelioma treated by surgical cytoreduction and hyperthermic intra-peritoneal chemotherapy (HIPEC). In Vivo 2008;22(1):153–7.

37. Comin CE, Novelli L, Boddi V, et al. Calretinin, thrombomodulin, CEA, and CD15: a useful combination of immunohistochemical markers for differentiating pleural

epithelial mesothelioma from peripheral pulmonary adenocarcinoma. Hum Pathol 2001;32(5):529–36.

38. Jacquet P, Sugarbaker PH. Current methodologies for clinical assessment of patients with peritoneal carcinomatosis. J Exp Clin Cancer Res 1996;15:49–58.

39. Yan TD, Deraco M, Elias D, et al. A novel tumor-node-metastasis (TNM) staging system of diffuse malignant peritoneal mesothelioma using outcome analysis of a multi-institutional database*. Cancer 2011;117(9):1855–63.

40. Antman K, Shemin R, Ryan L, et al. Malignant mesothelioma: prognostic variables in a registry of 180 patients, the Dana-Farber Cancer Institute and Brigham and Women's Hospital experience over two decades, 1965-1985. J Clin Oncol 1988; 6(1):147–53.

41. Chahinian AP, Antman K, Goutsou M, et al. Randomized phase II trial of cisplatin with mitomycin or doxorubicin for malignant mesothelioma by the Cancer and Leukemia Group B. J Clin Oncol 1993;11(8):1559–65.

42. Carteni G, Manegold C, Garcia GM, et al. Malignant peritoneal mesothelioma: results from the International Expanded Access Program using pemetrexed alone or in combination with a platinum agent. Lung Cancer 2009;64(2):211–8.

43. Simon GR, Verschraegen CF, Jaonne PA, et al. Pemetrexed plus gemcitabine as first-line chemotherapy for patients with peritoneal mesothelioma: final report of a phase II trial. J Clin Oncol 2008;26(21):3567–72.

44. Hesdorffer ME, Chabot JA, Keohan ML, et al. Combined resection, intraperitoneal chemotherapy, and whole abdominal radiation for the treatment of malignant peritoneal mesothelioma. Am J Clin Oncol 2008;31(1):49–54.

45. Markman M, Kelsen D. Efficacy of cisplatin-based intraperitoneal chemotherapy as treatment of malignant peritoneal mesothelioma. J Cancer Res Clin Oncol 1992;118(7):547–50.

46. Sugarbaker PH. Peritonectomy procedures. Ann Surg 1995;221(1):29–42.

47. Kusamura S, O'Dwyer ST, Baratti D, et al. Technical aspects of cytoreductive surgery. J Surg Oncol 2008;98(4):232–6.

48. Baratti D, Kusamura S, Cabras A, et al. Cytoreductive surgery with selective versus complete parietal peritonectomy followed by hyperthermic intraperitoneal chemotherapy in patients with diffuse malignant peritoneal mesothelioma: a controlled study. Ann Surg Oncol 2012;19(5):1416–24.

49. Baratti D, Kusamura S, Cabras AD, et al. Lymph node metastases in diffuse malignant peritoneal mesothelioma. Ann Surg Oncol 2010;17(1):45–53.

Current Status and Future Directions of Cytoreductive Surgery and Hyperthermic Intraperitoneal Chemotherapy in the Treatment of Ovarian Cancer

C. William Helm, MA, MBBChir

KEYWORDS

- Ovarian cancer • Epithelial ovarian cancer • Intraperitoneal chemotherapy • HIPEC
- Hyperthermia • Hyperthermic intraperitoneal chemotherapy

KEY POINTS

- Epithelial ovarian cancer (EOC) most often presents with disease that has metastasized. Optimal front-line therapy is associated with median overall 5-year survival of less than 50%.
- EOC is a peritoneal surface malignancy that remains within the peritoneal cavity for much of its life history. Recurrence is common, with 70% of cases having peritoneal disease.
- The incorporation of hyperthermic intraperitoneal chemotherapy (HIPEC) makes sound theoretic sense at the time of front-line treatment, for consolidation and for the treatment of recurrence.
- Studies increasingly report detailed adverse effect and outcome data associated with extensive cytoreductive surgery and HIPEC that allow more informed decision making for the patient and surgeon.
- More focused and randomized clinical trials are ongoing that will help to more precisely determine the role of HIPEC in treatment of EOC.

BACKGROUND

Section Key Points
1. Epithelial ovarian cancer (EOC) affects more than 200,000 women per year worldwide
2. It causes around 125,000 deaths per year worldwide
3. Most often the disease has spread from the ovaries at presentation
4. 5-year overall survival (OS) remains at less than 50%

Disclosures: None.
Division of Gynecologic Oncology, Department of Obstetrics, Gynecology and Women's Health, Saint Louis University School of Medicine, Suite 290, 6420 Clayton Road, St Louis, MO 63117, USA
E-mail address: chelm4@slu.edu

EOC is a peritoneal surface malignancy that remains confined to the peritoneal cavity and retroperitoneal lymph nodes for much of its natural history. Although originally thought to arise from the ovarian surface epithelium it is now considered likely that EOC arises from distal fallopian tube epithelium that becomes attached to the ovary during the time of ovulation.[1] This theory was initially prompted by the discovery of serous tubal intraepithelial carcinomas and occult invasive serous carcinomas, closely resembling ovarian serous carcinoma, in women with a genetic predisposition to ovarian cancer.[2]

Because both primary fallopian tube and primary peritoneal carcinoma are treated in similar fashion as EOC and have similar prognosis, they are all considered as EOC. The percentage contribution of each of these types of EOC is ovary 91.8%, peritoneum 5.3%, and fallopian tube 2.8%.[3]

EOC affects more than 200,000 women annually around the world, causing 125,000 deaths.[4] In the United States it affects more than 22,280 women annually and is responsible for 15,500 deaths.[5] The disease causes few symptoms initially and in most cases has already spread outside the pelvis with 50.2% being in International Federation of Gynecology and Obstetrics (FIGO) stage III (within the peritoneal cavity or involving para-aortic, pelvic, or inguinal lymph nodes) and 13% in FIGO stage IV (beyond the peritoneal cavity, including lung and liver parenchyma).[6]

EOC has a poor overall outcome, with only 46% to 49.7% of women with EOC surviving 5 years.[6,7] In addition, progress in reducing incidence and mortality has been slow.[7]

Low malignant potential (LMP), sometimes called borderline or atypical, proliferative tumors are a distinct form of EOC that occur at a younger age, at an earlier stage, with a less aggressive behavior, and much better prognosis than invasive EOC.[8] Ten-year relative OS for LMP carcinomas is 95% and, for stage I, II, III, and IV, it is 97%, 90%, 88%, and 69% respectively.[9] They have an overall 5-year survival of 87.3% compared with 49.7% for invasive EOC.[6] LMP tumors are not thought to respond to chemotherapy, although, in those tumors with invasive peritoneal implants or advanced disease, it is sometimes used.[9] There are no data on the use of hyperthermic intraperitoneal chemotherapy (HIPEC) for treatment of LMP tumors and it is not discussed further here. It is important that LMP carcinomas be identified in series reporting HIPEC therapy because their inclusion could skew outcomes.

CURRENT STATUS OF TREATMENT OF OVARIAN CANCER

Section Key Points
1. The amount of residual disease at the end of cytoreductive surgery is a major prognostic factor in EOC
2. Initial response to platinum chemotherapy defines treatment and prognosis at the time of recurrence
3. Front-line chemotherapy should include a combination of a platinum analogue and a taxane
4. The case for addition of bevacizumab to front-line therapy has not been proven

Discussion about the possible role of HIPEC in the treatment of ovarian cancer must involve an understanding of current standard treatments.

The Natural History Time Points of Ovarian Cancer

The natural history of EOC can be divided into treatment time points: front-line, front-line failure (persistent disease at the end of front-line treatment), consolidation (maintenance treatment given following a complete response to front-line treatment to reduce the time to recurrence), and recurrent disease. The current status of treatment and role of HIPEC at each time point are considered later.

The Importance of Initial Platinum Response to Prognosis in EOC

Prognosis for patients with EOC is defined by response to platinum[10–12] and disease can be divided into 2 distinct groups depending on prior response to platinum-containing chemotherapy. Those that are platinum sensitive, recur more than 6 months following a complete response to platinum-containing chemotherapy, whereas those that are platinum resistant, recur less than 6 months following response to treatment. Platinum-resistant tumors also include those that had only a partial response to front-line platinum (persistent disease) or no response (refractory disease).

Front-line Treatment

Standard front-line treatment of EOC involves the combination of cytoreductive surgery (CRS) and chemotherapy. The prognosis for patients with EOC was reported to be related to the amount of residual disease at the end of surgery: patients with the least disease survived longer.[13,14] This finding has been confirmed in multiple reports since then. Major current debate centers on the extent of CRS that is necessary and whether neoadjuvant chemotherapy (NAC; chemical cytoreduction given before CRS) is of benefit.

Extent of Surgery for EOC

Gynecologic oncology surgeons assess the extent of CRS by the greatest dimension of the largest lesion remaining at the end of CRS. At first, the consensus was that surgery leaving behind disease up to 2 cm in greatest dimension was optimal (as opposed to suboptimal) but over time this has reduced to 1 cm[15–17] Many gynecologic oncology surgeons currently believe that the goal should be to remove all visible disease.[18,19]

Surgery Before Chemotherapy or Vice Versa?

Most EOC is inherently sensitive to platinum chemotherapy and it has therefore been used to chemically reduce the volume of ascites and disease before CRS. Three or 4 cycles of a combination of NAC with platinum are considered optimal.[20] Not only can this improve a patient's performance status and ability to withstand a major surgery but CRS following a response to NAC is often of shorter duration, requires fewer procedures, and has less morbidity with quicker recovery for the patient.[21,22] It is associated with a higher chance of optimal cytoreduction than initial CRS.[23]

A systematic review of 26 studies including more than 1300 patients undergoing NAC found that the survival outcome was inferior to initial CRS followed by chemotherapy.[20] However, a randomized controlled trial (RCT) by the European Organization for Research and Treatment of Cancer (EORTC), including 632 women with mostly stage IIIC and stage IV disease receiving either initial CRS followed by intravenous (IV) chemotherapy or NAC followed by CRS then further IV chemotherapy, reported similar survival and progression-free survival (PFS) in both arms.[24]

There are proponents of both approaches. Some reserve NAC for those patients with medical comorbidities that would compromise their ability to withstand the stress of major surgery and/or patients with disease unlikely to be amenable to adequate CRS, whereas others use it more liberally.

Front-line Chemotherapy for Advanced EOC

The current primary treatment is front-line CRS followed by platinum and taxane combination chemotherapy. Carboplatin (Paraplatin) has replaced cisplatin (Platinol) as the IV platinum agent because of equal efficacy and reduced toxicity. A standard regimen includes IV carboplatin (dosed by the area under curve of 5–7.5 mg/mL/min) and IV paclitaxel (Taxol) (175 mg/m^2 over 3 hours) repeated every 3 weeks for 6 cycles or IV docetaxel (Taxotere) 75 mg/m^2 over 1 hour plus IV carboplatin AUC 5 over 1 hour every 21 days for 6 cycles provided the disease is responsive.[25–27] Results from treatment of front-line EOC with CRS followed by chemotherapy are given in **Table 1**.

Role of Normothermic Intraperitoneal Chemotherapy

Gynecologic Oncology Group (GOG) study 172 reported significantly improved PFS and OS for patients treated with a combination of IV and intraperitoneal (IP) chemotherapy following optimal CRS to no greater than 1 cm largest residual lesion size. The median OS for patients treated with combination IV/IP chemotherapy was 65.6 months versus 49.7 months for patients treated with CRS and IV chemotherapy only. A Cochrane Collaboration meta-analysis of all randomized studies using IP therapy for EOC reported a significant survival advantage for IP delivery.[28]

The problem with GOG 172 was that, despite the improved median OS, 65% of patients in the experimental arm experienced recurrence within the follow-up period of the study and only 42% of participants completed all 6 assigned courses of IP chemotherapy. Although many gynecologic oncologists in the United States offer women with small-volume residual disease following initial CRS a modified GOG 172 regimen, IP therapy has not been widely adopted in the oncology community. The reasons for this include the toxicity of the IP chemotherapy and the morbidity and problems associated with IP delivery.[29] The GOG is currently investigating the replacement of cisplatin IP with carboplatin IP.

The 65% recurrence rate in GOG 172 is similar to data reported previously. After a complete pathologic response confirmed at surgery following front-line treatment

Table 1
Selected reports of outcomes for front-line treatment of EOC

Residual Disease	Regimen*	Median PFS (mo)	Median OS (mo)
Suboptimal[a,104]	Day 1: paclitaxel 135 mg/m^2 over 24 h Day 1: cisplatin 75 mg/m^2 IV	14.1	26.3
Optimal[b,105]	Day 1: cisplatin 75 mg/m^2 IV at 1 mg/min Day 1: paclitaxel 135 mg/m^2 over 24 h	19.4	48.7
	Day 1: carboplatin AUC 7.5 IV Day 1: paclitaxel 175 mg/m^2 IV over 3 h	20.7	57.4
Optimal[b,106]	Day 1: paclitaxel 135 mg/m^2 IV over 24 h Day 2: cisplatin 75 mg/m^2 IV	18.3	49.7
	Day 1: paclitaxel 135 mg/m^2 IV over 24 h Day 2: cisplatin 100 mg/m^2 IP Day 8: paclitaxel 60 mg/m^2 IP	23.8	65.6

Abbreviation: IP, intraperitoneal.
  [a] Suboptimal, residual disease greater than 2 cm at CRS before chemotherapy.
  [b] Optimal, residual disease less than or equal to 1 cm.
  Cisplatin (Platinol), carboplatin (Paraplatin), paclitaxel (Taxol), docetaxel (Taxotere).
 * Cycles repeated every 21 d.

of stages III and IV EOC, 60% recurred in 5 years and 66% in 10 years.[30] This rate suggests that residual, and initially undetectable, disease is left behind at CRS.

Outcomes After Maximal Front-line CRS in EOC

Despite maximum efforts to resect EOC at surgery, overall 5 year survival for such patients is less than 50%.[31–33] Eisenkop and colleagues[31] reported a 5 year survival of 49% (median OS of 58.2 months) in 408 patients, most with advanced disease, 98.9% of whom underwent a complete CRS followed by standard chemotherapy. Benedetti-Panici and colleagues[32] reported a 5 year survival of 49.5% (median OS of 62.1 months) for patients with stage IIIB and C or IV treated with maximal CRS and systematic lymphadenectomy. For patients with no visible disease at the end of treatment, median OS may be as high as 106 months.[34]

Results for Latest Trials with Bevacizumab

Although there has been much excitement about studies of bevacizumab in front-line treatment the results have been disappointing and do not support the routine use of this agent. In GOG study 218, 1873 women with stage III (suboptimally debulked or optimally debulked with macroscopic disease) or stage IV disease were randomly assigned to bevacizumab during chemotherapy or, in addition, as consolidation therapy following chemotherapy for 15 months. After a median follow-up of 17.4 months, the addition of bevacizumab as consolidation was associated with a significantly improved median PFS of 14.1 versus 10.3 months with similar median OS (39.7 vs 39.3 months). There was no significant difference in PFS with bevacizumab given at the time of chemotherapy only. Also there was increased toxicity including severe hypertension and gastrointestinal perforation, hemorrhage, or fistula.[35] In another trial, ICON 7, 1528 women with high-risk early stage and advanced stage EOC were randomly assigned to 6 cycles of carboplatin/paclitaxel given every 3 weeks with or without bevacizumab, which was continued for 12 additional cycles. The restricted mean PFS was 21.8 months with bevacizumab versus 20.3 months without ($P = .004$). In an updated analysis, PFS (restricted mean) at 42 months was 24.1 months with bevacizumab versus 22.4 months without bevacizumab ($P = .04$).[36]

CURRENT STATUS OF HIPEC IN FRONT-LINE OVARIAN CANCER

Section Key Points:
1. The use of HIPEC in EOC makes theoretic sense in view of the high rates of recurrence following standard treatment
2. Experience reported in the literature is increasing
3. There are no RCTs to date
4. HIPEC should ideally be performed on a research protocol

Although the incorporation of HIPEC into the treatment of EOC makes sense at all the natural history time points, there have been no RCTs to compare efficacy against standard treatments. In view of the importance of having minimal tumor volume at the time of HIPEC treatment, the aim of CRS immediately before HIPEC should be to remove all visible disease or at least to achieve a residual lesion(s) size less than or equal to 2.5 mm.[37]

A phase I study including 5 women treated with HIPEC at the time of initial surgery was published in 1999[38] and since then several nonrandomized studies have been reported in this setting.[39–47] There are no RCTs and the studies are heterogeneous. Some have no survival data because of their phase I design or because of insufficient follow-up.[44,46] Outcomes in recent series are given in **Table 2**.

Table 2
PFS and OS for patients treated with initial CRS and HIPEC

Author	Year	N	PFS Median (mo)	PFS % 5-y Survival	OS Median (mo)	OS % 5-y Survival
Rufian et al[42]	2006	19	—	—	38[a]	37
Di Giorgio et al[45]	2008	18	25.5	—	27	—
Helm et al[48]	2010	26	24.8	19.7	41.7	33.3
Deraco et al[47]	2011	26	30	15.2	b	60.7

Abbreviation: HIPEC, hyperthermic intraperitoneal chemotherapy.
[a] Mean only given.
[b] Not reached.

Rufian and colleagues[42] reported on 19 patients with stage III disease treated with paclitaxel for 60 minutes at 41 to 43°C at the time of initial surgery. The mean 5-year OS was 37% but, for those patients with a resection to no macroscopic disease, the median OS was 66 months. In a multi-institutional phase II study, 26 women with stage III to IV EOC were prospectively treated with CRS and closed-abdomen HIPEC with cisplatin and doxorubicin.[47] Following surgery, they received systemic chemotherapy with carboplatin (AUC 6) and paclitaxel (175 mg/m^2) for 6 cycles. After a median follow-up of 25 months, 5 year OS was 60.7% and 5 year PFS 15.2% (median 30 months). Excluding a single perioperative death, all patients underwent systemic chemotherapy at a median of 46 days from HIPEC (range 29–75 days).

With the collaboration of 8 centers in the United States, the Hyperthermic Intraperitoneal Chemotherapy in Ovarian Cancer Registry (HYPERO) of patients treated with CRS and HIPEC was initiated.[48] In the initial report there were 20 patients treated with CRS and HIPEC who fitted entry criteria for GOG 172, having residual disease of less than 1 cm. There was no significant difference in the OS (HIPEC 57.5 months, GOG 172 65.6 months, and 2-year OS 66.4%: 82%) and 2-year PFS (47.6%: 53%).

CURRENT STATUS OF HIPEC FOLLOWING NAC

HIPEC given following NAC has the advantage of allowing lead time for preparation of the patient, the operating team, and the perfusion equipment and team. It is anticipated that the CRS before the HIPEC would also have the advantages described earlier for NAC but there are no data on this at present.

Reports in the literature for HIPEC after NAC are heterogeneous: the number of cycles varies and the data are difficult to evaluate. Steller and colleagues[38] included a single case and 3 other reports included only 17 patients in total.[41,49,50] de Bree[51] reported on 4 patients who had between 6 and 8 courses of chemotherapy before CRS.[51] In another nonrandomized series of 117 patients with different histologic types of ovarian cancer, 57 patients were treated with either (arm A) initial CRS followed by IV chemotherapy (6–8 cycles) followed by a further surgery combined with HIPEC, or (arm B) with 3 to 4 cycles of NAC followed by CRS and HIPEC.[52] Carboplatin and interferon-α were the agents given in combination as HIPEC. The historical control arm included 60 patients treated by traditional CRS followed by IV chemotherapy. There were 74 patients with stage III disease who received HIPEC in arms A or B. In the whole group, there was no significant difference in survival between the HIPEC groups and controls. However, within stage III, the median disease-free survival of 39 patients undergoing HIPEC was 26.4 months compared with 6.1 months for 39 historical controls. When only those patients within stage III with residual disease of less than 1 cm at the second CRS were considered, both the median disease-free survival and 5-year survivals were significantly better: 40.6 versus 13.2 months and 65.6% versus 40.7%. Although the difference in outcome seems impressive, the study contained some major confounding issues. It was nonrandomized, the control arm had an unusually poor survival of only 6.1 months, and there was no separate analysis of patients undergoing HIPEC at surgery following NAC or second-look laparotomy. In addition, the stage III control arm included patients with dysgerminoma, choriocarcinoma, and granulosa cell carcinoma, and the stage III group undergoing HIPEC included patients with choriocarcinoma, endodermal sinus tumor, and squamous cell carcinoma.

The initial HYPERO report included 19 patients who were treated by NAC followed by CRS. The median OS was 68.6 months with 2-year and 5-year survivals of 80.4 and 50.2 months. Although the numbers are too small to produce any meaningful conclusion, these survivals were not significantly different from the 26 patients treated with front-line surgery and HIPEC followed by chemotherapy, among whom the median OS was 41.7 months and 2-year and 5-year survivals 57.0 and 33.3 months.[48]

Current practice among surgeons using HIPEC seems to be split between those favoring NAC and FL. However, performing CRS and HIPEC after NAC might have an impact on reducing morbidity.

The Problem of Front-line Failure

Women with disease that persists following front-line platinum-containing therapy do poorly. A study of CRS and HIPEC in this setting was instituted by surgeons at the Instituto Tumori in Milano but closed early because of excessive morbidity and poor study accrual. This study confirmed the difficulty of finding active therapy in this setting. These patients have refractory disease and are unlikely to respond to any currently available therapy. In contrast, CRS and HIPEC might have a role for small-volume persistent disease such as that found in patients with a complete clinical response who undergo a second-look surgery if the disease is easily resectable.

CURRENT SITUATION WITH REGARD TO CONSOLIDATION

Section Key Points:
1. The recurrence rate following front-line treatment of EOC is high
2. There is no proven method of reducing this rate
3. IP consolidation makes sense because recurrence is often in the peritoneal cavity
4. HIPEC may have a role to play

There is a need for methods to reduce the high rate of recurrence following even complete pathologic responses to front-line therapy. Although there have been multiple trials of maintenance (consolidation) therapy, there is still no proven method. Efforts have included continuation of systemic chemotherapy beyond 6 cycles, use of intraperitoneal therapy, and experimental treatments including immunotherapy. However, a meta-analysis of RCTs found that there was no significant improvement in 5-year OS to justify its use (relative risk 1.07, 95% confidence interval 0.91–1.27).[53]

IV Chemotherapy for Consolidation

A randomized study investigating 3 versus 12 cycles of continued IV paclitaxel following a complete clinical response was closed early when a 7-month prolongation in median PFS was found in the 12-cycle arm but toxicity was increased.[54] In an update of the study, the median PFS for 12 versus 3 additional cycles was 22 versus 14 months but the median OS was not significantly different (53 vs 48 months).[55] An Italian study did not show any difference in PFS survival.[56]

IP Chemotherapy for Consolidation

There have been nonrandomized studies of additional IP normothermic chemotherapy. In a randomized study that closed early because of poor recruitment, recurrence occurred in 49% after 4 cycles of IP cisplatin compared with 55% of controls.[57] In a report of experience of normothermic IP at Memorial Hospital, New York, a subgroup of 89 patients with a complete pathologic response following front-line therapy treated for consolidation with agents including cisplatin and paclitaxel reported a median OS of 8.7 years.[58] In a phase II study from the same institution investigating the use of IP cisplatin and etoposide (VePosid) 39% of patients recurred compared with 54% of historical controls.[59,60]

CURRENT STATUS: HIPEC FOR CONSOLIDATION

There have been no randomized studies investigating HIPEC for consolidation, but those that have been performed suggest that HIPEC may have beneficial effects in this situation.

Among patients with initial stage III EOC, 68 underwent second-look laparotomy following completion of front-line therapy: 44 underwent HIPEC at this surgery (carboplatin n = 30, paclitaxel n = 14), and 24 patients used as historical controls did not.[61] All received further IV chemotherapy following the HIPEC. The 3 year PFS was 56.3% and 16.7% respectively ($P = .00028$) and the 5-year OS was 66.1% and 31.3% ($P = .0003$).

In another report, 51 patients with EOC who underwent initial CRS to less than 2 cm and received IV chemotherapy with cisplatin and cyclophosphamide (Cytoxan) were studied.[62] Of this group, 32 then received second-look laparotomy and HIPEC and 19 who did not formed the control group. Although not statistically significant, there was a trend toward a better outcome in the HIPEC group, with the median survivals being 64.4 and 46.4 months respectively.

There may be a problem with using oxaliplatin (Eloxatin) for consolidation. One of 2 recent studies reported a high frequency of bleeding after surgery leading to early closure.[63,64]

Just as there is no standard chemotherapeutic for consolidation therapy so there is no standard use of HIPEC. It would be useful to test this in clinical trials, although large numbers of patients are needed. It is a good time to use HIPEC because the CRS principally involves adhesiolysis provided there is no persistent disease to be resected or completion surgery to be performed.

CURRENT THERAPY FOR RECURRENT EOC

Section Key Points:
1. Recurrence following front-line treatment of ovarian cancer is common
2. 70% with recurrence will have peritoneal carcinomatosis (PC)
3. Systemic chemotherapy is not curative
4. Surgery followed by systemic chemotherapy may be beneficial in selected cases with localized disease, which is platinum sensitive with a long interval to recurrence

Although most EOC are inherently sensitive to platinum and most patients can achieve a complete clinical response at the end of FL therapy, most eventually recur[16] and the overall prognosis for women experiencing recurrence is poor.

IV Chemotherapy for Recurrence

Recurrent disease is mostly treated with systemic IV chemotherapy, with the type of agent(s) used being guided by the time interval from (1) completion and response to primary therapy to (2) recurrence.[10–12]

Median survival between 15 and 18 months is the norm in clinical trials of chemotherapy alone for recurrent EOC[65–68] and only a few studies report survival of close to 30 months.[66,69,70] For the subgroup with platinum-resistant and platinum-refractory disease, median survivals of about 12 months are reported.[71] Effective agents are needed particularly urgently for this group.

Surgery for Recurrence

Surgery has traditionally been reserved for a minority of patients with recurrence. Possible candidates would have single, or few, isolated recurrences in sites that are more easily resected, and with the recurrence occurring at a significant interval (12 months or more) from prior treatment. No randomized studies have been performed for CRS for recurrent disease with/without chemotherapy versus chemotherapy alone for recurrence. There are currently ongoing clinical trials investigating the role of surgery for recurrent disease. Median OS for CRS (followed by systemic chemotherapy) and CRS and HIPEC for recurrent EOC are given in **Table 3**.

Bristow and colleagues[66] reported a meta-analysis of studies that included more than 2000 women undergoing surgical treatment of recurrent disease with or without chemotherapy, and reported a mean weighted median postrecurrence survival of 30.3 months. The most important prognostic factor was the amount of residual disease at the end of surgery for recurrence. Another review reported that survival of 40 to 60 months was possible with CRS in selected patients.[72]

In a study of 250 women in German centers, the efficacy of CRS for women with recurrent EOC was investigated.[73] Patients with non-EOC and LMP tumors were excluded, and also patients undergoing primarily symptom-related and palliative surgery. In the 125 women with PC the treatment-free interval was less than 6 months in 17.6%. Complete resection of all visible disease was possible in 74% of those without PC and in only 26% with PC. The overall median survival was 29.5 months for all 250 patients but, for those with and without PC, it was 19.9 versus 45.3 months. Two-year survival for those with PC undergoing complete resection to no residual disease was not significantly different from those without PC undergoing a similar complete resection (77% vs 81%).

CURRENT STATUS OF HIPEC FOR RECURRENCE

Most women with recurrent EOC do not have the localized and easily resectable disease that would make them traditional surgical candidates. Two-thirds of those

Table 3 Median OS for surgery for recurrent EOC		
Author	**N**	**Median OS (mo)**
Bristow et al[66]	2019	30.3
Harter et al[73]	250	29.5
	125 without PC	45.3
	125 with PC	19.9
Helm et al[48]	83	23.5

Abbreviation: PC, peritoneal carcinomatosis.

with recurrence have PC.[74] HIPEC may have a significant role to play in conjunction with CRS in many patients with recurrent disease.

There are now multiple reports of the use of HIPEC for recurrent disease.[39,40,42,43,45,50,75–87] Despite the large numbers, the studies are difficult to compare and interpret because of their heterogeneity. Progression-free and OS durations are given in **Table 4**.

In the report by Rufian and colleagues,[42] patients aged less than or equal to 55 years who were reduced to no visible disease had a 5-year survival of 75%. In another study,[85] 14 patients undergoing CRS and HIPEC for recurrent EOC had 3-year and 5-year survivals of 64% and 50%, compared with those of 12 patients who underwent CRS alone: 57% and 17% respectively. These outcomes suggest that HIPEC is having a positive effect in this setting compared with the reports from Bristow and colleagues[66] and Harter and colleagues,[73] discussed earlier, and its role should be explored further.

In the HYPERO report,[48] despite 85% of the women treated for recurrence having PC and 29% being platinum resistant, the median OS was 23.5 months. It seems that this population was different from the one that would historically be treated with CRS for recurrence and again suggests an effect of HIPEC for patients with recurrent EOC with PC.

Prognostic factors for survival with HIPEC in recurrent EOC have included the interval from initial diagnosis to HIPEC,[77,83] the peritoneal carcinomatosis index (PCI),[43,50,77,81] the extent of CRS,[42,43,50,77,80–83,85] age,[42,77] preoperative performance status,[82] presence of lymph node metastasis,[42] and initial platinum response.[48]

MORTALITY AND MORBIDITY OF CRS AND HIPEC FOR EOC

All CRS is associated with morbidity and mortality and it is difficult to determine whether morbidity occurring after major CRS and HIPEC is caused by the surgery or the HIPEC. Mortality from any cause within 30 days of primary CRS for EOC in population-based series is 3.7% (range 2.5%–4.8%) and in single-center series has a mean of 2.5% (range 0%–6.7%).[88] The mortality for CRS alone in recurrent EOC was 1.4% (0%–3.4%).[72] Chua and colleagues[89] reviewed 19 studies including CRS and HIPEC at all time points of EOC and found mortalities between 0% and 10%. In the 141 patients undergoing CRS and HIPEC in the HYPERO registry, the mortality

Table 4				
PFS and OS for CRS and HIPEC for recurrent EOC				
			PFS	OS
Author	**Year**	**N**	**Median (mo)**	**Median (mo)**
Deraco et al[77]	2001	27	21.8	—
Zanon et al[81]	2004	30	b	28.1
Rufian et al[42]	2006	14	b	57[a]
Raspagliesi et al[82]	2006	40	23.9[a]	41.4[a]
Helm et al[83]	2007	18	10	31
Cotte et al[43]	2007	81	19.2	28.4
Helm et al[48]	2010	83	13.7	23.5
Fagotti et al[94]	2011	25	24	38

[a] Only mean given.
[b] Not available.

was 2.1%.[48] In a review of 13 publications, including 256 patients undergoing HIPEC for recurrent EOC, the mortality was 3.9% (10 of 256).[90]

MORBIDITY OF CRS AND HIPEC FOR EOC

Accurate data for the morbidity of HIPEC given at the time of initial surgery for EOC is best obtained from prospective studies designed to monitor and record morbidity. However, there is no standard classification used to report morbidity. The National Cancer Institute Common Terminology Criteria for Adverse Events (CTCAE)[91] are available and used by some, and there is increasing use of a surgical classification based on the interventions necessary to address the adverse effect.[92]

For the complications of CRS and HIPEC used as front-line treatments with and without NAC, a phase I study performed at the National Cancer Center of Korea reported adverse affects associated with CRS and HIPEC cisplatin 75 mg/m^2 at approximately 41.5°C for 90 minutes delivered using a closed method to 30 patients following CRS to less than 1 cm (16 patients at initial CRS and 14 at the time of ID) and following intestinal anastomoses.[46] Postoperative events were common but mostly grade I (self-limiting) or grade II, requiring only medical treatment for resolution. Grade 1 events occurred in 22 of 30 (73%), including transient nausea and vomiting, diarrhea, line sepsis, thrombocytopenia, and pleural effusion. One or more grade 2 events occurred in 27 patients (90%), including nausea and vomiting, cardiac arrhythmia, hypertension, diarrhea, pleural effusion, line sepsis, and increased creatinine. Twelve patients (40%) experienced 1 or more grade III complications that required invasive intervention, including anemia, pleural effusion, pneumothorax, fascial dehiscence, diarrhea, ileus, and pancreatic leakage. There were no grade IV events that would have required definitive urgent intervention such as reoperation or a return to the intensive care unit, and there were no deaths. It was discussed that most of these events could be the result of the CRS. The 3 cases of thrombocytopenia all occurred before postoperative day 3 and followed large blood transfusions. No case of leukopenia was reported and there was no intestinal/anastomotic leak. These data suggest that HIPEC can be delivered at the completion of initial CRS without significant additional toxicity.

In a more recent publication, Deraco and colleagues[47] reported a phase II multi-institutional study of front-line CRS and HIPEC using cisplatin and doxorubicin. Major complications according to CTCAE criteria occurred in 4 patients and postoperative death in 1. Four patients (15%) experienced 9 grade 3 to 5 complications. One patient developed grade 3 hematologic toxicity, pneumothorax, and pleural effusion, requiring operative drainage. She developed a subsequent abdominal abscess requiring reoperation and died of sepsis on the 39th postoperative day. Other major toxicities included abdominal abscess, sepsis, central line infection, colorectal anastomosis bleeding, and bladder fistula.

In a single-institution study, 41 patients with platinum-sensitive recurrent EOC underwent oxaliplatin-based HIPEC following optimal CRS, followed by IV docetaxel and oxaliplatin.[94] Severe complications (resulting in unplanned admission or a secondary surgical procedure) occurred in 15 of 43 procedures (34.8%), with a reoperation rate of 14% (6 of 43). Bleeding occurred in 16.3% (7/43) within 36 hours of surgery, 5 experienced hemoperitoneum, 3 rectal bleeding, and 1 both. Other major complications included a subphrenic abscess following pancreatic fistula that required open drainage, 2 large abscesses requiring hospital admission, 1 portal vein thrombosis, and 1 sepsis. Pleural effusion occurred in 19.5%. The complications were more frequent in the patients treated before September 2008 than after (73% vs 26.7%) and there were no perioperative deaths within 30 days. The complications of postoperative hemorrhage have previously been reported in association with HIPEC oxaliplatin.[63,93,95]

In a comprehensive review of 19 studies of CRS and HIPEC for EOC, the rate of complications was reported as grade 1 (no intervention required for resolution) 6% to 70%, grade II (medical treatments required for resolution) 3% to 50%, grade III (invasive intervention required for resolution) 0% to 40%, and grade IV (urgent definitive intervention such as returning to the operating room or intensive care unit) 0% to 15%.[89] Common postoperative complications included ileus, pleural effusion, infections (including wound infection), anastomotic leakage, fistula, bleeding, transient hepatitis, and thrombocytopenia.

In a review of 256 patients undergoing CRS and HIPEC for recurrent/persistent disease,[90] the frequency of severe toxicities included hematologic 4.3%, creatinemia (following cisplatin) 3.9%, wound infection 4.3%, anastomotic leak 1.6%, bowel perforation 2.3%, peritonitis 0.8%, and abscess formation 1.2%. Anastomotic leak remains a concern with HIPEC but the rate of leakage in the absence of a diverting stoma remains unknown and the performance of a fecal diversion remains a surgeon's prerogative and choice. Spontaneous intestinal perforations do occur and may reflect the effect of heated chemotherapy on bowel that has been traumatized, particularly during enterolysis.

The evidence shows that CRS and HIPEC can be performed together with manageable toxicity. The most important factor seems to be the number of bowel resections performed and the impact of HIPEC on anastomotic and serosal injury healing.

FUTURE DIRECTIONS

Despite the extensive use of HIPEC for EOC since the first report in 1994,[96] there is no defined standard for many parameters such as temperature of perfusate, duration of perfusion, agents to be used, and open or closed method. This needs to be corrected.

The need to perform randomized studies has been noted for several years. There are now at least 3 large, ongoing, randomized studies investigating HIPEC based in 3 different European countries. In a pioneering study based at the Netherlands Cancer Center, patients with primary EOC are treated with NAC and then submitted to CRS, at which time they are randomized to HIPEC with cisplatin or no further treatment (Principal Investigator, Dr Willemien Van Driel, 2012, personal communication). In the French CHIPOR study (available at http://clinicaltrials.gov/show/NCT01376752), patients with platinum-sensitive recurrent disease receive chemotherapy with carboplatin and liposomal doxorubicin or paclitaxel and then undergo CRS. Those whose disease is resected to no visible disease or no greater than 2.5 mm residual are randomized to HIPEC with cisplatin 75 mg/m^2 versus no HIPEC. In the Italian HORSE study (available at http://clinicaltrials.gov/show/NCT01539785), patients with platinum-sensitive recurrence will be randomized to CRS with HIPEC with cisplatin 75 mg/m^2 versus CRS alone.

These studies will help to answer questions about the role of HIPEC following NAC and in platinum-sensitive recurrence, including the efficacy of HIPEC, the specific morbidity attributable to HIPEC, and the indications for its use. However, other studies are needed of HIPEC at initial CRS, for consolidation, and to define treatment parameters. Continued efforts must be made to reduce any morbidity. All patients treated with HIPEC should optimally be on clinical research protocols or their data prospectively collected in registries such as the Hyperthermic Intraperitoneal Chemotherapy in Ovarian Cancer (HYPOVA) registry based at Saint Louis University, St Louis, Missouri (Principal Investigator, C. William Helm).

Future directions may include greater use of laparoscopic surgery in situations in which less CRS is needed, such as for consolidation, and in this regard repeated treatments with HIPEC given laparoscopically might be achievable. There is also a need to investigate the use of concomitant systemic chemotherapy[97] and early postoperative chemotherapy.[98]

From the clinical perspective, other forms of delivery of regional hyperthermia are worthy of continued research.[99,100] In addition, more laboratory research may enhance understanding of the effects and interactions of hyperthermia with chemotherapy agents at a molecular level and allow development of methods to improve efficacy.[101–103]

Interest in HIPEC in ovarian cancer has increased around the world and the spirit of cooperative research that has developed both within national borders and across borders will undoubtedly bring about progress in research and development of HIPEC that, hopefully, will improve the prognosis for women with EOC.

REFERENCES

1. Kurman RJ, Shih LM. Molecular pathogenesis and extraovarian origin of epithelial ovarian cancer—shifting the paradigm. Hum Pathol 2011;42:918–31.
2. Piek JM, van Diest PJ, Zweemer RP, et al. Dysplastic changes in prophylactically removed fallopian tubes of women predisposed to developing ovarian cancer. J Pathol 2001;195:451–6.
3. Goodman MT, Shvetsov YB. Incidence of ovarian, peritoneal, and fallopian tube carcinomas in the United States, 1995-2004. Cancer Epidemiol Biomarkers Prev 2009;18:132–9.
4. Parkin DM, Bray F, Ferlay J, et al. Global cancer statistics. CA Cancer J Clin 2002;2005(55):74–108.
5. American Cancer Society. Cancer facts & figures 2012. Atlanta (GA): American Cancer Society; 2012.
6. Heintz AP, Odicino F, Maisonneuve P, et al. Carcinoma of the ovary. FIGO 6th annual report on the results of treatment in gynecological cancer. Int J Gynaecol Obstet 2006;95(Suppl 1):S161–92.
7. Horner MJ, Ries LA, Krapcho M, et al, editors. SEER cancer statistics review, 1975-2006. Bethesda (MD): National Cancer Institute; 2009. Available at: http://seer.cancer.gov/csr/1975_2006/. based on November 2008 SEER data submission, posted to the SEER web site, 2009. Accessed August 18, 2012.
8. Seidman JD, Russell P, Kurman RJ. Surface epithelial tumors of the ovary. In: Kurman RJ, editor. Blaustein's pathology of the female genital tract. New York: Springer; 2002. p. 791–904.
9. Trimble CL, Kosary C, Trimble EL. Long-term survival and patterns of care in women with ovarian tumors of low malignant potential. Gynecol Oncol 2002;86:34–7.
10. Gore ME, Fryatt I, Wiltshaw E, et al. Treatment of relapsed carcinoma of the ovary with cisplatin or carboplatin following initial treatment with these compounds. Gynecol Oncol 1990;36:207–11.
11. Markman M, Rothman R, Hakes T, et al. Second-line platinum therapy in patients with ovarian cancer previously treated with cisplatin. J Clin Oncol 1991;9:389–93.
12. Vermorken JB. Second-line randomized trials in epithelial ovarian cancer. Int J Gynecol Cancer 2008;18(Suppl 1):59–66.
13. Munnell E. The changing prognosis and treatment in cancer of the ovary. Am J Obstet Gynecol 1968;100:790–5.

14. Griffiths CT. Surgical resection of tumor bulk in the primary treatment of ovarian carcinoma. Natl Cancer Inst Monogr 1975;42:101–4.

15. Hoskins WJ, Bundy BN, Thigpen JT, et al. The influence of cytoreductive surgery on recurrence-free interval and survival in small-volume stage III epithelial ovarian cancer: a Gynecologic Oncology Group study. Gynecol Oncol 1992;47:159–66.

16. Bristow RE, Tomacruz RS, Armstrong DK, et al. Survival effect of maximal cytoreductive surgery for advanced ovarian carcinoma during the platinum era: a meta-analysis. J Clin Oncol 2002;20:1248–59.

17. Eisenkop SM, Spirtos NM. What are the current surgical objectives, strategies, and technical capabilities of gynecologic oncologists treating advanced epithelial ovarian cancer? Gynecol Oncol 2001;82:489–97.

18. Eisenkop SM, Friedman RL, Wang HJ. Complete cytoreductive surgery is feasible and maximizes survival in patients with advanced epithelial ovarian cancer: a prospective study. Gynecol Oncol 1998;69:103–8.

19. Eisenhauer EL, Abu-Rustum NR, Sonoda Y, et al. The addition of extensive upper abdominal surgery to achieve optimal cytoreduction improves survival in patients with stages IIIC-IV epithelial ovarian cancer. Gynecol Oncol 2006; 103:1083–90.

20. Bristow RE, Eisenhauer EL, Santillan A, et al. Delaying the primary surgical effort for advanced ovarian cancer: a systematic review of neoadjuvant chemotherapy and interval cytoreduction. Gynecol Oncol 2007;104:480–90.

21. Surwit E, Childers J, Atlas I, et al. Neoadjuvant chemotherapy for advanced ovarian cancer. Int J Gynecol Cancer 1996;6:356–61.

22. Huober J, Meyer A, Wagner U, et al. The role of neoadjuvant chemotherapy and interval laparotomy in advanced ovarian cancer. J Cancer Res Clin Oncol 2002; 128:153–60.

23. Kang S, Nam BH. Does neoadjuvant chemotherapy increase optimal cytoreduction rate in advanced ovarian cancer? Meta-analysis of 21 studies. Ann Surg Oncol 2009;16:2315–20.

24. Vergote I, Trope CG, Amant F, et al. Neoadjuvant chemotherapy or primary surgery in stage IIIC or IV ovarian cancer. N Engl J Med 2010;363:943–53.

25. du Bois A, Quinn M, Thigpen T, et al. 2004 consensus statements on the management of ovarian cancer: final document of the 3rd International Gynecologic Cancer Intergroup Ovarian Cancer Consensus Conference (GCIG OCCC 2004). Ann Oncol 2005;16(Suppl 8):viii7–12.

26. NCCN guidelines version 2. 2012: epithelial ovarian cancer/fallopian tube cancer/ primary peritoneal cancer. 2012. Available at: http://www.nccn.org/professionals/physician_gls/f_guidelines.asp. Accessed June 2, 2012.

27. Helm CW, Edwards RP. Ovarian cancer treatment protocols. 2011. Available at: http://emedicine.medscape.com/article/2006723-overview. Accessed May 28, 2012.

28. Jaaback K, Johnson N. Intraperitoneal chemotherapy for the initial management of primary epithelial ovarian cancer. Cochrane Database Syst Rev 2006;(1): CD 005340.

29. Helm CW. Ports and complications for intraperitoneal chemotherapy delivery [review]. BJOG 2012;119:150–9.

30. Rubin SC, Randall TC, Armstrong KA, et al. Ten-year follow-up of ovarian cancer patients after second-look laparotomy with negative findings. Obstet Gynecol 1999;93:21–4.

31. Eisenkop SM, Spirtos NM, Friedman RL, et al. Relative influences of tumor volume before surgery and the cytoreductive outcome on survival for patients

with advanced ovarian cancer: a prospective study. Gynecol Oncol 2003;90: 390–6.

32. Panici PB, Maggioni A, Hacker N, et al. Systematic aortic and pelvic lymphade-nectomy versus resection of bulky nodes only in optimally debulked advanced ovarian cancer: a randomized clinical trial. J Natl Cancer Inst 2005;97:560–6.

33. Chi DS, Eisenhauer EL, Zivanovic O, et al. Improved progression-free and over-all survival in advanced ovarian cancer as a result of a change in surgical para-digm. Gynecol Oncol 2009;114:26–31.

34. Chi DS, Eisenhauer EL, Lang J, et al. What is the optimal goal of primary cyto-reductive surgery for bulky stage IIIC epithelial ovarian carcinoma (EOC)? Gy-necol Oncol 2006;103:559–64.

35. Burger RA, Brady MF, Bookman MA, et al. Phase III trial of bevacizumab (BEV) in the primary treatment of advanced epithelial ovarian cancer (EOC), primary peritoneal cancer (PPC), or fallopian tube cancer (FTC): A Gynecologic Oncology Group study. 2010;28:5s (Suppl; abstr LBA1). Abstract available at: http://www.asco.org/ASCOv2/Meetings/Abstracts?&vmview=abst_detail_view& confID=74&abstractID=52788. Accessed June 3, 2012.

36. Perren TJ, Swart AM, Pfisterer J, et al. A phase 3 trial of bevacizumab in ovarian cancer. N Engl J Med 2011;365:2484–96.

37. Helm CW, Bristow RE, Kusamura S, et al. Hyperthermic intraperitoneal chemo-therapy with and without cytoreductive surgery for epithelial ovarian cancer. J Surg Oncol 2008;98:283–90.

38. Steller MA, Egorin MJ, Trimble EL, et al. A pilot phase I trial of continuous hyper-thermic peritoneal perfusion with high-dose carboplatin as primary treatment of patients with small-volume residual ovarian cancer [Erratum appears in Cancer Chemother Pharmacol 1999;44(1):90]. Cancer Chemother Pharmacol 1999;43: 106–14.

39. Look M, Chang D, Sugarbaker PH. Long-term results of cytoreductive surgery for advanced and recurrent epithelial ovarian cancers and papillary serous carcinoma of the peritoneum. Int J Gynecol Cancer 2004;14:35–41.

40. Piso P, Dahlke MH, Loss M, et al. Cytoreductive surgery and hyperthermic intra-peritoneal chemotherapy in peritoneal carcinomatosis from ovarian cancer. World J Surg Oncol 2004;2:21–7.

41. Yoshida Y, Sasaki H, Kurokawa T, et al. Efficacy of intraperitoneal continuous hyperthermic chemotherapy as consolidation therapy in patients with advanced epithelial ovarian cancer: a long-term follow-up. Oncol Rep 2005;13:121–5.

42. Rufian S, Munoz-Casares FC, Briceno J, et al. Radical surgery-peritonectomy and intraoperative intraperitoneal chemotherapy for the treatment of peritoneal carcinomatosis in recurrent or primary ovarian cancer. J Surg Oncol 2006;94: 316–24.

43. Cotte E, Glehen O, Mohamed F, et al. Cytoreductive surgery and intraperitoneal chemo-hyperthermia for chemo-resistant and recurrent advanced epithelial ovarian cancer: prospective study of 81 patients [see comment]. World J Surg 2007;31:1813–20.

44. Lentz SS, Miller BE, Kucera GL, et al. Intraperitoneal hyperthermic chemo-therapy using carboplatin: a phase I analysis in ovarian carcinoma. Gynecol On-col 2007;106:207–10.

45. Di Giorgio A, Naticchioni E, Biacchi D, et al. Cytoreductive surgery (peritonec-tomy procedures) combined with hyperthermic intraperitoneal chemotherapy (HIPEC) in the treatment of diffuse peritoneal carcinomatosis from ovarian cancer. Cancer 2008;113:315–25.

46. Lim MC, Kang S, Choi J, et al. Hyperthermic intraperitoneal chemotherapy after extensive cytoreductive surgery in patients with primary advanced epithelial ovarian cancer: interim analysis of a phase II study. Ann Surg Oncol 2009;16: 993–1000.

47. Deraco M, Kusamura S, Virze S, et al. Cytoreductive surgery and hyperthermic intraperitoneal chemotherapy as upfront therapy for advanced epithelial ovarian cancer: multi-institutional phase-II trial. Gynecol Oncol 2011;122:215–20.

48. Helm CW, Richard SD, Pan J, et al. Hyperthermic intraperitoneal chemotherapy in ovarian cancer: first report of the HYPER-O registry. Int J Gynecol Cancer 2010;20:61–9.

49. Di Giorgio A, Cardi M, Sammartino P. Peritonectomy and hyperthermic intraperitoneal chemotherapy (HIPEC) for ovarian peritoneal carcinomatosis: an argued role. Gynecol Oncol 2010;117:146–7.

50. Reichman TW, Cracchiolo B, Sama J, et al. Cytoreductive surgery and intraoperative hyperthermic chemoperfusion for advanced ovarian carcinoma. J Surg Oncol 2005;90:51–6.

51. de Bree E, Rosing H, Beijnen JH, et al. Pharmacokinetic study of docetaxel in intraoperative hyperthermic i.p. chemotherapy for ovarian cancer. Anticancer Drugs 2003;14:103–10.

52. Ryu KS, Kim JH, Ko HS, et al. Effects of intraperitoneal hyperthermic chemotherapy in ovarian cancer. Gynecol Oncol 2004;94:325–32.

53. Mei L, Chen H, Wei DM, et al. Maintenance chemotherapy for ovarian cancer [review]. Cochrane Database Syst Rev 2010;(9):CD007414.

54. Markman M, Liu PY, Wilczynski S, et al. Phase III randomized trial of 12 versus 3 months of maintenance paclitaxel in patients with advanced ovarian cancer after complete response to platinum and paclitaxel-based chemotherapy: a Southwest Oncology Group and Gynecologic Oncology Group trial [see comment]. J Clin Oncol 2003;21:2460–5.

55. Markman M, Liu PY, Moon J, et al. Impact on survival of 12 versus 3 monthly cycles of paclitaxel (175 mg/m^2) administered to patients with advanced ovarian cancer who attained a complete response to primary platinum-paclitaxel: follow-up of a Southwest Oncology Group and Gynecologic Oncology Group phase 3 trial. Gynecol Oncol 2009;114:195–8.

56. Pecorelli S, Favalli G, Gadducci A, et al. Phase III trial of observation versus six courses of paclitaxel in patients with advanced epithelial ovarian cancer in complete response after six courses of paclitaxel/platinum-based chemotherapy: final results of the After-6 protocol 1. J Clin Oncol 2009;27:4642–8.

57. Piccart MJ, Floquet A, Scarfone G, et al. Intraperitoneal cisplatin versus no further treatment: 8-year results of EORTC 55875, a randomized phase III study in ovarian cancer patients with a pathologically complete remission after platinum-based intravenous chemotherapy. Int J Gynecol Cancer 2003;2: 196–203.

58. Barakat RR, Sabbatini P, Bhaskaran D, et al. Intraperitoneal chemotherapy for ovarian carcinoma: results of long-term follow-up. J Clin Oncol 2002;20:694–8.

59. Barakat RR, Almadrones L, Venkatraman ES, et al. A phase II trial of intraperitoneal cisplatin and etoposide as consolidation therapy in patients with stage II-IV epithelial ovarian cancer following negative surgical assessment. Gynecol Oncol 1998;69:17–22.

60. Tournigand C, Louvet C, Molitor JL, et al. Long-term survival with consolidation intraperitoneal chemotherapy for patients with advanced ovarian cancer with pathological complete remission. Gynecol Oncol 2003;91:341–5.

61. Bae JH, Lee JM, Ryu KS, et al. Treatment of ovarian cancer with paclitaxel- or carboplatin-based intraperitoneal hyperthermic chemotherapy during secondary surgery. Gynecol Oncol 2007;106:193–200.
62. Gori J, Castano R, Toziano M, et al. Intraperitoneal hyperthermic chemotherapy in ovarian cancer. Int J Gynecol Cancer 2005;15:233–9.
63. Pomel C, Ferron G, Lorimier G, et al. Hyperthermic intra-peritoneal chemotherapy using oxaliplatin as consolidation therapy for advanced epithelial ovarian carcinoma. Results of a phase II prospective multicentre trial. CHIPOVAC study. Eur J Surg Oncol 2010;36:589–93.
64. Frenel JS, Leux C, Pouplin L, et al. Oxaliplatin-based hyperthermic intraperitoneal chemotherapy in primary or recurrent epithelial ovarian cancer: a pilot study of 31 patients. J Surg Oncol 2011;103:10–6.
65. Bolis G, Scarfone G, Giardina G, et al. Carboplatin alone vs carboplatin plus epidoxorubicin as second-line therapy for cisplatin- or carboplatin-sensitive ovarian cancer. Gynecol Oncol 2001;81:3–9.
66. Bristow RE, Puri I, Chi DS, et al. Cytoreductive surgery for recurrent ovarian cancer: a meta-analysis. Gynecol Oncol 2009;112:265–74.
67. Pfisterer J, Plante M, Vergote I, et al. Gemcitabine plus carboplatin compared with carboplatin in patients with platinum-sensitive recurrent ovarian cancer: an intergroup trial of the AGO-OVAR, the NCIC CTG, and the EORTC GCG. J Clin Oncol 2006;24:4699–707.
68. Gordon AN, Tonda M, Sun S, et al. Long-term survival advantage for women treated with pegylated liposomal doxorubicin compared with topotecan in a phase 3 randomized study of recurrent and refractory epithelial ovarian cancer. Gynecol Oncol 2004;95:1–8.
69. Cantu MG, Buda A, Parma G, et al. Randomized controlled trial of single-agent paclitaxel versus cyclophosphamide, doxorubicin, and cisplatin in patients with recurrent ovarian cancer who responded to first-line platinum-based regimens. J Clin Oncol 2002;20:1232–7.
70. Parmar MK, Ledermann JA, Colombo N, et al. Paclitaxel plus platinum-based chemotherapy versus conventional platinum-based chemotherapy in women with relapsed ovarian cancer: the ICON4/AGO-OVAR-2.2 trial. Lancet 2003; 361:2099–106.
71. Naumann RW, Coleman RL. Management strategies for recurrent platinum-resistant ovarian cancer [review]. Drugs 2011;71:1397–412.
72. Munkarah AR, Coleman RL. Critical evaluation of secondary cytoreduction in recurrent ovarian cancer. Gynecol Oncol 2004;95:273–80.
73. Harter P, Hahmann M, Lueck HJ, et al. Surgery for recurrent ovarian cancer: role of peritoneal carcinomatosis: exploratory analysis of the DESKTOP I Trial about risk factors, surgical implications, and prognostic value of peritoneal carcinomatosis. Ann Surg Oncol 2009;16:1324–30.
74. Ferrandina G, Legge F, Salutari V, et al. Impact of pattern of recurrence on clinical outcome of ovarian cancer patients: clinical considerations. Eur J Cancer 2006;42:2296–302.
75. van der Vange N, van Goethem AR, Zoetmulder FA, et al. Extensive cytoreductive surgery combined with intra-operative intraperitoneal perfusion with cisplatin under hyperthermic conditions (OVHIPEC) in patients with recurrent ovarian cancer: a feasibility pilot. Eur J Surg Oncol 2000;26: 663–8.
76. Cavaliere F, Perri P, Di Filippo F, et al. Treatment of peritoneal carcinomatosis with intent to cure. J Surg Oncol 2000;74:41–4.

77. Deraco M, Rossi CR, Pennacchioli E, et al. Cytoreductive surgery followed by intraperitoneal hyperthermic perfusion in the treatment of recurrent epithelial ovarian cancer: a phase II clinical study. Tumori 2001;87:120–6.

78. Panteix G, Beaujard A, Garbit F, et al. Population pharmacokinetics of cisplatin in patients with advanced ovarian cancer during intraperitoneal hyperthermia chemotherapy. Anticancer Res 2002;22:1329–36.

79. de Bree E, Romanos J, Michalakis J, et al. Intraoperative hyperthermic intraperitoneal chemotherapy with docetaxel as second-line treatment for peritoneal carcinomatosis of gynaecological origin. Anticancer Res 2003;23:3019–27.

80. Chatzigeorgiou K, Economou S, Chrysafis G, et al. Treatment of recurrent epithelial ovarian cancer with secondary cytoreduction and continuous intraoperative intraperitoneal hyperthermic chemoperfusion (CIIPHCP). Zentralbl Gynakol 2003;125:424–9.

81. Zanon C, Clara R, Chiappino I, et al. Cytoreductive surgery and intraperitoneal chemohyperthermia for recurrent peritoneal carcinomatosis from ovarian cancer. World J Surg 2004;28:1040–5.

82. Raspagliesi F, Kusamura S, Campos Torres JC, et al. Cytoreduction combined with intraperitoneal hyperthermic perfusion chemotherapy in advanced/recurrent ovarian cancer patients: the experience of National Cancer Institute of Milan. Eur J Surg Oncol 2006;32:671–5.

83. Helm CW, Randall-Whitis L, Martin RS 3rd, et al. Hyperthermic intraperitoneal chemotherapy in conjunction with surgery for the treatment of recurrent ovarian carcinoma. Gynecol Oncol 2007;105:90–6.

84. Harrison LE, Bryan M, Pliner L, et al. Phase I trial of pegylated liposomal doxorubicin with hyperthermic intraperitoneal chemotherapy in patients undergoing cytoreduction for advanced intra-abdominal malignancy [see comment]. Ann Surg Oncol 2008;15:1407–13.

85. Munoz-Casares FC, Rufian S, Rubio MJ, et al. The role of hyperthermic intraoperative intraperitoneal chemotherapy (HIPEC) in the treatment of peritoneal carcinomatosis in recurrent ovarian cancer. Clin Transl Oncol 2009;11: 753–9.

86. Cavaliere F, Giannarelli D, Valle M, et al. Peritoneal carcinomatosis from ovarian epithelial primary: combined aggressive treatment. In Vivo 2009;23:441–6.

87. Carrabin N, Mithieux F, Meeus P, et al. Hyperthermic intraperitoneal chemotherapy with oxaliplatin and without adjuvant chemotherapy in stage IIIC ovarian cancer. Bull Cancer 2010;97(4):E23–32.

88. Gerestein CG, Damhuis RA, Burger CW, et al. Postoperative mortality after primary cytoreductive surgery for advanced stage epithelial ovarian cancer: a systematic review [review]. Gynecol Oncol 2009;114:523–7.

89. Chua TC, Robertson G, Liauw W, et al. Intraoperative hyperthermic intraperitoneal chemotherapy after cytoreductive surgery in ovarian cancer peritoneal carcinomatosis: systematic review of current results. J Cancer Res Clin Oncol 2009; 135:1637–45.

90. Helm CW. The role of hyperthermic intraperitoneal chemotherapy (HIPEC) in ovarian cancer. Oncologist 2009;14:683–94.

91. Criteria NCICT for adverse events (CTCAE) version 4.0. Available at: http://evs.nci.nih.gov/ftp1/CTCAE/CTCAE_4.03_2010-06-14_QuickReference_5x7.pdf. Accessed June 3, 2012.

92. Dindo D, Demartines N, Clavien PA. Classification of surgical complications: a new proposal with evaluation in a cohort of 6336 patients and results of a survey. Ann Surg 2004;240:205–13.

93. Marcotte E, Sideris L, Drolet P, et al. Hyperthermic intraperitoneal chemotherapy with oxaliplatin for peritoneal carcinomatosis arising from appendix: preliminary results of a survival analysis. Ann Surg Oncol 2008;15:2701–8.

94. Fagotti A, Costantini B, Vizzielli G, et al. HIPEC in recurrent ovarian cancer patients: morbidity-related treatment and long-term analysis of clinical outcome. Gynecol Oncol 2011;122:221–5.

95. Ceelen WP, Peeters M, Houtmeyers P, et al. Safety and efficacy of hyperthermic intraperitoneal chemoperfusion with high-dose oxaliplatin in patients with peritoneal carcinomatosis. Ann Surg Oncol 2008;15:535–41.

96. Loggie BW, Sterchi JM, Rogers AT, et al. Intraperitoneal hyperthermic chemotherapy for advanced gastrointestinal and ovarian cancers. Reg Cancer Treat 1994;2:78–81.

97. Van der Speeten K, Stuart OA, Mahteme H, et al. Pharmacokinetic study of perioperative intravenous ifosfamide. Int J Surg Oncol 2011;2011:185092.

98. Sugarbaker PH, Graves T, DeBruijn EA, et al. Early postoperative intraperitoneal chemotherapy as an adjuvant therapy to surgery for peritoneal carcinomatosis from gastrointestinal cancer: pharmacological studies. Cancer Res 1990;50: 5790–4.

99. Pietzner K, Schmuck RB, Fotopoulou C, et al. Long term combination treatment with bevacizumab, pegylated liposomal doxorubicin and regional abdominal hyperthermia in platinum refractory ovarian cancer: a case report and review of the literature [review]. Anticancer Res 2011;31:2675–7.

100. Jones E, Alvarez Secord A, Prosnitz LR, et al. Intra-peritoneal cisplatin and whole abdomen hyperthermia for relapsed ovarian carcinoma. Int J Hyperthermia 2006;22:161–72.

101. Muenyi CS, States VA, Masters JH, et al. Sodium arsenite and hyperthermia modulate cisplatin-DNA damage responses and enhance platinum accumulation in murine metastatic ovarian cancer xenograft after hyperthermic intraperitoneal chemotherapy (HIPEC). J Ovarian Res 2011;4:9–19.

102. Muenyi CS, Pinhas AR, Fan TW, et al. Sodium arsenite ± hyperthermia sensitizes p53-expressing human ovarian cancer cells to cisplatin by modulating platinum-DNA damage responses. Toxicol Sci 2012;127:139–49.

103. States JC. Inhibition of HSP90 greatly enhances the efficacy of platinum-based therapies for ovarian cancer including hyperthermia. Abstract presented at Seventh International Symposium on Regional Cancer Therapies, Captiva Island (FL): February 2012.

104. Muggia FM, Braly PS, Brady MF, et al. Phase III randomized study of cisplatin versus paclitaxel versus cisplatin and paclitaxel in patients with suboptimal stage III or IV ovarian cancer: a gynecologic oncology group study. J Clin Oncol 2000;18:106–15.

105. Ozols RF, Bundy BN, Greer BE, et al. Phase III trial of carboplatin and paclitaxel compared with cisplatin and paclitaxel in patients with optimally resected stage III ovarian cancer: a Gynecologic Oncology Group study [see comment]. J Clin Oncol 2003;21:3194–200.

106. Armstrong DK, Bundy B, Wenzel L, et al. Intraperitoneal cisplatin and paclitaxel in ovarian cancer. N Engl J Med 2006;354:34–43.

Randomized Clinical Trials for Colorectal Cancer Peritoneal Surface Malignancy

Itzhak Avital, MD[a,b], Björn L.D.M. Brücher, MD, FRCS (Engl)[c],
Aviram Nissan, MD[d], Alexander Stojadinovic, MD[b,e,f],*

KEYWORDS

- Carcinomatosis • Colorectal cancer • Prospective • Randomized • Clinical trials • HIPEC
- CRS • Oxaliplatin and mitomycin

KEY POINTS

- Peritoneal carcinomatosis (PC) from colorectal cancer (CRC) treated with chemotherapy alone results in median survival of 5 to 13 months.
- Approximately 55% of high-risk patients (patients presenting with synchronous PC, ovarian metastases, perforated primary CRC, and emergency presentation of CRC with bleeding or obstructing lesions) develop PC.
- Early PC is generally undetectable by conventional cross-sectional or functional imaging.
- Cytoreductive surgery (CRS) and hyperthermic intraperitoneal chemotherapy (HIPEC) for early CRCPC results in median survival of 22 to 63 months and 5-year survival of ~50%.
- Efforts are under way to identify patients at high risk for carcinomatosis or those with early peritoneal disease dissemination and to intervene at a time in the natural history of the disease when treatment-related benefit is highest with multimodality therapy, including CRS/HIPEC/chemotherapy.

Disclosure of any commercial interest: The authors have no disclosures that are relevant to the preparation or publication of this manuscript.

Support: This clinical research effort was supported, in part, by the United States Military Cancer Institute, Washington, DC and the Henry M. Jackson Foundation, Rockville, MD.

[a] Bon Secours Cancer Institute, Peritoneal Surface Malignancies Center of Excellence, 5855 Bremo Street, Suite 405, Richmond, VA 23226, USA; [b] Uniformed Services University of the Health Sciences, Bethesda, MD, USA; [c] Theodor-Billroth-Academy®, Josephsburgstrasse 6, 81673 Munich, Germany; [d] Department of Surgery, Rabin Medical Center, 39 Jabotinski Street, 49100 Petah Tikvah, Israel; [e] Department of Surgery, Walter Reed National Military Medical Center, 8901 Wisconsin Avenue, Bethesda, MD 20889, USA; [f] GI Cancer Program, United States Military Cancer Institute, 8901 Wisconsin Avenue, Bethesda, MD 20889, USA

* Corresponding author. Department of Surgery, Walter Reed National Military Medical Center, 8901 Wisconsin Avenue, Building 9, Room 1272, Bethesda, MD 20889-5600.

E-mail address: stojadinovicmd2011@gmail.com

Surg Oncol Clin N Am 21 (2012) 665–688
http://dx.doi.org/10.1016/j.soc.2012.07.004
1055-3207/12/$ – see front matter Published by Elsevier Inc.

surgonc.theclinics.com

INTRODUCTION: NATURE OF THE PROBLEM

Peritoneal carcinomatosis (PC) is a frequently occurring event in the natural history of malignancy of colorectal cancer (CRC) origin (upwards of 40% of all patients with CRC), and is associated with marked deterioration in quality of life (QOL) and limited overall survival (OS).[1–3] Despite advances in early detection of CRC, peritoneal disease spread continues to be a common mode of disease progression, because 8% of patients with CRC have synchronous peritoneal spread of disease at time of primary resection, and up to 25% of patients with recurrent CRC have disease confined to the peritoneal cavity.[4,5] In about 30% of patients with CRC, peritoneal spread is the main reason for death.[6]

CLINICAL PRESENTATION AND COURSE

PC represents a formidable treatment challenge in oncology. Once considered a variant of systemic spread of disease, CRCPC was treated with palliative systemic chemotherapy alone, with surgery reserved only for palliation of disease-related or treatment-related secondary events such as bowel obstruction and ascites. Systemic multidrug chemotherapy has not altered significantly the natural history of CRCPC, as patients suffer disease progression and functional deterioration. This situation is attributable to visceral obstruction, malignant ascites, and cancer cachexia over a limited median survival of 5 to 9 months.[7,8]

Novel first-line 5-fluorouracil (5-FU)/leucovorin (LV)-based cytotoxic chemotherapeutic regimens to treat metastatic (liver and lung) CRC, including oxaliplatin (FOLFOX) and irinotecan (IFL, FOLFIRI) with or without targeted antibody therapy using bevacizumab (IFL/bevacizumab) or cetuximab (Erbitux), have increased response rates (25%–55%) and median OS (from 12 to 24 months) significantly greater than what has been the benchmark regimen over the past 4 decades (5-FU or 5-FU/LV).[9–17] However, long-term survival for patients with systemic disease spread remains poor, and the outcomes for patients with advanced disease confined to peritoneal surfaces treated with these modern agents, indeterminate.

RELEVANT ANATOMY/PATHOPHYSIOLOGY

The biology of PC is distinctive, unlike hematogenous metastasis. Insights into the natural history of peritoneal tumor dissemination have engendered novel multimodality treatment approaches to this challenging clinical problem. Tumor dissemination across peritoneal surfaces occurs through established mechanisms of direct tumor extension, transcoelomic tumor cell spread in peritoneal fluid, and malignant peritoneal seeding from surgical manipulation of the tumor; this form of malignant disease dissemination can occur in the absence of regional or distant nodal or systemic metastases.[18–23] Another possibility is hematogenous spread to the peritoneal surfaces, although evidence for this theoretic possibility does not exist.

Confinement of disease to the parietal peritoneal surface, in the absence of systemic metastasis, has served as the basis for undertaking surgical eradication of disease through aggressive surgical cytoreduction, or cytoreductive surgery (CRS). However, surgery alone has not achieved significant improvement in survival in patients with PC, because microscopic or grossly apparent disease inevitably remains after even aggressive CRS.[4,24]

THERAPEUTIC OPTIONS

That viable tumor cells become sequestered in avascular intraperitoneal adhesions explains partly the resistance to and ineffectiveness of systemic therapy alone for

PC.[25] The presence of an anatomic barrier, the peritoneal-plasma partition, has enabled administration of high local concentrations of chemotherapy at the peritoneal surface in excess of systemically administered agents when drug delivery is intraperitoneal.[26–31] For example, high-molecular-weight agents such as mitomycin C (334 Da), and oxaliplatin (397 Da) have favorable pharmacokinetic profiles (area under curve (AUC), peritoneal fluid relative to plasma: mitomycin C, 75:1; oxaliplatin, 25:1) permitting dose-dense intraperitoneal therapy over prolonged periods with rapid tissue concentration (in residual tumor deposits and peritoneum), but limited systemic absorption or toxicity.[32–34] This unique therapeutic approach addresses the problem of systemic chemotherapy resistance and, with its reduced systemic toxicity, provides distinct pharmacologic advantage over systemic drug delivery.[35,36]

Intraperitoneal hyperthermia, shown to be technically feasible, was integrated into the treatment paradigm of CRS and intraperitoneal chemotherapy for PC to increase tissue penetration, direct killing of free tumor cells, and augment cytotoxicity of the delivered antineoplastic agent.[37,38] Another advantage is the homogenous distribution of the intraperitoneal chemotherapy. Hyperthermia itself is cytotoxic to tumor cells based on established mechanisms involving inhibition of nuclear matrix-mediated functions essential to DNA replication, transcription, and repair.[39,40] However, it is the combined antitumor effect of heat and intraperitoneal chemotherapy that serves as the basis for the currently practiced treatment approach to PC.[37,41] The abdomen in this concept is seen as a localized compartment, and thus CRCPC without metastatic disease is considered locally advanced disease.

Although hyperthermic intraperitoneal chemotherapy (HIPEC) permits high local drug concentrations to exposed peritoneal surface tumors, 1 important limiting factor is the narrow depth of tissue penetration by the delivered cytostatic agent.[42] Depth of drug peritoneal penetration is limited to 3 mm or less from the parietal peritoneal surface.[43,44] Hence, the efficacy of HIPEC is inversely proportional to the volume of residual disease; thereby, therapeutic benefit is maximized when all grossly apparent disease is resected (complete cytoreduction, CCR0).

This situation makes aggressive cytoreduction logical and imperative, which is conducted with the intent to eradicate macroscopic deposits of tumor and optimize the efficacy of HIPEC in obliterating minimal residual disease. Optimal therapeutic synergy is achieved when intraperitoneal heated chemotherapy is administered immediately after maximal cytoreduction, thereby minimizing trapping of viable peritoneal tumor cells in fibrin and postoperative adhesions, and maximizing kill of tumor cells shed during resection.[45] Adhesions have to be divided during CRS to facilitate uniform distribution of perfusate, maximize direct contact of drug with residual peritoneal tumor cells, and harness the advantage of thermochemotherapeutic antitumor synergism.[36,46–48]

PC of CRC origin has long been considered a preterminal condition. A multicenter prospective study determined median survival in this group of patients to be 5 months.[7] A retrospective analysis of more than 3000 patients with CRC reported median OS of 7 months in patients with CRCPC.[5] The trimodality therapeutic paradigm to PC consisting of CRS plus HIPEC followed by systemic chemotherapy has shown promising oncological outcomes.

CLINICAL OUTCOMES

A multicenter registry study of more than 500 patients with CRCPC treated with CRS plus HIPEC reported median OS of 19.2 months, and 3-year and 5-year OS rates of 39% and 19%, respectively.[3] For patients with no macroscopic residual disease after cytoreduction (CCR0), 3-year and 5-year OS was 47% and 31%, with median survival of 32.4 months (**Fig. 1**), similar to outcomes after complete resection of CRC liver metastases. Treatment with adjuvant systemic chemotherapy after cytoreduction and perioperative thermochemotherapy was an independent predictor of improved survival on multivariate analysis. This study, although retrospective in nature, suggested that improved outcomes are indeed possible with a combined modality treatment approach incorporating CRS, regional/compartmental intraperitoneal chemotherapy with or without adjuvant systemic therapy in patients who could otherwise expect limited survival ranging from 5 to 8 months.[4,5,7] OS in another large international registry study was consistent with that reported in previous smaller phase II studies of combined CRS and perioperative HIPEC for CRCPC.[49–60]

Thus far there is only 1 prospective randomized trial providing level I data, and supporting CRS plus HIPEC for patients with CRCPC. It was a single-institution, randomized controlled trial (RCT) (phase III) trial that showed the superiority of this combined modality approach for patients with colorectal PC over adjuvant systemic therapy, with or without surgical palliation.[2] One hundred and five patients with CRCPC were randomly assigned to receive standard, 5-FU/LV, systemic chemotherapy (standard of care) or CRS plus HIPEC with mitomycin C (35 mg/m^2 at 41° C for 90 minutes). After a median follow-up time of 22 months, median survival was increased significantly in the CRS/HIPEC arm of the study (22.4 vs 12.9 months; hazard ratio = 0.55: 95% confidence interval [CI], 0.32–0.95; P = .032). The analysis was conducted on an intent-to-treat basis and study design required randomization before operation such that only 37% underwent CCR0, which is an imperative if benefit is to be achieved with HIPEC. Another point of contention is the mixed population of high-grade and low-grade CRCs. Subsequently, Verwaal and colleagues[61] reported the long-term outcomes of this trial. At a median follow-up of 8 years (range: 72–115 months), 4 of 51 patients were still alive in the standard therapy arm (2 with and 2 without disease); in the CRS plus HIPEC arm, 5 patients remained alive (2 with and 3 without disease). The

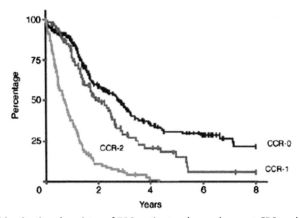

Fig. 1. A multi-institutional registry of 506 patients who underwent CRS and HIPEC for colorectal carcinomatosis reported a 1-year, 3-year, and 5-year survival of 72%, 39%, and 19%, respectively, with a median survival of 19 months. Patients with complete CRS (CCR0) achieved the highest survival. The patients who underwent CCR0 resection achieved a 1-year, 3-year, and 5-year survival of 87%, 47%, and 31%. (*From* Glehen O, Kwiatkowski F, Sugarbaker PH, et al. Cytoreductive surgery combined with perioperative intraperitoneal chemotherapy for the management of peritoneal carcinomatosis from colorectal cancer: a multi-institutional study. J Clin Oncol 2004;22(16):3288; with permission.)

median progression-free survival (PFS) was 7.7 months and 12.6 months in the standard therapy and CRS plus HIPEC arms, respectively ($P = .02$). The median disease-specific survival was 12.6 and 22.2 months in the standard and CRS plus HIPEC arms, respectively ($P = .028$). Based on these data, approximately 5 patients need to undergo CRS plus HIPEC for 1 patient to experience survival advantage at 3 years.

Study subjects in Verwaal and colleagues[2,61] RCT with extensive carcinomatosis having incomplete CRS also underwent HIPEC. This was the first RCT to report OS benefit in patients with CRCPC treated with CRS and HIPEC when compared with palliative chemotherapy.[2,61] However, the study used a dated systemic therapy regimen in the form of 5-FU (400 mg/m^2 intravenous [IV] bolus) and LV (80 mg/m^2 IV) administered weekly for 26 weeks or until progression, intolerable toxicity or death, with or without palliative surgery.

COMPLICATIONS AND CONCERNS

The absolute OS benefit of ~10 months in the Dutch RCT conducted by Verwaal and colleagues[2,61] was offset by considerable treatment-related morbidity (grade 4 morbidity = 45%) and mortality (8%) in the CRS/HIPEC arm. A significant proportion of treatment-associated complications (median operative blood loss 4000 mL; small bowel fistula, 15%; operative site infection, 6%; renal failure, 6%; pancreatitis, 2%) have been hypothesized to be caused by the high dose of intraperitoneal hyperthermic mitomycin C, which was administered in the context of this RCT. Reductions in intraperitoneal mitomycin C doses have been recommended on that basis.

Others have reported significantly lesser treatment-related morbidity (23%–35%) and mortality (0%–4%) with HIPEC using reduced mitomycin C doses.[46,57,62] The Dutch RCT reported benefit of CRT with HIPEC for patients with CRCPC, and it challenged the predominant therapeutic nihilism that has been the accepted norm for patients with this disease.[2,61] The actual contribution of the HIPEC to the observed survival benefit, despite the considerable cost in terms of treatment-related morbidity evident in that trial, remains in question; however, acceptable therapeutic toxicity has been reported in other studies with lower doses of intraperitoneal mitomycin C without apparent compromise in treatment efficacy.[46]

Modern systemic therapy with combination cytotoxic and biologic agents has resulted in unprecedented median OS exceeding 20 months for stage IV CRC. However, the most common mode of distant disease spread in these studies has been hematogenous dissemination. Patients with PC with metastatic disease confined to the peritoneal surface treated with complete (CCR0) cytoreduction and HIPEC have showed median survival exceeding 40 months (range 28–60 months).[3,49–60] Based on these data, Elias and colleagues[63] reported on a series that follows patients with CRCPC without systemic dissemination treated with current standard of care systemic chemotherapy regimens of FOLFOX (5-FU, LV, and oxaliplatin) and FOLFIRI (5-FU, LV, and irinotecan). Based on the inability to perform a randomized trial, Elias and colleagues[63] performed a comparative study that case-matched controls to CRS and HIPEC to answer 2 questions. First, what is the natural history of patients with PC treated with modern regimens? Second, do patients treated with CRS and HIPEC benefit in terms of survival? The investigators reported a median survival for the standard group and the CRS/HIPEC group of 23.9 months and 62.7 months, respectively ($P<.05$). The 2-year survival was 65% and 81%; 5-year survival was 13% and 51%, respectively (**Fig. 2**). With the caveat that this was not a prospective randomized trial, patients with CRCPC have benefited from improved multiagent systemic regimens. However, the benefit of modern systemic

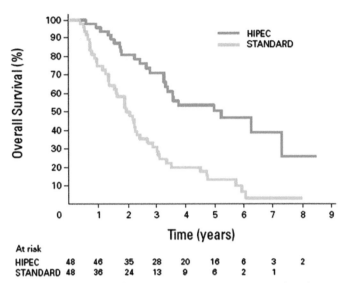

Fig. 2. OS in patients with PC without systemic metastases treated with CRS + HIPEC + systemic therapy (*blue*) versus current standard of care with systemic chemotherapy alone (*yellow*). Median OS was 23.9 (*STANDARD*) versus 62.7 months (*HIPEC*). Two-year survival was 65% versus 81% and 5-year survival 13% versus 51% in the STANDARD and HIPEC groups, respectively. (*From* Elias D, Lefevre JH, Chevalier J, et al. Complete cytoreductive surgery plus intraperitoneal chemohyperthermia with oxaliplatin for peritoneal carcinomatosis of colorectal origin. J Clin Oncol 2009;27(5):683; with permission.)

chemotherapy incorporating combinations of 5-FU, LV, oxaliplatin, irinotecan, capecitabine, bevacizumab and cetuximab for patients with CRCPC without distant metastases is not fully understood. Oxaliplatin-based and irinotecan-based regimens are not without complications. For a full discussion, please see the section on HIPEC with oxaliplatin.

CURRENT STANDARD TREATMENT APPROACH FOR ADVANCED CRC

Approximately 40% of patients present initially with metastatic CRC, and the majority are treated with palliative multiagent systemic therapy, because the extent of disease precludes complete surgical resection in most of these patients.[64] For more than 40 years a thymidylate synthase-inhibiting fluoropyrimidine analogue, 5-FU, has been the prevailing active cytotoxic chemotherapeutic agent used in combination with a biomodulating agent, LV. However, the clinical benefit with the standard first-line regimen of 5-FU/LV for advanced CRC has been a modest response rate of ~20%, and median OS ~12 months.[65]

New agents emerged, which advanced significantly the treatment of metastatic CRC. Various combinations of 5-FU/LV and the topoisomerase I inhibitor, irinotecan, the third-generation platinum analogue, oxaliplatin, and the oral fluoropyrimidine, capecitabine, have nearly doubled the median OS (20–22 months) for patients with advanced disease. Novel targeted agents such as the recombinant humanized monoclonal antibody to vascular endothelial growth factor (VEGF), bevacizumab, and the antibody targeting epidermal growth factor receptor, cetuximab, have expanded the therapeutic options and improved oncological outcomes even further, with median OS exceeding 2 years when all active agents are administered over the course of the patient's disease.

Three pivotal RCTs showed the superiority of irinotecan (CPT-11) in combination with 5-FU/LV over 5-FU/LV alone (either bolus [Mayo regimen] or infusional 5-FU/LV) in advanced CRC in terms of treatment response rate (RR: 39%–62% vs 21%–34%) and PFS (6.7–8.5 vs 4.3–6.4 months), and in 2 of these studies, OS (14.8–20.1 vs 12.6–16.9 months).[9,10,66] These trials established combination weekly infusional 5-FU/LV + irinotecan, 5-fluorouracil and leucovorin (IFL) as a new standard first-line therapy for metastatic CRC in the year 2000.

Three RCTs that compared oxaliplatin with an infusional 5-FU/LV backbone with infusional 5-FU/LV alone as first-line therapy for metastatic colorectal adenocarcinoma reported significant improvement in RR (49%–53% vs 16%–22%) and PFS (7.8–9.0 vs 5.3–6.2 months).[11,67] The availability of effective second-line (salvage) systemic chemotherapy and modest study group sample size may have limited showing a statistically significant OS benefit with first-line 5-FU/LV + oxaliplatin (OS: 16.2–19.9 vs 14.7–19.4 months).[11,67]

The North Central Cancer Treatment Group (NCCTG N9741) trial, which compared IFL (control group), irinotecan (125 mg/m^2) and bolus FU (500 mg/m^2) plus LV (20 mg/m^2) on days 1, 8, 15, and 22 every 6 weeks with FOLFOX4, oxaliplatin (85 mg/m^2 on day 1) + infusional FU (400 mg/m^2 IV bolus followed by 600 mg/m^2 continuous 22-hour infusions on days 1 and 2 every 2 weeks) + LV (200 mg/m^2), with IROX, irinotecan (200 mg/m^2) and oxaliplatin (85 mg/m^2) every 3 weeks, established FOLFOX4 as front-line therapy for metastatic CRC.[13] Significant improvement in treatment response, PFS, and OS was reported with FOLFOX4 (RR 45%, PFS 8.7 months, OS 19.5 months) compared with IFL (RR 31%, PFS 6.9 months, OS 15.0 months) and IROX (RR 35%, PFS 6.5 months, OS 17.4 months) in that study.

The FOLOX4 regimen had significantly lower grade 3+ toxicity (including nausea, vomiting, diarrhea, dehydration, and febrile neutropenia) than IFL, but was more commonly associated with neuropathy and neutropenia.[13] This NCCTG trial emphasized the importance of infusional rather than bolus 5-FU administration in combination with irinotecan and oxaliplatin to optimize the tolerability of triple combination therapy. The superior treatment efficacy and safety profile seen with FOLFOX4 in the NCCTG N9741 trial made it the new first-line standard of care for advanced colorectal carcinoma.

Two phase III trials have shown comparable efficacy of FOLFOX and infusional/bolus 5-FU/LV + irinotecan (FOLFIRI) for first-line treatment of stage IV CRC, pointing out that treatment selection largely depends on anticipated adverse event profile (gastrointestinal [GI] toxicity with FOLFIRI vs sensory neuropathy with FOLFOX).[14,16] FOLFIRI, which incorporates infusional 5-FU, has superseded IFL, which uses bolus 5-FU, because IFL has significant dose-limiting toxicity (diarrhea, dehydration, and myelosuppression) and inferior clinical outcomes.[68] One trial has emphasized the findings of a preceding meta-analysis of 7 randomized phase III trials in advanced CRC, specifically, multidrug triple combination (FOLFOX, FOLFIRI) first-line chemotherapy and administration of all 3 active cytotoxic agents (5-FU, irinotecan and oxaliplatin) over the course of the disease represents the optimal treatment strategy, because it translates into significant OS benefit.[69]

Bevacizumab is a recombinant humanized monoclonal antibody targeting the VEGF-A receptor, which alone has not shown activity against CRC; however, when combined with present-day cytotoxic agents, it has proved highly efficacious. The randomized TREE1 and TREE2 trials compared mixed FOLFOX, bolus 5-FU/LV/oxaliplatin and capecitabine/oxaliplatin (CAPOX) with or without bevacizumab.[69] The addition of bevacizumab enhanced the efficacy of each individual combination by increasing treatment response, PFS, and OS (**Table 1**).

Table 1
Summary of TREE1 and TREE2 trials comparing mixed FOLFOX (mFOLFOX), bolus 5-FU/LV/oxaliplatin (bFOL) and capecitabine/oxaliplatin (CAPOX) with or without bevacizumab

Outcome	mFOLFOX		bFOL		CAPOX	
	No Bevacizumab	Plus Bevacizumab	No Bevacizumab	Plus Bevacizumab	No Bevacizumab	Plus Bevacizumab
RR (%)	41	52	20	39	27	46
PFS (mo)	8.7	9.9	6.9	8.3	5.9	10.3
(95% CI)	(6.5–9.8)	(7.9–11.7)	(4.2–8.0)	(6.6–9.9)	(5.1–7.4)	(8.6–12.5)
OS (mo)	19.2	26.0	17.9	20.7	17.2	27.0

The TREE1/TREE2 trials showed the significant added benefit of bevacizumab (5 mg/kg) when combined with standard first-line FOLFOX for advanced CRC, not only in terms of increased treatment response (52% vs 41%) and PFS (9.9 vs 8.7 months) but also OS (26.0 vs 19.2 months).[69]

The Eastern Cooperative Oncology Group (ECOG) 3200 trial substantiated the added benefit of FOLFOX4 + bevacizumab.[70] Bevacizumab-naive and oxaliplatin-naive patients with advanced CRC previously treated with 5-FU+irinotecan were randomized to receive FOLFOX4, high-dose bevacizumab (10 mg/kg) alone, or FOLFOX4 + bevacizumab. The addition of bevacizumab to second-line FOLFOX significantly increased treatment RR, PFS, and OS (**Table 2**). Phase III trial data strongly support bevacizumab as an integral component of first-line triple combination therapy (FOLFOX or FOLFIRI) for metastatic CRC.[69,70] FOLFOX + bevacizumab are now recommended as standard first-line therapy for advanced unresectable CRC by the National Comprehensive Cancer Network.[71] In addition, CAPOX has been added as a potential regimen in this trial, because it is one of the acceptable standard first-line chemotherapy regimens for metastatic disease according to the latest NCCN guidelines.

THE NEED FOR EVIDENCE-BASED APPROACHES TO THERAPY FOR COMBINED MODALITY THERAPY (CRS + HIPEC + SYSTEMIC THERAPY)

A standardized, evidence-based approach is lacking for patients with peritoneal surface malignancy from CRC origin. A collaborative trial with surgical quality assurance and modern multidrug systemic therapy incorporating critical assessment of disease burden, determinants of CCR, treatment-related toxicity, QOL, and survival, although imperative, is unlikely to be achieved. The Dutch RCT, although not perfect, has provided the basis for further study, which should use a new reference study arm. If future randomized trials are undertaken for CRCPC origin, then appropriate study selection will be key, which should be limited to selected patients having potentially curable regionally advanced CRC confined to the parietal peritoneal surface.

Table 2
Benefit of adding bevacizumab to first-line treatment of metastatic CRC

	Bevacizumab (n = 243)	FOLFOX4 (n = 290)	FOLFOX4 + Bevacizumab (n = 289)	FOLFOX4 + Bevacizumab vs FOLFOX4 P =
RR (%)	3.0	9.2	21.8	<0.001
PFS (mo)	3.5	5.5	7.4	<0.001
OS (mo)	10.2	10.7	12.5	0.002

As systemic therapy for CRC continues to improve, an increasing number of patients fail in the peritoneum despite adequate control of lymphatic and hematogenous dissemination of disease. Peritoneal surface disease is difficult to detect with cross-sectional imaging modalities routinely implemented for this patient population. Patients with peritoneal surface malignancy from GI cancers almost uniformly succumb to advanced locoregional disease in the form of intractable ascites, malignant visceral obstruction, and cancer cachexia. The natural history of peritoneal carcinomatosis from GI malignancies is inexorably lethal, with median OS of approximately 5 months,[7] because patients with disease confined to the peritoneum remain at increased risk of synchronous occult hematogenous metastases. Hence, multiagent systemic therapy is recommended under these circumstances.

Although systemic therapy improves outcome in patients with hematogenous disease spread, improvements are needed to control peritoneal surface malignancy, which is known to be relatively resistant to systemic agents, principally because of the presence of a peritoneal-plasma partition. Moreover, the results of surgical resection alone for peritoneal dissemination of colon cancer have been disappointing given the difficulty in clearing surgically all microscopic disease foci. The infusion of chemotherapy into the peritoneal cavity provides distinct pharmacokinetic advantages. The addition of hyperthermia potentiates the effect of intraperitoneal chemotherapy through antitumor synergism, without systemic drug absorption.[45–48]

Mitomycin C has been studied most extensively for HIPEC in patients with PC of GI origin. Mitomycin C has also shown consistent pharmacokinetics, favorable toxicity profile, and invariable hyperthermia-facilitated tumor cytotoxicity, which is enhanced under conditions of tumor hypoxia; furthermore, mitomycin C contributes to improved outcomes after optimal cytoreduction.[37,43,48,52,55,58,72,73] Hence, the delivery of intraperitoneal heated chemotherapy has the advantage of dose-dense regional delivery of cytotoxic agents, with little systemic toxicity.

We have witnessed a milestone development in the treatment of metastatic CRC. Median OS has been doubled through the use of all active agents over the patient's disease course, from 12 months with 5-FU to nearly 24 months with infusional 5-FU-LV in combination with oxaliplatin or irinotecan, and biologic agents such as bevacizumab and cetuximab. These modern-day multidrug systemic regimens have proven benefit with hematogenous disease spread; however, the role of modern systemic therapy in patients with colorectal carcinoma confined to the peritoneal cavity remains undefined. It is anticipated that these newer agents will prove effective in clearing clinically unapparent systemic circulating tumor cells that place the patient at high risk of distant dissemination of disease after cytoreduction and HIPEC. However, the most common site of metastatic disease in the studies of modern multiagent systemic regimens was hematogenous dissemination. The benefit of modern systemic chemotherapy incorporating 5-FU, LV, oxaliplatin (FOLFOX), bevacizumab, and cetuximab for patients with advanced CRC confined to the peritoneal surface is unknown. Level I evidence strongly supports adding the biologic agent, bevacizumab, to standard first-line triple combination chemotherapy (FOLFOX or FOLFIRI) for advanced CRC (see **Table 2**).[68,70,71]

CRS, HIPEC, and systemic chemotherapy are not competitive therapies, and current practice patterns in selected specialty centers reflect the acceptance in some parts of the oncological community that all 3 modalities have a role in the multidisciplinary approach to appropriately selected patients with CRCPC origin. Given that the benefit of current systemic therapy regimens for limited peritoneal disease of CRC origin remains to be determined, an RCT was proposed to compare standard multiagent systemic therapy with combined modality therapy (CRS + HIPEC + systemic therapy;

US Military Cancer Institute (USMCI) and American College of Surgeons Oncology Group (ACOSOG)-National Cancer Institute (NCI)/Cancer Therapy Evaluation Program (CTEP) protocol, USMCI 8214/ACOSOG Z6091). The control arm of the RCT was intended to assess response to modern-day systemic agents for documented disease confined to the peritoneal surface. The trial emphasized the importance of exposing patients with metastatic colon cancer to all active agents over the course of disease irrespective of sequence of drug administration. Because current clinical experience suggests contemporary systemic chemotherapy is associated with prolonged survival among patients with CRCPC compared with historical controls, it was postulated that adding CRS to modern systemic chemotherapy regimens could significantly improve oncological outcomes.

The NCI/CTEP protocol USMCI 8214/ACOSOG Z6091 comparing standard systemic therapy with CRS + HIPEC + standard systemic therapy in patients with limited peritoneal dissemination of colon adenocarcinoma recognized the importance of: (1) surgical standardization and quality control; (2) multimodality treatment of patients with CRC having resectable dissemination of peritoneal disease, absent apparent hematogenous or distant nodal disease spread, who are considered suitable candidates for aggressive local-regional therapy: CRS with HIPEC; and (3) the potential challenges of a systemic-chemotherapy-only treatment arm apparent in previous unsuccessful randomized designs. The potential favorable synergy of modern systemic and regional therapies, along with the preference of the larger oncological community to treat advanced CRC with or without CRCPC with upfront systemic therapy, as well as the expectations of patients with CRCPC origin, made it necessary to: (1) include patients who received previous first-line systemic therapy for metastatic CRC; and (2) to allow crossover from the systemic therapy control arm to the multimodality treatment arm at time of disease progression (**Fig. 3**).[74] Despite this situation, the trial failed to meet accrual goals and closed, calling into question the feasibility of conducting such an RCT to assess the efficacy of combined modality therapy in patients with limited PC of CRC. if definitive level I evidence is absent, some experts in CRS regard combined modality therapy for limited CRCPC as the current standard of care.[1,75] For example, in France, this therapeutic paradigm has already been incorporated into the French guidelines. In Germany, it will be integrated in to the treatment guidelines as a therapeutic option in 2012.

Efforts are under way to identify patients at high risk for carcinomatosis or those with early peritoneal disease dissemination and to intervene at a time in the natural history of the disease when treatment-related benefit is highest with multimodality therapy, including CRS/HIPEC/chemotherapy. Recognizing that ~55% of high-risk patients (patients presenting with synchronous PC, ovarian metastases, perforated primary CRC, and emergency presentation of CRC with bleeding or obstructing lesions) develop CRCPC, and that early PC is undetectable by conventional cross-sectional or functional imaging, others have taken a different approach to establish level I evidence for CRS/HIPEC in limited PC of CRC origin.

RCT EVALUATING MANDATORY SECOND-LOOK SURGERY WITH CRS/HIPEC VERSUS STANDARD OF CARE IN PATIENTS AT HIGH RISK OF DEVELOPING CRC PERITONEAL METASTASES

In the United States, approximately 108,070 patients are diagnosed with colon cancer and 40,740 patients with rectal cancer per year.[76] Nearly 50,000 patients die from CRC per year. Initially, PC commonly occurs without systemic dissemination. In 1 study of 3019 patients reviewed with CRC, 349 (13%) had carcinomatosis.[5] A total of 214

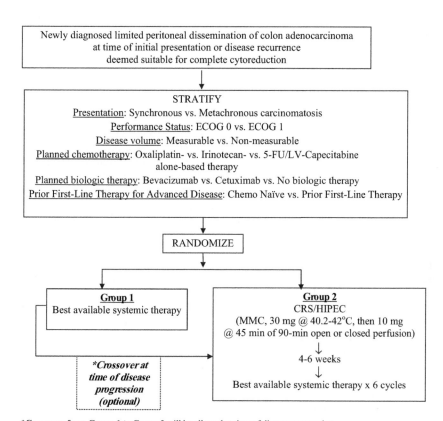

Fig. 3. Study schema for NCI/CTEP Protocol USMCI 8214/ACOSOG Z6091 comparing standard systemic therapy with CRS + HIPEC + standard systemic therapy in patients with limited peritoneal dissemination of colon adenocarcinoma.

(61%) patients had synchronous disease, and 135 (39%) patients had metachronous disease. Nearly 60% of synchronous PC was limited to the peritoneal cavity, and 64% of these patients had localized disease to 1 quadrant.[5] Overall, recurrences are limited to the peritoneum in 25% of patients with CRC. It is estimated that in the United States, approximately 8000 patients are diagnosed yearly with synchronous PC.

The median survival of patients with PC without systemic dissemination was 7 months with 5-FU and LV regimens for the 3019 patients reported earlier.[5] Another study evaluated prospectively 45 patients with PC, who achieved a median OS of 6 months.[4] A total of 118 patients in a French registry showed a median OS of 5.2 months,[7] although multiple reports show an increased survival with current chemotherapeutic regimens.[10–12,15,16,77]

PC is usually detected late in the course of disease secondary to late presentation of symptoms and difficulty, with detection based on imaging techniques (computed tomography [CT], magnetic resonance imaging, or fluorodeoxyglucose positron emission tomography [FDG-PET]) and tumor markers. The only reliable means of detection is repeat laparotomy, but this operation cannot be justified in all patients with CRC. Attempts have been made to identify a high-risk group of patients who may benefit from CRS.[78–80] Patients with synchronous limited PC at initial operation, synchronous ovarian metastases, perforated primary tumors, and T4 lesions that required adjacent organ resection and emergency presentation for obstructing/bleeding lesions who underwent surgery have been identified as high-risk patients who may benefit from second-look surgery.[78] Sixty-two percent of patients with limited PC at presentation, 75% of patients with ovarian metastases, 15% of patients with perforated CRC, and 59% of patients with T4 lesions that required resection of adjacent organs develop PC.[5]

CRS and HIPEC initially were used as the treatment of appendiceal malignancy and malignant peritoneal mesothelioma.[81–83] In 2006, this procedure was declared the standard of care by the NCI for ovarian PC based on the results of a phase III study.[84] In the past decade, 2 RCTs, 1 nonrandomized comparative study, and 11 observational studies have been reported for CRCPC origin, and summarized (**Table 3**) in a comprehensive review article by Yan and colleagues.[46] Most of the patients from the nonrandomized reviews are incorporated into a 2004 summary of a multi-institutional registry from 28 international institutions for CRC.[3]

As discussed earlier, Verwaal and colleagues[2,61] performed an RCT of CRS and HIPEC versus systemic chemotherapy, which reported a significant OS benefit with increase in median survival of 22 months versus 12 months and 2-year survival of 44% versus 22%, respectively (**Fig. 4**). Even although this RCT shows a clear benefit, the systemic therapy used in that study, 5-FU/LV, is an outdated regimen compared with current treatment with FOLFOX or FOLFIRI. Regardless, patients who underwent intent-to-treat randomization and received CRC + HIPEC achieved a significant OS advantage ($P = .032$). For patients who received an R0 resection, the 2-year survival was 60%.

As mentioned earlier, diligent attempts have been made to accrue to an RCT with current regimens, but the trials failed to accrue secondary to patient unwillingness to be enrolled in the control arm, among other reasons. A trial at the NCI attempted to accrue patients to a trial comparing CRS with or without HIPEC, but this trial failed to accrue as well. CRS and HIPEC have been compared with hepatectomy for CRC metastases and liver transplantation as procedures adopted as standard of care without being compared with nonoperative standards of care in the context of RCTs.

Given the impact on survival with CRS and HIPEC, Elias and colleagues[78] performed a prospective study to analyze the outcomes with second-look laparotomy for patients at high risk for peritoneal recurrence. As stated earlier, high-risk included previous limited PC, resected ovarian metastases, and perforated primary lesions. All patients were clinically without evidence of disease based on symptoms, tumor markers, CT, and FDG-PET. Every patient had appropriate primary tumor resection with adjuvant FOLFOX or FOLFIRI as the current standard of care. Six months after chemotherapy (approximately 1 year after initial operation), second-look laparotomy was performed. Patients with detectable disease underwent CRS and HIPEC with both intraperitoneal oxaliplatin and irinotecan with IV 5-FU and LV.[78]

Macroscopic PC was found in 55% of the patients (16/29) who were asymptomatic with negative evaluation.[78] All of the patients with recurrence were treated with CRS and HIPEC. No postoperative mortality occurred. Postoperative complications occurred in 38% of the patients. Extra-abdominal complications included: grade 3 hematologic toxicity (n = 2); pneumonia (n = 2), central line infection (n = 1), and urinary tract infection (n = 4). Fourteen percent of patients (n = 2) required intra-abdominal abscess drainage. With a median follow-up of 27 months, of 16 patients with recurrent disease, 8 (50%) were without evidence of disease, 4 (25%) relapsed with PC (2 with distant metastases), and 4 (25%) developed visceral metastases. Most importantly, this study revealed that high-risk patients with CRS have recurrences that are detected only at laparotomy despite appropriate clinical, serum tumor marker, and diagnostic imaging surveillance.[78]

Cisplatin was the initial drug of choice for intraperitoneal administration both at the NCI and at other cancer centers.[85–88] However, cisplatin has been replaced by

Table 3
Summary of 2 RCTs, 1 nonrandomized comparative study, and 11 observational studies reported for PC of CRC origin

Treatment Center	Group	No. of Patients	Median Survival (mo)	Survival Rates (%)				NED (%)	AWD (%)	DFD (%)
				1-y	2-y	3-y	5-y			
Amsterdam[a,50]	IPHC	54	22	67	44	—	—	—	—	—
	No IPHC	51	13	56	22	—	—	—	—	—
Villejuif[33]	EPIC	16	—	—	60	—	—	—	—	—
	No EPIC	19	—	—	60	—	—	—	—	—
Uppsala[b,53]	EPIC	18	32	—	60	—	28	—	—	—
	No EPIC	18	14	—	10	—	5	—	—	—
Multi-institutional[30]	Overall	506	19	72	—	39	19	27	—	—
	CCR0	271	32	87	—	47	31	36	—	—
Washington[26]	CCR0	70	33	88	—	44	32	—	—	—
Lyon[28]	Overall	53	13	55	32	—	11	—	—	—
	CCR0	23	33	85	54	—	22	—	—	—
Villejuif[34]	CCR0	30	60	—	73	53	49	27	—	—
Amsterdam[40]	Overall	117	22	75	—	28	19	—	—	—
	CCR0	59	43	94	—	56	43	—	—	—
Winston-Salem[43]	Overall	77	16	56	—	25	17	32	—	—
	CCR0	37	28	77	—	42	35	—	—	—
Rome[45]	Overall	14	—	—	64	—	—	—	—	—
Columbus[46]	Overall	15	—	—	—	—	—	7	—	—
Padova[47]	Overall	46	18	—	31	—	—	9	17	48
Belgrade[48]	Overall	•18	15	—	—	—	—	56	17	17
Sydney[49]	Overall	30	29	72	64	—	—	—	—	—
	CCR0	21	—	85	71	—	—	—	—	—

Abbreviations: AWD, alive with disease; CCR0, patients with CCR included; overall, all patients included; DFD, died as a result of disease; EPIC, early postoperative intraperitoneal chemotherapy; IPHC, intraperitoneal hyperthermic chemotherapy; NED, no evidence of disease.

[a] P = .032.

[b] P = .01.

Data from Yan TD, Black D, Savady R, et al. Systematic review on the efficacy of cytoreductive surgery combined with perioperative intraperitoneal chemotherapy for peritoneal carcinomatosis from colorectal carcinoma. J Clin Oncol 2006;24:4011–9.

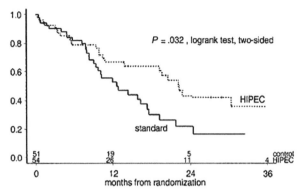

Fig. 4. Dutch RCT of CRS and HIPEC versus systemic chemotherapy and palliative surgery, which reported a significant OS benefit with increase in median survival of 22 months versus 12 months and 2-year survival of 44% versus 22%, in CRS + HIPEC versus systemic therapy and palliative surgery, respectively. (*From* Verwaal VJ, Ruth S, Bree E, et al. Randomized trial of cytoreduction and hyperthermic intraperitoneal chemotherapy versus systemic chemotherapy and palliative surgery in patients with peritoneal carcinomatosis of colorectal cancer. J Clin Oncol 2003;21(20):3741; with permission.)

oxaliplatin, a third-generation platinum complex with a diaminocyclohexane carrier group and an oxalate ligand, because the renal and hepatic toxicities seen with cisplatin rarely if ever occur with oxaliplatin. In addition, oxaliplatin has been shown to be more effective in CRC than cisplatin, and is currently the most studied intraperitoneal drug.[32,89,90] Oxaliplatin is also potentiated by hyperthermia and it works at all stages of cell division.[86,91] Oxaliplatin has shown major activity against CRC as a systemic agent.

Given that FOLFOX has the highest efficacy among various regimens for CRC, it has been used increasingly as an intraperitoneal regimen.[67,92] In addition, oxaliplatin has been tested and is used for ovarian and gastric carcinomatosis.

HIPEC WITH OXALIPLATIN

Several trials have been performed with intraperitoneal oxaliplatin. In 1 trial, the pharmacokinetics of heated intraperitoneal oxaliplatin were tested for 20 patients.[32] The trial by Elias and colleagues[89] established the dose of 460 mg/2L/m^2 without significant toxicity, including no neurotoxicity, nephrotoxicity, or neutropenia during phase I dose escalation. The tissue concentration studies revealed that at this dose, the bathed tissue concentration was 17.8-fold higher than the nonbathed tissue concentration and the peritoneal instillate concentration exceeded that of plasma 25-fold. Half the drug was absorbed in the first 40 minutes. The plasma concentration peaked at 30 minutes, then rapidly decreased (**Fig. 5**). Total volume of 2 L/m^2 was established and higher volumes led to decrease in concentration of the drug. This trial recommended doses of 5-FU (400 mg/m^2) and LV (20 mg/m^2) administered intravenously 20 minutes before HIPEC. A second trial studied the pharmacokinetics of oxaliplatin with hypo-osmotic solutions in 16 patients. Again, half the dose of oxaliplatin was absorbed within 40 minutes; however, no dosing changes were recommended (specifically, hypo-osmotic not recommended). A phase II study of 24 patients who received HIPEC with oxaliplatin showed an overall 2-year survival rate of 50%.[90] Another trial incorporated irinotecan, which increased the hematologic toxicities significantly and therefore was not used in this trial.[93]

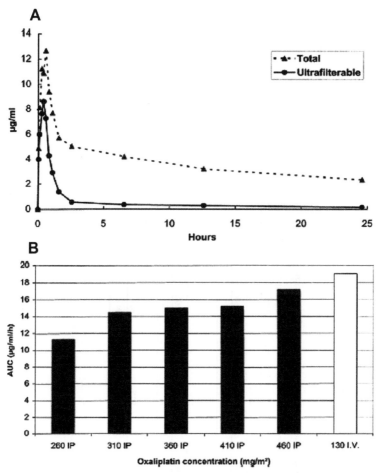

Fig. 5. Pharmacokinetics of intraperitoneal oxaliplatin. (*A*) Oxaliplatin pharmacokinetics in plasma after heated intraperitoneal chemotherapy. Oxaliplatin dose: 460 mg/m² in 21/m² of 5% dextrose. (*B*) Plasma AUC variations of ultrafiltered platinum versus peritoneal concentration of heated oxaliplatin. (*From* Elias D, Bonnay M, Puizillou JM, et al. Heated intraoperative intraperitoneal oxaliplatin after complete resection of peritoneal carcinomatosis: pharmacokinetics and tissue distribution. Ann Oncol 2002;13(2):270; with permission.)

MORBIDITY AND MORTALITY FOR HIPEC WITH OXALIPLATIN

Twenty consecutive patients in a phase I study[32] were evaluated for the HIPEC regimen proposed for in the NCI/National Institutes of Health RCT, Evaluating Mandatory Second Look Surgery with HIPEC and CRS Versus Standard of Care in Subjects at High Risk of Developing CRC Peritoneal Metastases (CC Protocol 10-C-0037A; P09582). No mortality occurred in the phase I study. Complications included intestinal fistulas (n = 2), percutaneous drainage of abscesses (n = 3), pneumonia (n = 3), urinary tract infection (n = 3), and central venous catheter infections (n = 2). Neither renal failure nor neutropenia occurred. However, using the same regimen for PC as in gastric cancer resulted in more than 50% postoperative neutropenia and thrombocytopenia at postoperative day number 5 (US/NCI experience). In the trial evaluating second-look surgery by

Table 4
Morbidity and mortality associated with CRS and intraperitoneal chemotherapy for PC of CRC origin

Treatment Center	No. of Patients	Morbidity (%)	Hematologic Toxicity (%)	Blood Loss (mm³)	Operation Time (h)	Reoperation (%)	Mortality (%)	Hospital Stay (d)
Amsterdam[50]	54	—	19	3900	8.1	—	8	29
Multi-institutional[39]	506	23	2.4	—	—	11	4	—
Lyon[28]	53	23	—	—	—	4	4	15
Villejuif[34]	30	37	—	940	7.6	—	0	—
Amsterdam[40]	117	—	—	—	—	—	6	—
Winston-Salem[43]	77	30	19	—	9.0	—	12	10
Columbus[46]	15	—	7	—	—	—	—	—
Padova[47]	46	35	9	—	7.7[a]	6	0	11[a]
Belgrade[48]	18	44	—	919	5.5	—	0	14[a]
Sydney[49]	30	43	—	—	9	10	0	21

[a] Mean.
Data from Yan TD, Black D, Savady R, et al. Systematic review on the efficacy of cytoreductive surgery combined with perioperative intraperitoneal chemotherapy for peritoneal carcinomatosis from colorectal carcinoma. J Clin Oncol 2006;24:4011–9.

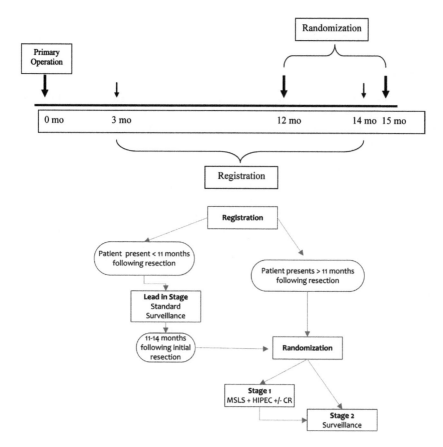

Fig. 6. Trial schema for RCT evaluating mandatory second-look surgery with HIPEC and CRS versus standard of care in subjects at high risk of developing colorectal peritoneal metastases. (*From* Ripley RT, Davis JL, Kemp CD, et al. Prospective randomized trial evaluating mandatory second look surgery with HIPEC and CRS vs standard of care in patients at high risk of developing colorectal peritoneal metastases. Trials 2010;11:62; with permission.)

Elias and colleagues,[78] mortality was 0% (0/20) and morbidity (grade II–IV) was 38%. Extra-abdominal complications (all grade II) were hematologic (n = 2), lung infections (n = 2), catheter-related infections (n = 1), and urinary tract infections (n = 4). Two patients required percutaneous drainage of intra-abdominal abscesses. Mean hospital stay was 16.4 days. Yan and colleagues[46] reviewed the available data for perioperative outcomes in studies evaluating efficacy of CRS combined with perioperative intraperitoneal chemotherapy for CRCPC (see **Table 3; Table 4**). Morbidity ranged from 23% to 44%. Hematologic toxicity ranged from 2% to 19%. Median operative blood loss was 940 mL to 3900 mL. Reoperation occurred in 4% to 11%. Overall mortality was 0% to 12%. In the study including irinotecan,[93] univariate analyses were performed for factors associated with grade 3 to 5 complications. Intra-abdominal complications were correlated with number of organs resected ($P = .07$), but not with anastomoses ($P = .54$), bulk of tumor (peritoneal score) ($P = .49$), duration of surgery ($P = .10$), or operative blood loss ($P = .55$). Extra-abdominal complications were correlated with number of resected organs ($P = .001$), peritoneal score ($P = .0008$), duration of surgery ($P = .0001$), and blood loss ($P = .0001$). QOL was reported in 2 studies by the same investigators.[94,95]

Nearly two-thirds of patients had a short-term decrease in QOL, but it returned to baseline within 3 to 6 months after surgery. Seventeen patients reported QOL at greater than 3 years, and more than 90% of patients had minimal to no limitations.

SUMMARY

For approximately 50% of patients who develop PC from CRC, a CCR0 resection (peritopneal carcinomatosis index [PCI] = 0) may potentially be curative. Patients with high-risk primary CRC have an incidence of PC greater than 50%, which cannot be detected preoperatively and at an early stage using standard imaging platforms. The NCI trialists hypothesized that conducting CRS and HIPEC when indicated to patients who are at high risk for recurrence of CRC at 1 year after curative resection will lead to improved survival compared with patients who receive standard of care follow-up. They anticipate that this situation will be seen in patients who have visible disease on laparotomy and undergo CRS and in patients with microscopic disease only who do not undergo CRS but receive HIPEC. This theory was the basis for the RCT evaluating mandatory second-look surgery with HIPEC and CRS versus standard of care in patients at high risk of developing CRC peritoneal metastases. The study can be summarized as outlined in **Fig. 6**; see **Table 4**):

Objectives

Primary objective

- To compare the OS of patients at high risk for developing CRCPC who undergo MSLS (mandatory second-look laparotomy) + HIPEC and CRS versus similar patients who receive standard of care

Secondary objectives

- To determine recurrence-free survival in both arms
- To investigate selection criteria for patients who might benefit from a strategy of MSLS with CRS + HIPEC

Eligibility

- Patients who have undergone curative resection for CRC, and who are at high risk for recurrence
- Patients who show no evidence of disease at the time of enrollment
- Patients with ECOG ≤0 to 2 and suitable candidates for laparotomy, HIPEC, and CRS

Design

- Patients with CRC at high risk for developing PC who underwent curative surgery and subsequently received standard of care and remained with no evidence of disease for 12 months after primary surgery will be randomized into MSLS/CRS/HIPEC or continuing standard of care.
- HIPEC will be performed using oxaliplatin/5-FU/LV.
- Up to 100 patients will be enrolled to allow for 35 evaluable patients in each arm; accrual is expected to last 5 years.

REFERENCES

1. Chua TC, Esquivel J, Pelz JO, et al. Summary of current therapeutic options for peritoneal metastases from colorectal cancer. J Surg Oncol 2012. [Epub ahead of print]. http://dx.doi.org/10.1002/jso.23189.

2. Verwaal V, Ruth S, Bree E, et al. Randomized trial of cytoreduction and hyperthermic intraperitoneal chemotherapy versus systemic chemotherapy and palliative surgery in patients with peritoneal carcinomatosis of colorectal cancer. J Clin Oncol 2003;21:3737–43.

3. Glehen O, Kwiatkowski F, Sugarbaker PH, et al. Cytoreductive surgery combined with perioperative intraperitoneal chemotherapy for the management of peritoneal carcinomatosis from colorectal cancer: a multi-institutional study. J Clin Oncol 2004;22:3284–92.

4. Chu DZ, Lang NP, Thompson C, et al. Peritoneal carcinomatosis in nongynecologic malignancy: a prospective study of prognostic factors. Cancer 1989; 63(2):364–7.

5. Jayne DG, Fook S, Loi C, et al. Peritoneal carcinomatosis from colorectal cancer. Br J Surg 2002;89:1545–50.

6. Brücher BL, Piso P, Verwaal V, et al. Peritoneal carcinomatosis: cytoreductive surgery and HIPEC–overview and basics. Cancer Invest 2012;30(3):209–24.

7. Sadeghi B, Arvieux C, Glehen O, et al. Peritoneal carcinomatosis from nongynecologic malignancies: results of the EVOCAPE 1 multicentric prospective study. Cancer 2000;88:58–63.

8. Jacquet P, Vidal-Jove J, Zhu B, et al. Peritoneal carcinomatosis from gastrointestinal malignancy: natural history and new prospects for management. Acta Chir Belg 1994;94(4):191–7.

9. Saltz LB, Cox JV, Blanke C, et al. Irinotecan plus fluorouracil and leucovorin for metastatic colorectal cancer. Irinotecan Study Group. N Engl J Med 2000; 343(13):905–14.

10. Douillard JY, Cunningham D, Roth AD, et al. Irinotecan combined with fluorouracil compared with fluorouracil alone as first-line treatment for metastatic colorectal cancer: a multicentre randomised trial. Lancet 2000;355(9209):1041–7.

11. Giacchetti S, Perpoint B, Zidani R, et al. Phase III multicenter randomized trial of oxaliplatin added to chronomodulated fluorouracil-leucovorin as first-line treatment of metastatic colorectal cancer. J Clin Oncol 2000;18(1):136–47.

12. Rothenberg ML, Oza AM, Bigelow RH, et al. Superiority of oxaliplatin and fluorouracil-leucovorin compared with either therapy alone in patients with progressive colorectal cancer after irinotecan and fluorouracil-leucovorin: interim results of a phase III trial. J Clin Oncol 2003;21(11):2059–69.

13. Goldberg RM, Sargent DJ, Morton RF, et al. A randomized controlled trial of fluorouracil plus leucovorin, irinotecan, and oxaliplatin combinations in patients with previously untreated metastatic colorectal cancer. J Clin Oncol 2004;22(1):23–30.

14. Tournigand C, Andre T, Achille E, et al. FOLFIRI followed by FOLFOX6 or the reverse sequence in advanced colorectal cancer: a randomized GERCOR study. J Clin Oncol 2004;22(2):229–37.

15. Hurwitz H, Fehrenbacher L, Novotny W, et al. Bevacizumab plus irinotecan, fluorouracil, and leucovorin for metastatic colorectal cancer. N Engl J Med 2004; 350(23):2335–42.

16. Colucci G, Gebbia V, Paoletti G, et al. Phase III randomized trial of FOLFIRI versus FOLFOX4 in the treatment of advanced colorectal cancer: a multicenter study of the Gruppo Oncologico Dell'Italia Meridionale. J Clin Oncol 2005;23(22):4866–75.

17. Goldberg RM, Sargent DJ, Morton RF, et al. Randomized controlled trial of reduced-dose bolus fluorouracil plus leucovorin and irinotecan or infused fluorouracil plus leucovorin and oxaliplatin in patients with previously untreated metastatic colorectal cancer: a North American Intergroup Trial. J Clin Oncol 2006; 24(21):3347–53.

18. Willet CG, Tepper JE, Cohen AM, et al. Failure patterns following curative resection of colonic carcinoma. Surgery 1984;200:685–90.
19. Eggermont AM, Steller EP, Sugarbaker PH. Laparotomy enhances intraperitoneal tumor growth and abrogates the antitumor effects of IL-2 and lymphokine-activated killer cells. Surgery 1987;102:71–8.
20. Averbach AM, Jacquet P, Sugarbaker PH. Surgical technique and colorectal cancer: impact on local recurrence and survival. Tumori 1995;81:65–71.
21. Schott A, Vogel I, Krueger U, et al. Isolated tumor cells are frequently detected in peritoneal cavity of gastric and colonic cancer patients and serve as a new prognostic marker. Ann Surg 1998;227:372–9.
22. Carmignani CP, Sugarbaker TA, Bromley CM, et al. Intraperitoneal cancer dissemination: mechanisms of the patterns of spread. Cancer Metastasis Rev 2003;22:465–72.
23. Glehen O, Osinsky D, Beaujard AC, et al. Natural history of peritoneal carcinomatosis from nongynecologic malignancies. Surg Oncol Clin North Am 2003;12:729–39.
24. Loggie BW, Fleming RA, McQuellon RP, et al. Cytoreductive surgery with intraperitoneal chemotherapy for disseminated peritoneal cancer of gastrointestinal origin. Am Surg 2000;66(6):561–8.
25. Stewart JH, Shen P, Levine EA. Intraperitoneal hyperthermic chemotherapy for peritoneal surface malignancy: current status and future directions. Ann Surg Oncol 2005;12(10):756–77.
26. Speyer JL, Collins JM, Dedrick RL, et al. Phase I and pharmacological studies of 5-fluorouracil administrated intraperitoneally. Cancer Res 1980;40:567–72.
27. Flessner MF, Dedrick RL, Schultz JS. A distributed model of peritoneal-plasma transport: analysis of experimental data in the rat. Am J Physiol 1985;248:F413–24.
28. Dedrick RL. Theoretical and experimental basis of intraperitoneal chemotherapy. Semin Oncol 1985;12(3 Suppl 4):1–6.
29. Dedrick RL. Interspecies scaling of regional drug delivery. J Pharm Sci 1986;75:1047–52.
30. Kuzuya T, Yamauchi M, Ito A, et al. Pharmacokinetic characteristics of 5-flourourcil and mitomycin C in intraperitoneal chemotherapy. J Pharm Pharmacol 1994;46:685–9.
31. Dedrick RL, Flessner MF. Pharmacokinetic problems in peritoneal drug administration: tissue penetration and surface exposure. J Natl Cancer Inst 1997;89:480–7.
32. Elias D, Bonnay M, Puizillou JM, et al. Heated intra-operative intraperitoneal oxaliplatin after complete resection of peritoneal carcinomatosis: pharmacokinetics and tissue distribution. Ann Oncol 2002;13(2):267–72.
33. Elias D, Matsuhisa T, Sideris L, et al. Heated intra-operative intraperitoneal oxaliplatin plus irinotecan after complete resection of peritoneal carcinomatosis: pharmacokinetics, tissue distribution and tolerance. Ann Oncol 2004;15(10):1558–65.
34. Sugarbaker PH, Stuart OA, Carmignani CP. Pharmacokinetic changes induced by the volume of chemotherapy solution in patients treated with hyperthermic intraperitoneal mitomycin C. Cancer Chemother Pharmacol 2006;57(5):703–8.
35. Sugarbaker PH, Graves T, DeBruijn EA, et al. Rationale for early postoperative intraperitoneal chemotherapy (EPIC) in patients with advanced gastrointestinal cancer. Cancer Res 1990;50:5790–4.
36. Katz M, Barone R. The rationale of perioperative intraperitoneal chemotherapy in the treatment of peritoneal surface malignancies. Surg Oncol Clin North Am 2003;12:673–88.
37. Teicher BA, Kowal CD, Kennedy KA, et al. Enhancement by hyperthermia of the in vitro cytotoxicity of mitomycin C toward hypoxic tumor cells. Cancer Res 1981;41(3):1096–9.

38. El-Kareh AW, Secomb TW. A theoretical model for intraperitoneal delivery of cisplatin and the effect of hyperthermia on drug penetration distance. Neoplasia 2004;6(2):117–27.

39. VanderWaal R, Thampy G, Wright WD, et al. Heat-induced modifications in the association of specific proteins with the nuclear matrix. Radiat Res 1996; 145(6):746–53.

40. Roti Roti JL, Kampinga HH, Malyapa RS, et al. Nuclear matrix as a target for hyperthermic killing of cancer cells. Cell Stress Chaperones 1998;3(4):245–55.

41. Pelz JO, Doerfer J, Hohenberger W, et al. A new survival model for hyperthermic intraperitoneal chemotherapy (HIPEC) in tumor-bearing rats in the treatment of peritoneal carcinomatosis. BMC Cancer 2005;5(1):56.

42. van Ruth S, Verwaal VJ, Hart AA, et al. Heat penetration in locally applied hyperthermia in the abdomen during intra-postoperative hyperthermic intraperitoneal chemotherapy. Anticancer Res 2003;23:1501–8.

43. Kerr DJ, Kaye SB. Aspects of cytotoxic drug penetration, with particular reference to anthracyclines. Cancer Chemother Pharmacol 1987;19:1–5.

44. Los G, Mutsaers PH, van der Vijgh WJ, et al. Direct diffusion of cis-diamminedichloroplatinum(II) in intraperitoneal rat tumors after intraperitoneal chemotherapy: a comparison with systemic chemotherapy. Cancer Res 1989; 49:3380–4.

45. Zoetmulder FA. Cancer cell seeding during abdominal surgery: experimental studies. In: Sugarbaker PH, editor. Peritoneal carcinomatosis: principles of management. Boston: Kluwer Academic Press; 1996. p. 155–62.

46. Yan TD, Black D, Savady R, et al. Systematic review on the efficacy of cytoreductive surgery combined with perioperative intraperitoneal chemotherapy for peritoneal carcinomatosis from colorectal carcinoma. J Clin Oncol 2006;24:4011–9.

47. Hahn GM, Braun J, Har-Kedar I. Thermochemotherapy: synergism between hyperthermia (42–43 degrees) and adriamycin (of bleomycin) in mammalian cell inactivation. Proc Natl Acad Sci U S A 1975;72:937–40.

48. Barlogie B, Corry PM, Drewinko B. In vitro thermochemotherapy of human colon cancer cells with cis-dichlorodiammineplatinum (II) and mitomycin C. Cancer Res 1980;40:1165–8.

49. Fujimura T, Yonemura Y, Fujita H, et al. Chemohyperthermic peritoneal perfusion for peritoneal dissemination in various intraabdominal malignancies. Int Surg 1999;84:60–6.

50. Cavaliere F, Perri P, Di Filippo F, et al. Treatment of peritoneal carcinomatosis with intent to cure. J Surg Oncol 2000;74:41–4.

51. Pestieau SR, Sugarbaker PH. Treatment of primary colon cancer with peritoneal carcinomatosis: comparison of concomitant vs delayed management. Dis Colon Rectum 2000;43:1341–6.

52. Beaujard AC, Glehen O, Caillot JL, et al. Intraperitoneal chemohyperthermia with mitomycin C for digestive tract cancer patients with peritoneal carcinomatosis. Cancer 2000;88:2512–9.

53. Culliford A, Brooks AD, Sharma S, et al. Surgical debulking and intraperitoneal chemotherapy for established peritoneal metastases from colon and appendix cancer. Ann Surg Oncol 2001;8:787–95.

54. Elias D, Blot F, El Otmany A, et al. Curative treatment of peritoneal carcinomatosis arising from colorectal cancer by complete resection and intraperitoneal chemotherapy. Cancer 2001;92:71–6.

55. Witkamp AJ, de Bree E, Kaag MM, et al. Extensive cytoreductive surgery followed by intra-operative hyperthermic intraperitoneal chemotherapy with

mitomycin-C in patients with peritoneal carcinomatosis of colorectal origin. Eur J Cancer 2001;37:979–84.

56. Cavaliere F, Perri P, Rossi CR, et al. Indications for integrated surgical treatment of peritoneal carcinomatosis of colorectal origin: experience of the Italian Society of Locoregional Integrated Therapy in Oncology. Tumori 2003;89:21–3.

57. Pilati P, Mocellin S, Rossi CR, et al. Cytoreductive surgery combined with hyperthermic intraperitoneal intraoperative chemotherapy for peritoneal carcinomatosis arising from colon adenocarcinoma. Ann Surg Oncol 2003;10:508–13.

58. Shen P, Levine EA, Hall J, et al. Factors predicting survival after intraperitoneal hyperthermic chemotherapy with mitomycin C after cytoreductive surgery for patients with peritoneal carcinomatosis. Arch Surg 2003;138:26–33.

59. Elias D, Pocard M. Treatment and prevention of peritoneal carcinomatosis from colorectal cancer. Surg Oncol Clin North Am 2003;12:543–59.

60. Glehen O, Mithieux F, Osinsky D, et al. Surgery combined with peritonectomy procedures and intraperitoneal chemohyperthermia in abdominal cancers with peritoneal carcinomatosis: a phase II study. J Clin Oncol 2003;21:799–806.

61. Verwaal VJ, van Ruth S, Witkamp A, et al. Long-term survival of peritoneal carcinomatosis of colorectal origin. Ann Surg Oncol 2005;12(1):65–71.

62. Glehen O, Cotte E, Schreiber V, et al. Intraperitoneal chemohyperthermia and attempted cytoreductive surgery in patients with peritoneal carcinomatosis of colorectal origin. Br J Surg 2004;91:747–54.

63. Elias D, Lefevre JH, Chevalier J, et al. Complete cytoreductive surgery plus intraperitoneal chemohyperthermia with oxaliplatin for peritoneal carcinomatosis of colorectal origin. J Clin Oncol 2009;27(5):681–5.

64. American Cancer Society. Cancer facts & figures. 2006. Available at: http://www.cancer.org. Accessed June 15, 2012.

65. Meta-Analysis Group in Cancer. Modulation of fluorouracil in patients with advanced colorectal cancer: an updated meta-analysis. J Clin Oncol 2004;22:3766–75.

66. Kohne CH, van Cutsem E, Wills J, et al. Phase III study of weekly high-dose infusional fluorouracil plus folinic acid with or without irinotecan in patients with metastatic colorectal cancer: European Organisation for Research and Treatment of Cancer Gastrointestinal Group Study 40986. J Clin Oncol 2005;23(22):4856–65.

67. de Gramont A, Figer A, Seymour M, et al. Leucovorin and fluorouracil with or without oxaliplatin as first-line treatment in advanced colorectal cancer. J Clin Oncol 2000;18(16):2938–47.

68. Fuchs C, Marshall J, Mitchell E, et al. A randomized trial of first-line irinotecan/fluoropyrimidine combinations with or without celecoxib in metastatic colorectal cancer (BICC-C). J Clin Oncol 2006;24(18S):3506 [2006 ASCO Annual Meeting Proceedings Part I].

69. Hochster HS, Hart LL, Ramanathan RK, et al. Safety and efficacy of oxaliplatin/fluoropyrimidine regimens with or without bevacizumab as first-line treatment of metastatic colorectal cancer (mCRC): final analysis of the TREE-Study. J Clin Oncol 2006;24(18S):3510 [2006 ASCO Annual Meeting Proceedings Part I].

70. Giantonio B, Catalano D, Meropol NJ, et al. High-dose bevacizumab improves survival when combined with FOLFOX4 in previously treated advanced colorectal cancer: results from the Eastern Cooperative Oncology Group study E3200. J Clin Oncol 2005;23(16S):2 [2005 ASCO Annual Meeting Proceedings].

71. National Comprehensive Cancer Network Clinical Practice Guidelines in Oncology. Colon Cancer. Version.1.2007. Available at: http://www.nccn.org/professionals/physician_gls/PDF/colon.pdf. Accessed June 15, 2012.

72. Wallner KE, Banda M, Li GC. Hyperthermic enhancement of cell killing by mitomycin C in mitomycin C-resistant Chinese hamster ovary cells. Cancer Res 1987;47:1308–12.
73. Shen P, Hawksworth J, Lovato J, et al. Cytoreductive surgery and intraperitoneal hyperthermic chemotherapy with mitomycin C for peritoneal carcinomatosis from nonappendiceal colorectal carcinoma. Ann Surg Oncol 2004;11(2):178–86.
74. Elias D, Delperro JR, Sideris L, et al. Treatment of peritoneal carcinomatosis from colorectal cancer: impact of complete cytoreductive surgery and difficulties in conducting randomized trials. Ann Surg Oncol 2004;11:518–21.
75. Yan TD, Morris DL. Cytoreductive surgery and perioperative intraperitoneal chemotherapy for isolated colorectal peritoneal carcinomatosis: experimental therapy or standard of care? Ann Surg 2008;248(5):829–35.
76. Jemal A, Siegel R, Ward E, et al. Cancer statistics. CA Cancer J Clin 2008;58(2):71–96.
77. Hurwitz HI, Fehrenbacher L, Hainsworth JD, et al. Bevacizumab in combination with fluorouracil and leucovorin: an active regimen for first-line metastatic colorectal cancer. J Clin Oncol 2005;23(15):3502–8.
78. Elias D, Goere D, Di Pietrantonio D, et al. Results of systematic second-look surgery in patients at high risk of developing colorectal peritoneal carcinomatosis. Ann Surg 2008;247(3):445–50.
79. Willett C, Tepper JE, Cohen A, et al. Obstructive and perforative colonic carcinoma: patterns of failure. J Clin Oncol 1985;3(3):379–84.
80. Slanetz CA Jr. The effect of inadvertent intraoperative perforation on survival and recurrence in colorectal cancer. Dis Colon Rectum 1984;27(12):792–7.
81. Sugarbaker PH, Graves T, DeBruijn EA, et al. Early postoperative intraperitoneal chemotherapy as an adjuvant therapy to surgery for peritoneal carcinomatosis from gastrointestinal cancer: pharmacological studies. Cancer Res 1990;50(18):5790–4.
82. Sugarbaker PH. New standard of care for appendiceal epithelial neoplasms and pseudomyxoma peritonei syndrome? Lancet Oncol 2006;7(1):69–76.
83. Feldman AL, Libutti SK, Pingpank JF, et al. Analysis of factors associated with outcome in patients with malignant peritoneal mesothelioma undergoing surgical debulking and intraperitoneal chemotherapy. J Clin Oncol 2003;21(24):4560–7.
84. Armstrong DK, Bundy B, Wenzel L, et al. Intraperitoneal cisplatin and paclitaxel in ovarian cancer. N Engl J Med 2006;354(1):34–43.
85. Elias D, Antoun S, Goharin A, et al. Research on the best chemohyperthermia technique of treatment of peritoneal carcinomatosis after complete resection. Int J Surg Investig 2000;1(5):431–9.
86. Elias D, Detroz B, Debaene B, et al. Treatment of peritoneal carcinomatosis by intraperitoneal chemo-hyperthermia: reliable and unreliable concepts. Hepatogastroenterology 1994;41(3):207–13.
87. Sugarbaker PH. Intraperitoneal chemotherapy and cytoreductive surgery for the prevention and treatment of peritoneal carcinomatosis and sarcomatosis. Semin Surg Oncol 1998;14(3):254–61.
88. Yonemura Y, Fujimura T, Nishimura G, et al. Effects of intraoperative chemohyperthermia in patients with gastric cancer with peritoneal dissemination. Surgery 1996;119(4):437–44.
89. Elias D, El Otmany A, Bonnay M, et al. Human pharmacokinetic study of heated intraperitoneal oxaliplatin in increasingly hypotonic solutions after complete resection of peritoneal carcinomatosis. Oncology 2002;63(4):346–52.

90. Elias D, Sideris L, Pocard M, et al. Efficacy of intraperitoneal chemohyperthermia with oxaliplatin in colorectal peritoneal carcinomatosis. Preliminary results in 24 patients. Ann Oncol 2004;15(5):781–5.

91. Rietbroek RC, van der Vaart PJ, Haveman J, et al. Hyperthermia enhances the cytotoxicity and platinum-DNA adduct formation of lobaplatin and oxaliplatin in cultured SW 1573 cells. J Cancer Res Clin Oncol 1997;123(1):6–12.

92. Becouarn Y, Ychou M, Ducreux M, et al. Phase II trial of oxaliplatin as first-line chemotherapy in metastatic colorectal cancer patients. Digestive Group of French Federation of Cancer Centers. J Clin Oncol 1998;16(8):2739–44.

93. Elias D, Goere D, Blot F, et al. Optimization of hyperthermic intraperitoneal chemotherapy with oxaliplatin plus irinotecan at 43 degrees C after compete cytoreductive surgery: mortality and morbidity in 106 consecutive patients. Ann Surg Oncol 2007;14(6):1818–24.

94. McQuellon RP, Loggie BW, Fleming RA, et al. Quality of life after intraperitoneal hyperthermic chemotherapy (IPHC) for peritoneal carcinomatosis. Eur J Surg Oncol 2001;27(1):65–73.

95. McQuellon RP, Loggie BW, Lehman AB, et al. Long-term survivorship and quality of life after cytoreductive surgery plus intraperitoneal hyperthermic chemotherapy for peritoneal carcinomatosis. Ann Surg Oncol 2003;10(2):155–62.

Early Intervention for Treatment and Prevention of Colorectal Carcinomatosis
A Plan for Individualized Care

Paul H. Sugarbaker, MD, FRCS

KEYWORDS

- Cytoreductive surgery • HIPEC • Colorectal cancer • Carcinomatosis
- Intraperitoneal chemotherapy • Second look surgery

KEY POINTS

- Peritoneal metastases from colorectal cancer can be cured, similar to lymph nodal metastases, liver metastases, and pulmonary metastases.
- The extent of disease, in large part, determines the success that can be expected with cytoreductive surgery and perioperative chemotherapy treatments.
- Cytoreductive surgery and hyperthermic intraperitoneal chemotherapy can be used as part of the management of primary colorectal cancer presenting with peritoneal metastases.
- The hyperthermic intraperitoneal chemotherapy treatments must evolve so that they are capable of preserving the surgical complete response that is achieved with cytoreductive surgery.

INTRODUCTION

Currently, the standard of care for advanced primary colorectal cancer involves treatments that are nearly identical for all patients. A routine surgery is followed by a routine systemic chemotherapy. A routine follow-up by physical examination and computed tomography (CT) then occurs. If symptoms or CT findings suggest a localized recurrence, a palliative surgery is followed by second-line chemotherapy. This plan fails to recognize that the primary disease is a complex process and that the anatomic sites of initial treatment failure vary greatly between individuals **Fig. 1** diagrams the directions for metastases when primary surgery fails. The goal of this report is to establish new guidelines for the individualized management of those patients who are likely to have progression of resection site disease and/or carcinomatosis as the initial site of treatment failure.

The author has nothing to disclose.
Program in Peritoneal Surface Malignancy, Washington Cancer Institute, 106 Irving Street, Northwest, Suite 3900, Washington, DC 20010, USA
E-mail address: Paul.Sugarbaker@medstar.net

Surg Oncol Clin N Am 21 (2012) 689–703
http://dx.doi.org/10.1016/j.soc.2012.07.009
1055-3207/12/$ – see front matter
surgonc.theclinics.com

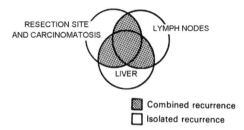

RESECTION SITE
AND CARCINOMATOSIS

LYMPH NODES

LIVER

▨ Combined recurrence
☐ Isolated recurrence

Fig. 1. Treatment failures in the surgical treatment of primary colorectal cancer. Ring diagram shows that hematogenous metastases and cancer seeding can occur in isolation or in combination with other sites of surgical treatment failure. High-density seeding at the resection site causes a layering of cancer; low-density seeding at a distance results in peritoneal carcinomatosis. *From* Sugarbaker PH. Second-look surgery for colorectal cancer: revised selection factors and new treatment options for greater success. Int J Surg Oncol 2011;2011:915,078. Epub 2010 Dec 5.

RATIONALE FOR A NEW STRATEGY OF EARLY INTERVENTION

The combination of cytoreductive surgery with perioperative chemotherapy has become a treatment option for selected patients with peritoneal dissemination of colorectal cancer.[1] It is well documented that the results of treatment vary greatly with the clinical status of the patient. Quantitative prognostic indicators have been established that allow the oncologist to inform the patient regarding the likelihood of long-term benefit.[2] One of these prognostic indicators is the completeness of cytoreduction (CC) score; for colorectal cancer a complete cytoreduction indicates that the surgery was effective in clearing all visible evidence of disease (CC-0) or left behind only a few minute deposits of cancer that are expected to be eradicated by perioperative local-regional chemotherapy (CC-1). Complete cytoreduction includes both CC-0 and CC-1 cytoreduction. A necessary (but not sufficient) requirement for long-term benefit is complete cytoreduction. A potentially curative treatment for colorectal peritoneal dissemination does not occur in the absence of a complete cytoreduction.[3]

A second useful quantitative prognostic indicator is the peritoneal cancer index (PCI). This prognostic indicator scores both the distribution and extent of carcinomatosis in 13 abdominal and pelvic regions to arrive at a quantitative assessment of the extent of carcinomatosis.[2] The PCI predicts the likelihood of an incomplete cytoreduction; also, it predicts long-term survival even though the cytoreduction is complete.[4] A low PCI, indicating a limited extent of carcinomatosis, is associated with an improved prognosis. Elias and colleagues, in a French collaborative study of 523 patients, reported a 50% survival rate at 5 years with PCI of 6 or less, 27% rate with PCI between 7 and 19, and less than 10% rate with PCI greater than 19. He suggested that an attempt at complete cytoreduction with a PCI greater than 20 should occur only under special circumstances, such as a young and fit patient.[5]

These 2 prognostic indicators taken together indicate that the extent of carcinomatosis has a profound effect on the outcome when this manifestation of metastatic disease is treated with cytoreductive surgery and perioperative chemotherapy. A reliable concept worthy of pursuit states that the likelihood of long-term survival will continue to improve as extent of disease as measured by PCI decreases. The clinical correlate of this concept is that definitive treatment early in the natural history of carcinomatosis can be expected to optimize survival benefit.

Support for this concept of early intervention with a small volume of carcinomatosis can be found in the oncology literature.[6] Recently, Elias and colleagues reported on a new plan for early intervention in patients with a high risk for local-regional recurrence after primary colon cancer surgery with small volume peritoneal seeding, ovarian metastases, or perforation through the primary cancer.[7] After treatment with systemic chemotherapy, the patients were taken back to the operating room for a "systematic second look surgery." Return for reoperation occurred within 1 year. At exploration, Elias found cancer present in 16 (55%) of the 29 patients who had repeat surgical intervention. All patients with progressive disease were treated with cytoreductive surgery and perioperative intraperitoneal chemotherapy. At 27-month median follow-up, the survival of patients with cancer found at second look was 50%. The high incidence of prolonged survival in this group of patients with early definitive intervention supports the concept of maximal benefit in patients with minimal disease.

This concept of increasing benefits with reduced extent of disease may be a valid concept throughout oncology. It is the basic hypothesis that drives the TNM system. Certainly, it operates definitively with colorectal liver metastases. The greater the number of deposits resected from the liver, the poorer is the prognosis; this is true even though an R0 liver resection is achieved.[8] Perhaps it is not surprising that this concept of increasing benefits with a lesser extent of disease is important for interpreting the results of treatment with colorectal carcinomatosis.

An important clinical question concerns the rational application of this concept to the management of colorectal cancer, especially patients with carcinomatosis. Currently, the results of treatment of a population of carcinomatosis patients are guarded – often not accepted, because the risks of treatment are perceived to exceed its benefits. In current practice, these patients must submit to a major surgical intervention with an extended hospitalization and long convalescence. Unfortunately, within a few months or years, a majority (estimated at 70%) recur within the abdomen or pelvis, have no further treatment options, and go on to die.

If cytoreductive surgery and perioperative hyperthermic chemotherapy represent an accepted treatment modality, and the author believes that it is, then its application should be modified to maximize benefits. It is possible that the concept of early intervention for carcinomatosis treatment can be brought into the management strategies for colorectal carcinomatosis. This can be done by integrating the concepts of second-look surgery, treatments with cytoreductive surgery and perioperative intraperitoneal chemotherapy, and risk of local-regional disease progression.

HISTORICAL REVIEW OF SECOND-LOOK SURGERY FOR COLORECTAL CANCER

In 1948, Wangensteen at the University of Minnesota initiated a new plan he hoped would improve the management of intra-abdominal cancer.[9] He reasoned that surgery was the only effective tool by which to cure primary gastrointestinal cancer; therefore, more radical cancer surgery could be an adjuvant treatment used to extirpate isolated sites of disease progression and thereby improve survival. He identified lymph node–positive disease at the time of primary cancer resection as an indication for a systematic plan of reoperation. In selected patients at 6- to 8-month intervals, surgical reexploration of the abdomen and pelvis was performed. Reoperations were scheduled until no cancer was found or until the disease was beyond surgical control. Initially, patients were only taken to surgery in an asymptomatic state; however, as the clinical results from the reoperative treatment strategies evolved, patients with symptoms from recurrent disease were included in the series.

Table 1 presents the results of second-look surgery for colon cancer after 20 years of data accumulation. In 36 patients who had Cancer progression documented

Table 1
Second-look surgery in patients with cancer of the colon

	Second-Look Negative	Second-Look Positive	Symptomatic Look
Number of patients	62	36	47
Operative deaths	2%–3.2%[a]	6%–17%	7%–15%
Recurrent cancer[b]	12%–19%	24%–67%	33%–70%
Living and well, last look negative	41	4	4
Living and well, last look positive	–	0	3
Living with residual	1	0	0
Dead from other than cancer	10	2	0
Total converted	–	6%–17%	7%–15%

[a] One patient had residual cancer and died at fifth look.
[b] Considered failures in negative-look group.
  Data from Griffen WO, Humphrey L, Sosin H. The prognosis and management of recurrent abdominal malignancies. Curr Probl Surg 1969;1–43.

(positive second look), 6 (17%) patients were "converted" from a second look positive to a long-term disease-free status. In 47 patients who had a symptomatic second look, 7 (15%) patients were converted by reoperative surgery to long-term survival. In their review of these data from the second-look approach, Griffin and colleagues concluded that "significant patient survival resulted from the second look approach in patients with cancer of the colon. This effort should be continued and extended."[10]

Benefits for patients "converted" from a positive second look to long-term survival were offset, at least in part, by the impact this management plan had on the entire group of patients. Extensive surgical procedures to remove recurrent disease led to an operative mortality of 17% in the patients who had a positive second look. Also, in the patients with the symptomatic second look, there was a 15% operative mortality. In interpreting these mortality statistics, one must realize that this high operative mortality occurred in patients identified as having progressive disease. These patients would presumably have gone on to die of this disease in the near future. However, their lives were cut short as a result of the second-look surgery.

Perhaps most worrisome for the surgeon performing planned second-look procedures were the 2 (3.2%) patients who died postoperatively after a negative exploration. These patients dying with a negative second-look result may have been long-term survivors in the absence of this aggressive surgical treatment strategy.

There have been efforts to expand the indications for second-look surgery. In the mid-1970s, a collaborative effort of the Peter Bent Brigham Hospital and the Mallory Gastrointestinal Laboratory searched for clinical relationships between the carcinoembryonic antigen (CEA) and the natural history of surgically treated colorectal cancer. Sugarbaker and colleagues determined that serial CEA assays determined at 3-month intervals after a colon or rectal cancer resection would detect occult recurrent disease approximately 6 months before clinical signs and symptoms.[11] These results led to a clinical study to use CEA as a surveillance test for recurrent colon or rectal cancer after a potentially curative cancer resection. Steele and colleagues reported on a prospective study of 75 patients who had CEA assays performed at approximately 2-month intervals. Fifteen of 18 tumor recurrences were first diagnosed by increasing CEA values despite no other evidence of progressive disease. In 4 of these 15 patients, complete resection of recurrent cancer with a potential for cure was reported. Long-term follow-up of the total number of patients "converted" from recurrent disease to long-term survival was not available.[12]

Attiyeh and Sterns presented data on 32 patients who underwent second-look surgery for "a significant CEA elevation" following a curative resection for adenocarcinoma of the large bowel.[13] The total number of patients from whom these 32 with an increasing CEA blood test were selected was not available. These 32 patients underwent a total of 37 exploratory procedures with 16 (43%) of 37 potentially curative resections. Again, the number of patients "converted" from recurrent disease to long-term survival was not available from this report.

Additional data regarding the possible benefits of second look surgery in colorectal cancer patients comes from the prospective evaluation of this strategy reported in 1985.[14] Minton and colleagues initiated a multi-institutional study. They prospectively collected data on 400 patients operated on at 31 different institutions. Their results emphasize that the surgeons performing the second-look surgery had advanced training in reoperative surgery. These 400 patients had 43 CEA-directed reoperations and 32 symptomatic second-look reoperations. At 5 years after the second-look surgery, 22 (29%) of 75 patients remained disease free. Minton and colleagues, as a result of their study, recommended meticulous clinical surveillance of Dukes' stage C2 cancer following primary colorectal cancer resection, CEA determinations at 1- to 2-month intervals postoperatively, and second-look surgery before serial CEA testing exceeded 11 ng/mL.

As a result of these efforts to use postoperative monitoring of CEA in patients at high risk for recurrence of colon and rectal cancer, a standard of practice has evolved in patients surgically treated for colorectal cancer. If a progressive increase in the CEA blood test occurs, patients should be considered for reoperation. Radiologic tests should be performed to show that the elevated CEA determination occurs in the absence of systemic disease or unresectable disease within the abdomen or pelvis. Minton and colleagues should be credited with establishing a strong rationale for meticulous follow-up of patients with colorectal cancer and a reasonable likelihood of benefit from second-look surgery.

Goldberg and coworkers collected data in a prospective follow-up of 1247 patients with resected stage 2 or stage 3 colon cancer[15]; 548 patients had recurrence of colon cancer and second-look surgery was attempted in 222 (41%) patients. In 109 (20%) patients, potentially curative surgery resulted. In patients who came to curative intent second-look surgery, recurrent disease was identified by radiologic follow-up in 36 patients, serial CEA tests in 41 patients, and symptoms in 27 patients. The 5-year disease-free survival of these 109 patients was 23%. The surgical mortality was 2%. These authors concluded that early reoperation as a result of careful postoperative follow-up testing of patients with colon cancer may identify recurrent disease in some and that the second-look surgery can result in a long-term disease-free survival.

PATHOBIOLOGY OF COLORECTAL CANCER RECURRENCE AFTER SURGICAL RESECTION

Sugarbaker and coworkers suggested that peritoneal carcinomatosis and local failure are caused by the same mechanism.[16,17] Surgical trauma causing dissemination of cancer cells from the primary malignancy is an unfortunate but common occurrence with the cancer resection. Free intracoelomic cancer cells can result from surgical trauma to the primary tumor, blood or lymph contaminated by cancer cells being spilled into the resection site or free peritoneal cavity, or cancer cells disseminated before or at the time of cancer resection from full-thickness invasion of the bowel wall. These spilled cancer cells can accumulate at the resection site, usually in high density, and result in local recurrence. They can accumulate at lower density at distant sites within the peritoneal cavity as peritoneal carcinomatosis. For example, in a rectal cancer, the hollow of the sacrum would be favored by gravity for accumulation of the largest number of cancer cells. Consequently, if the primary rectal cancer is traumatized during its resection, the patient will suffer a local recurrence. The confines of the pelvis make full exposure difficult so that surgical trauma to the primary cancer is a great danger. Only a few cells may escape from the traumatized primary cancer but they would be expected to adhere, implant, and then vascularize within the adjacent tissues. By this theory, the resection site of a cancer is at great risk for progressive disease.

However, not all the cancer cells disseminated from the primary malignancy must implant locally. Some may gain access to the free peritoneal cavity. Cancer cells within intraperitoneal blood clot may later become manifest as recurrences within abdominal adhesions. Free cancer cells will move along with peritoneal fluid to distant sites such as the pelvis, beneath the right hemidiaphragm, or in the right and left paracolic sulci. With small amounts of intraperitoneal fluid, peritoneal seeding may be restricted to structures proximal to the resection site. With larger amounts of ascites fluid or with mucinous cancer cells, distant spread of carcinomatosis will occur.[17]

It is known that cancer cells may enter the portal venous system and cause liver metastases. Similarly, cancer cells present within venous blood spilled at the time of primary cancer resection may find their way into the free peritoneal cavity. These free cancer cells may cause resection site recurrence and/or carcinomatosis.

CYTOREDUCTIVE SURGERY AND HYPERTHERMIC INTRAPERITONEAL CHEMOTHERAPY AS NEW TREATMENT OPTIONS AVAILABLE FOR SECOND-LOOK SURGERY

Second-look surgery may have a greater likelihood of success now than in the past. The knowledgeable use of systemic chemotherapy has reduced the proportion of patients who die as a result of progression of systemic micrometastatic disease. The surgical technology for liver resection of colorectal metastases has evolved during the past 2 decades; liver secondary tumors are resected if the patient can be made clinically disease-free by liver surgery with minimal morbidity and almost no mortality.[18] Also, surgical technologies for complete removal of local recurrence and peritoneal seeding within the abdomen and pelvis have become available. The combination of visceral resections, peritonectomy procedures, and hyperthermic intraperitoneal chemotherapy offers a treatment option that may be successful in as many as 50% of patients with carcinomatosis.[1,3,5,19] As established earlier in this report, the more limited the extent of carcinomatosis, the greater is the benefit from definitive treatment.

Extended lymph node dissections are now advocated so that all possible sites for lymphatic dissemination from colon or rectal cancer are eradicated.[20] Although segmental resections of a colon cancer may have been popular a decade ago, new data strongly support the surgical removal of all regional lymph nodes that drain the primary cancer. Countless lymphatic channels must be transected in a colon or rectal cancer resection. Cancer cells in lymphatic channels may be lost into the abdominal or pelvic space. A logical conclusion from this hypothesis is that the risk of local recurrence is greater in patients with colorectal cancers that show lymph node metastases.[21] In primary colorectal cancer resection and in reoperative surgery, wide dissection of the colorectal mesentery to the superior mesenteric artery and vein on the right or aorta on the left is indicated. This extended lymph node dissection should result in few surgical treatment failures within lymph nodes (see **Fig. 1**).

NEW INDICATIONS FOR SECOND-LOOK SURGERY

The most modern concept in primary colorectal cancer resection demands complete clearance of the primary malignancy and total containment of the malignant process during the colon or rectal cancer resection.[22,23] Unfortunately, there are groups of patients for whom even the most knowledgeable and skillful efforts to deal definitively with the primary cancer will fail.[24] Some patients (approximately 20%) will show peritoneal dissemination of the primary cancer at the time of initial diagnosis.[25] Other patients who are at high risk for dissemination of cancer cells as either local-regional recurrence or peritoneal carcinomatosis can be identified through a careful evaluation of the clinical presentation of the primary cancer and a study of the pathology report. Patients who present with peritoneal dissemination, even if it is very limited and is removed at the time of primary cancer resection, will consistently show progression of carcinomatosis. The high-risk patients include those with perforated cancers, mucinous T3 and all T4 cancers, cancers with adjacent organ involvement, cancers with ovarian involvement, cancers with positive peritoneal cytology, and cancers that are ruptured intraoperatively. Any patient who has free cancer cells identified within the peritoneal space at the time of colon or rectal cancer resection is known to have a high incidence of local and regional cancer recurrence.[26] **Table 2** lists the patients at high risk for progression of local-regional disease or peritoneal carcinomatosis. These patients can be identified as eligible for a planned second-look surgery on the basis of their clinical presentation and their pathology reports.

One requirement of colorectal cancer surgery that is currently not a standard of practice should be to thoroughly evaluate patients for this revised second-look approach. A cytologic examination of the peritoneal surface of the primary tumor (optimally a "touch prep") should occur before a colorectal cancer resection. Also, aspiration of fluid for a cytologic study of the space beneath the right lobe of the liver and from the pelvis should occur. Finally, a cytologic study of the whole abdomen

Table 2
Patients with primary colorectal cancer who are at high risk for local-regional recurrence and/or peritoneal carcinomatosis

	Estimated Survival at 5 y
Visible evidence of peritoneal carcinomatosis	0
Ovarian cysts showing adenocarcinoma suggested to be of gastrointestinal origin	0
Positive cytologic results either before or after cancer resection	20
Adjacent organ involvement or cancer-induced fistula	20
Obstructed cancer	20
Perforated cancer	9
T3 mucinous cancer	30
T4 cancer or a positive "touch prep" of the primary cancer	0
Cancer mass ruptured with the resection	0
Positive lateral margins of excision	0
N2 lymph nodal disease	30

The outcome of these patients should be improved by using cytoreductive surgery and perioperative hyperthermic chemotherapy. The categories for high risk and their estimated survival in the absence of cytoreductive surgery and perioperative chemotherapy are listed.

From Sugarbaker PH. Second-look surgery for colorectal cancer: revised selection factors and new treatment options for greater success. Int J Surg Oncol 2011;2011:915,078. Epub 2010 Dec 5.

following the completion of the colorectal cancer resection is important. Patients with cytologically positive colon or rectal cancer are at high risk for death from progressive disease.[26] These patients with a positive "touch prep" from the surface of the primary cancer or positive cytology are identified as high risk for local-regional recurrence and eligible for second-look surgery.

IMPLEMENTATION OF A NEW SECOND-LOOK TREATMENT STRATEGY

With a group of patients with colorectal cancer who are identified who are at high risk for local-regional recurrence and with new and more effective liver resection and peritoneal surface treatment strategies available, an expanded application of second-look surgery should be implemented. This comprehensive treatment plan would include 3 groups of patients: (1) patients at high risk for recurrence on the basis of surgical and pathologic findings, (2) patients who have symptoms or signs on follow-up that suggest disease progression, and (3) patients who show a progressive increase in CEA levels. However, to keep the morbidity and mortality associated with this reoperative surgery at a minimum, ineligibility requirements for this group of patients should be enumerated. **Box 1** lists those patients who are not considered reasonable candidates for the revised second-look strategy. Patients with more than 4 liver metastases or liver metastases that cannot be resected are ineligible.[27,28] Of course, patients who have a poor performance status or serious medical conditions and are not likely to survive or recover from the second-look surgery should not be included. Patients who have had a low rectal cancer with recurrence at the resection site are not good candidates for cytoreductive surgery and hyperthermic intraperitoneal chemotherapy and are poor candidates for reoperation.[4] And patients who have unresectable systemic disease (especially disease in the bone marrow or numerous pulmonary metastases) are not candidates for second-look surgery. The most modern radiologic technologies for detecting systemic disease should be used before a reoperative event.

Box 1
Ineligibility requirements in patients considered for second-look surgery

Major

Liver metastases >4

Performance status >2

Serious medical condition

    Renal failure with creatinine >3

    Cardiac failure with ejection fraction <50%

    Malnutrition

Radiologic study showing systemic disease

Minor

Obesity

Low rectal cancer

Intestinal obstruction from progressive cancer or an interval of >1 year between primary cancer resection and second-look surgery

From Sugarbaker PH. Second-look surgery for colorectal cancer: revised selection factors and new treatment options for greater success. Int J Surg Oncol 2011;2011:915,078. Epub 2010 Dec 5.

The final ineligibility requirement listed in **Box 1** concerns the interval between primary cancer resection and the second look. In patients at high risk for local-regional recurrence who are to have a planned reoperative intervention, the surgery should occur within 1 year of the primary cancer resection. This restriction is an attempt for this clinical pathway to identify patients with disease recurrence that has a limited progression within the abdomen and pelvis. For those patients with peritoneal carcinomatosis, it seeks to identify patients with a PCI of less than 10. As discussed earlier in this report, there is no doubt that one of the most important requirements for success with cytoreductive surgery and hyperthermic intraperitoneal chemotherapy is a low PCI.

Criteria for Repeat Surgical Intervention in Patients with Colorectal Cancer

This plan for early reintervention for colorectal carcinomatosis is based on clinical data regarding the natural history of this disease. This is in contrast to current standard of care for recurrent colorectal cancer surgery that is initiated because the patient is symptomatic or a defect is identified on CT. In the new individualized approach to early intervention, these standard criteria are judged to be woefully insufficient and inaccurate parameters of disease recurrence for reoperative treatment. A long delay and, as a consequence, extensive disease are usually the findings at surgical exploration. The large extent of disease makes even the most aggressive intervention with perioperative chemotherapy unlikely to provide long-term benefit.

ALGORITHM FOR REVISED SECOND-LOOK SURGERY

Before the second-look surgery, patients undergo radiologic tests to rule out systemic disease. CT scanning of chest, abdomen, and pelvis is suggested. Also, a positron-emission tomography scan is necessary. A colonoscopy to examine the entire colon for second primary tumors and suture line recurrence is a requirement.[29]

Fig. 2 presents an algorithm for second-look surgery in 3 groups of patients. There are those patients who have limited carcinomatosis identified at the time of primary colon or rectal cancer resection and those patients whose clinical symptoms and signs and pathology report indicate that they are at high risk for local and regional recurrence. In this group, the maximum interval between primary colorectal cancer resection and the planned second look should be 1 year. At any time in their follow-up, patients with a progressive increase in CEA level, symptoms of progression, or radiologic evidence of disease progression will be considered for a second-look surgery.

Note in **Fig. 2** that patients with a negative second-look surgery will not have a simple "open and close" laparotomy. These patients are considered at high risk for recurrent disease. In an attempt to protect them from local-regional relapse after their full reexploration, they will have a greater and lesser omentectomy, oophorectomy, and hyperthermic intraperitoneal chemotherapy procedure. It is possible that a limited surgery plus perioperative chemotherapy will improve the outlook in these patients with a negative second look and add little to the expected low morbidity and mortality.

In patients who have a positive second-look surgery, there will be cytoreductive surgery that involves the necessary peritonectomy procedures and visceral resections.[30] Following surgery to remove all visible evidence of disease, hyperthermic intraperitoneal chemotherapy is performed.[1,5]

EVALUATION OF THE REVISED SECOND-LOOK SURGERY

The evaluation of this clinical project must be prospective and thorough. The primary endpoint for the study is the percentage of patients "converted" from a positive second look to long-term survival. A secondary endpoint would be the percentage

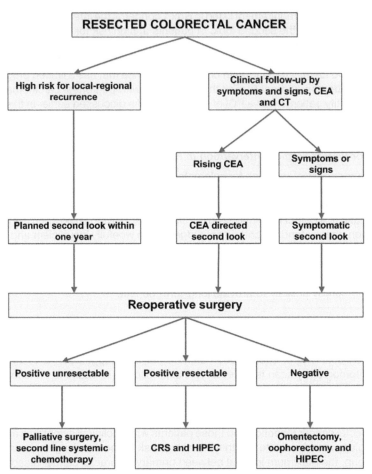

Fig. 2. Algorithm for a planned second-look surgery in patients at high risk for local-regional cancer recurrence. CRS, cytoreductive surgery; HIPEC, hyperthermic intraperitoneal chemotherapy. *From* Sugarbaker PH. Second-look surgery for colorectal cancer: revised selection factors and new treatment options for greater success. Int J Surg Oncol 2011;2011:915,078. Epub 2010 Dec 5.

of patients who have a positive second-look surgery compared with those who have a negative second-look surgery. A third endpoint is a comprehensive morbidity and mortality assessment of both positive and negative second-look surgeries. At the end of data accumulation, a summary of the credits and debits of this approach using the revised second-look surgery will become available (**Box 2**).

TIMING OF REOPERATIVE SURGERY, PROACTIVE OR PALLIATIVE

A large proportion of a person's health care costs occur within the last 6 months of life. For gastrointestinal cancer, recurrence within the abdomen and pelvis that is allowed to progress to intestinal obstruction, fistula, or abscess brings about a clinical situation that requires extensive and expensive health care. Clear guidelines for reoperative colorectal cancer surgery to prevent this devastating clinical situation are not

---

Box 2
Evaluation of revised guidelines for planned second-look surgery, CEA-directed second-look surgery, and symptomatic second-look surgery

Credits

1. Percentage of patients "converted" from disease recurrence to 5-year survival

2. Median time to recurrence and median survival of patients with a positive second-look surgery who are resected

3. Median time to recurrence and median survival of patients with a negative second-look surgery

Debits

1. Percentage of patients with a negative second-look surgery

2. Morbidity and mortality of patients with a negative second-look surgery

3. Morbidity and mortality of patients with a positive second-look surgery

4. Cost of reoperative surgery

5. Cost of follow-up program

From Sugarbaker PH. Second-look surgery for colorectal cancer: revised selection factors and new treatment options for greater success. Int J Surg Oncol 2011;2011:915,078. Epub 2010 Dec 5.

---

available. Can a planned reoperative surgical procedure add a reasonable length of good-quality life? Which patients will profit from a surgical intervention and which patients should be told that further surgery is not an option? If a second- or third-look surgical intervention is beneficial, *when* should it be performed? Early, before symptoms occur, or later, after patients have lost gastrointestinal function? If the revised guidelines suggested in this report for second-look surgery are placed into practice, can local-regional failure be prevented in a significant proportion of patients and thereby significantly reduce health care costs? This group of patients at high risk for loss of local control may benefit in terms of quality of life and improved survival by proactive early intervention rather than palliative surgery after symptoms of local-regional disease have occurred.

Introducing Hyperthermic Intraperitoneal Chemotherapy into the Treatment of Primary Colorectal Cancer

If a patient with primary colorectal cancer with small volume carcinomatosis or a patient with primary colorectal cancer and a high risk of local-regional recurrence (see **Table 2**) is operated on at an institution that delivers treatments for carcinomatosis, definitive cytoreductive surgery with perioperative intraperitoneal chemotherapy should be considered as part of the management of the primary colorectal cancer. There is evidence from the literature that local-regional chemotherapy as a planned part of a colorectal cancer is of benefit and improves survival.

Pestieau and Sugarbaker reported on 5 patients with carcinomatosis with a diagnosis made at the time of primary colon cancer resection.[31] These patients had a small volume of disease not evident by clinical signs or radiologic studies before colon resection. All 5 patients survived 5 years, with 2 patients manifesting late recurrences and eventually dying of systemic disease. When a small extent of carcinomatosis was definitively treated along with resection of the primary cancer, the outcome was favorable.

Tentes and colleagues[32] explored the use of hyperthermic intraperitoneal chemotherapy in patients with T3 and T4 colon cancer. The authors observed a 100% 5-year survival rate in 40 treated patients compared with 69% in a group of historical control patients (P = .011).

Definitive evaluation of the success of perioperative chemotherapy in primary colorectal cancer requires that patients are separated into those with established peritoneal carcinomatosis and those who are at high risk for local-regional recurrence. The operative intervention in both groups would be followed by adjuvant systemic chemotherapy.

In patients who present with stage IV disease (biopsy-documented carcinomatosis), the expected 5-year survival without special treatments is near zero. Any improvement in this statistic could be attributed to cytoreductive surgery and perioperative chemotherapy. In this group of patients, the level of evidence to support combined treatment is level IB. A properly designed randomized trial supports the intervention.[33] Scientific evidence suggests that the treatment should be offered to all eligible patients. Also, no evidence for an adequate alternative treatment exists.[34] Data accumulation within a well-designed phase II study is necessary.

The patients with primary colorectal cancer at high risk for recurrence present a more difficult evaluation. The most perfect evaluation would be to randomize eligible patients in the operating theater to receive or not receive cytoreductive surgery and perioperative chemotherapy. However, copious data regarding survival of patients with poor prognosis colorectal cancer exist. Patients with colorectal cancer with free perforation through the primary tumor has an approximate 9% survival at 5 years.[25] A walled-off perforation carries a slightly improved prognosis of 25%. Patients with positive cytology survive at a rate of 20% to 40% at 5 years.[35,36] An improvement in survival, if it exists, should be documented for each type of patient at high risk for local-regional recurrence. A precise strategy for stratification of these patients is an important aspect of the nonrandomized clinical trial.

Some modifications in the surgical management of colorectal cancer need to occur to initiate this prospective evaluation of carcinomatosis prevention or early treatment. The requirements are listed on **Box 3**. The preoperative clinical and radiologic workup for the primary colorectal cancer will suggest that most patients do not fulfill the requirements for the treatment as listed in **Table 2**. However, a proportion, estimated at 20%, will be found at the time of laparoscopic or open exploration to be at high risk for local-regional recurrence. For these patients to be included in carcinomatosis treatments, all patients to undergo primary colorectal cancer resection should sign a consent for perioperative chemotherapy.

For most of the criteria for protocol eligibility listed in **Table 2**, the operating surgeon should make the determination for carcinomatosis treatment and identify the category

---

Box 3
Modifications in the surgical management of primary colorectal cancer required to clinically test the concept of early intervention in carcinomatosis

1. All patients going to surgery for colon or rectal cancer resection must sign a consent for perioperative chemotherapy treatment.

2. Hyperthermic chemotherapy must be available on short notice in the operating theater.

3. A collaborative interaction in the operating suite between surgeon and pathologist must exist to identify patients with T3 mucinous, T4, and N2 lymph nodal disease.

4. An intraoperative, postoperative, and 5-year follow-up data retrieval system must be implemented. A comprehensive morbidity and mortality assessment for the hospitalization is necessary.

of high risk. In some patients, an experienced pathologist must be available to cut the specimen; a frozen section will be necessary to establish mucinous T3 or T4 primary cancer.

Finally, the clinical pathway cannot provide useful data unless there is careful clinical monitoring. The collection of intraoperative data, postoperative morbidity and mortality data, and 5-year follow-up data is necessary.

SUMMARY

A new management plan for patients at high risk for intra-abdominal colorectal cancer recurrence is suggested. There are 3 criteria by which to select patients for second-look surgery: (1) a high risk of local-regional recurrence of cancer, (2) an increasing CEA blood test level, or (3) symptoms and signs of disease recurrence. Accumulated data show that early reoperative intervention may convert a second-look–positive patient into a long-term survivor. New cytoreductive surgical techniques including peritonectomy and perioperative chemotherapy will be used to eradicate abdominal and pelvic recurrence. Also, improved techniques for management of limited liver metastases in combination with peritoneal carcinomatosis are appropriate. From this literature review, the credits and debits for an expanded second-look approach to colorectal cancer were formulated. The major credit will be the proportion of patients converted from a positive second-look surgery to a long-term survivor. The debits will be morbidity and mortality of the second-look surgery for all patients and the cost of the interventions. Important will be morbidity and mortality of those patients who have a negative second-look surgery. A projected incidence of a positive versus a negative second-look surgery is 50%. The projected survival of patients with a positive second-look surgery converted to a disease-free status is 50% at 5 years.

At institutions where perioperative chemotherapy is readily available for carcinomatosis treatments, it should be used as a planned part of the primary colon and rectal cancer resection in selected patients. This individualized treatment would be appropriate for the same group of patients identified at high risk for local-regional recurrence and the planned second-look surgery. The results of treatment compared with historical controls would be used to evaluate a pilot study.

REFERENCES

1. Deraco M, Elias D, Glehen O, et al. Peritoneal surface malignancy. In: DeVita VT, Lawrence T, Rosenberg SA, editors. Cancer: principles and practice of oncology. 9th edition. Lippincott Williams and Wilkins; 2011. p. 2081–9.
2. Jacquet P, Sugarbaker PH. Current methodologies for clinical assessment of patients with peritoneal carcinomatosis. J Exp Clin Cancer Res 1996;15:49–58.
3. Sugarbaker PH, Jablonski KA. Prognostic features of 51 colorectal and 130 appendiceal cancer patients with peritoneal carcinomatosis treated by cytoreductive surgery and intraperitoneal chemotherapy. Ann Surg 1995;221:124–32.
4. da Silva RG, Sugarbaker PH. Analysis of prognostic factors in seventy patients having a complete cytoreduction plus perioperative intraperitoneal chemotherapy for carcinomatosis from colorectal cancer. J Am Coll Surg 2006;203: 878–86.
5. Elias D, Gilly F, Boutitie F, et al. Peritoneal colorectal carcinomatosis treated with surgery and perioperative intraperitoneal chemotherapy: retrospective analysis of 523 patients from a multicentric French study. J Clin Oncol 2010;28:63–8.

6. Sugarbaker PH, Graves T, DeBruijn EA, et al. Early postoperative intraperitoneal chemotherapy as an adjuvant therapy to surgery for peritoneal carcinomatosis from gastrointestinal cancer: pharmacologic studies. Cancer Res 1990;50:5790–4.

7. Elias D, Goere D, Di Pietrantonio D, et al. Results of systemic second-look surgery in patients at high risk of developing colorectal peritoneal carcinomatosis. Ann Surg 2008;247:445–50.

8. Hughes KS, Scheele J, Sugarbaker PH. Surgery for colorectal cancer metastatic to the liver: optimizing the results of treatment. Surg Clin North Am 1989;69:339–59.

9. Wangensteen OH. Cancer of the colon and rectum; with special reference to earlier recognition of alimentary tract malignancy; secondary delayed re-entry of the abdomen in patients exhibiting lymph node involvement; subtotal primary excision of the colon; operation in obstruction. Wis Med J 1949;48:591–7.

10. Griffen WO, Humphrey L, Sosin H. The prognosis and management of recurrent abdominal malignancies. Curr Probl Surg 1969;1–43.

11. Sugarbaker PH, Zamcheck N, Moore FD. Assessment of serial carcinoembryonic antigen (CEA) assays in postoperative detection of recurrent colorectal cancer. Cancer 1976;38:2310–5.

12. Steele G Jr, Zamcheck N, Wilson R, et al. Results of CEA-initiated second-look surgery for recurrent colon cancer. Am J Surg 1980;139:544–8.

13. Attiyeh FF, Stearns MW Jr. Second-look laparotomy based on CEA elevations in colorectal cancer. Cancer 1981;47:2119–25.

14. Minton JP, Hoehn JL, Gerber DM, et al. Results of a 400-patient carcinoembryonic antigen second-look colorectal cancer study. Cancer 1985;55:1284–90.

15. Goldberg RM, Fleming TR, Tangen CM, et al. Surgery for recurrent colon cancer: strategies for identifying resectable recurrence and success rates after resection. Ann Intern Med 1998;129:27–35.

16. Sugarbaker PH, Gianola FJ, Speyer JL, et al. Prospective randomized trial of intravenous versus intraperitoneal 5 fluorouracil in patients with advanced primary colon or rectal cancer. Surgery 1985;98:414–21.

17. Sugarbaker PH. Observations concerning cancer spread within the peritoneal cavity and concepts supporting an ordered pathophysiology. In: Sugarbaker PH, editor. Peritoneal carcinomatosis: principles of management. Boston: Kluwer; 1996. p. 79–100.

18. Alexander HR, Allegra CJ, Lawrence TS. Metastatic cancer to the liver. In: DeVita VT Jr, Hellman S, Rosenberg SA, editors. Cancer: principles and practice of oncology. 6th edition. Philadelphia: JB Lippincott; 2001. p. 2690–713.

19. Yan TD, Black D, Savady R, et al. Systematic review on the efficacy of cytoreductive surgery combined with perioperative intraperitoneal chemotherapy for peritoneal carcinomatosis from colorectal carcinoma. J Clin Oncol 2006;24:4011–9.

20. Swanson RS, Compton CC, Stewart AK, et al. The prognosis of T3N0 colon cancer is dependent on the number of lymph nodes examined. Ann Surg Oncol 2003;10:65.

21. Rich T, Gunderson LL, Galdabini J, et al. Clinical and pathologic factors influencing local failure after curative resection of carcinoma of the rectum and rectosigmoid. Cancer 1983;52:1317–27.

22. West NP, Morris EJ, Rotimi O, et al. Pathology grading of colon cancer surgical resection and its association with survival: a retrospective observational study. Lancet Oncol 2008;9:857–65.

23. Bokey EL, Chapuis PH, Dent OF, et al. Surgical technique and survival in patients having a curative resection for colon cancer. Dis Colon Rectum 2003;46:860–6.

24. Sugarbaker PH. Successful management of microscopic residual disease in large bowel cancer. Cancer Chemother Pharmacol 1999;43(Suppl):S15–25.

25. Sugarbaker PH, Gunderson LL, Wittes RE. Colorectal cancer. In: DeVita VT Jr, Hellman S, Rosenberg SA, editors. Cancer: principles and practice of oncology, vol. 1, 2nd editiion. Philadelphia: JB Lippincott; 1985. p. 795–866.
26. Rekhraj S, Aziz O, Prabhudesai S, et al. Can intra-operative intraperitoneal free cancer cell detection techniques identify patients at higher recurrence risk following curative colorectal cancer resection: a meta-analysis. Ann Surg Oncol 2007;15:60–8.
27. Elias D, Sideris L, Pocard M, et al. Results of R0 resection for colorectal liver metastases associated with extrahepatic disease. Ann Surg Oncol 2004;11: 274–80.
28. Elias D, Liberale G, Vernerey D, et al. Hepatic and extrahepatic colorectal metastases: when resectable, their localization does not matter, but their prognostic features of 51 colorectal and 130 appendiceal cancer patients with peritoneal carcinomatosis treated by cytoreductive surgery and intraperitoneal chemotherapy. Ann Surg 1995;221:124–32.
29. Sugarbaker PH. Monitoring after resection of upper and lower gastrointestinal cancer. In: Wanebo HJ, editor. Surgery for gastrointestinal cancer: a multidisciplinary approach. Philadelphia: Lippincott-Raven; 1997. p. 87–95.
30. Sugarbaker PH. Peritonectomy procedures. Surg Oncol Clin N Am 2003;12: 703–27.
31. Pestieau SR, Sugarbaker PH. Treatment of primary colon cancer with peritoneal carcinomatosis: a comparison of concomitant versus delayed management. Dis Colon Rectum 2000;43:1341–8.
32. Tentes AA, Spiliotis ID, Korakianitis OS, et al. Adjuvant perioperative intraperitoneal chemotherapy in locally advanced colorectal carcinoma: preliminary results. (in press).
33. Verwaal VJ, van Ruth S, de Bree E, et al. Randomized trial of cytoreduction and hyperthermic intraperitoneal chemotherapy versus systemic chemotherapy and palliative surgery in patients with peritoneal carcinomatosis of colorectal cancer. J Clin Oncol 2003;21:3737–43.
34. Glasziou P, Chalmers I, Rawlins M, et al. When are randomised trials unnecessary? picking signal from noise. BMJ 2007;334:349–51.
35. Lennon AM, Mulcahy HE, Hyland JMP, et al. Peritoneal involvement in stage II colon cancer. Am J Clin Pathol 2003;119:108–13.
36. Schott A, Vogel I, Krueger U, et al. Isolated tumor cells are frequently detectable in the peritoneal cavity of gastric and colorectal cancer patients and serve as a new prognostic marker. Ann Surg 1998;227:372–9.

Index

Note: Page numbers of article titles are in **boldface** type

surgonc.theclinics.com

United States Postal Service

Statement of Ownership, Management, and Circulation
(All Periodicals Publications Except Requestor Publications)

1. Publication Title	2. Publication Number	3. Filing Date
Surgical Oncology Clinics of North America	0 1 2 - 5 6 5	9/14/12

4. Issue Frequency	5. Number of Issues Published Annually	6. Annual Subscription Price
Jan, Apr, Jul, Oct	4	$263.00

7. Complete Mailing Address of Known Office of Publication (Not printer) (Street, city, county, state, and ZIP+4®)

	Contact Person
Elsevier Inc. 360 Park Avenue South New York, NY 10010-1710	Stephen Bushing
	Telephone (Include area code) 215-239-3688

8. Complete Mailing Address of Headquarters or General Business Office of Publisher (Not printer)

Elsevier Inc., 360 Park Avenue South, New York, NY 10010-1710

9. Full Names and Complete Mailing Addresses of Publisher, Editor, and Managing Editor (Do not leave blank)

Publisher (Name and complete mailing address)

Kim Murphy, Elsevier, Inc., 1600 John F. Kennedy Blvd. Suite 1800, Philadelphia, PA 19103-2899

Editor (Name and complete mailing address)

Jessica McCool, Elsevier, Inc., 1600 John F. Kennedy Blvd. Suite 1800, Philadelphia, PA 19103-2899

Managing Editor (Name and complete mailing address)

Barbara Cohen-Kligerman, Elsevier, Inc., 1600 John F. Kennedy Blvd. Suite 1800, Philadelphia, PA 19103-2899

10. Owner (Do not leave blank. If the publication is owned by a corporation, give the name and address of the corporation immediately followed by the names and addresses of all stockholders owning or holding 1 percent or more of the total amount of stock. If not owned by a corporation, give the names and addresses of the individual owners. If owned by a partnership or other unincorporated firm, give its name and address as well as those of each individual owner. If the publication is published by a nonprofit organization, give its name and address.)

Full Name	Complete Mailing Address
Wholly owned subsidiary of	1600 John F. Kennedy Blvd., Ste. 1800
Reed/Elsevier, US holdings	Philadelphia, PA 19103-2899

11. Known Bondholders, Mortgagees, and Other Security Holders Owning or Holding 1 Percent or More of Total Amount of Bonds, Mortgages, or Other Securities. If none, check box ☐ None

Full Name	Complete Mailing Address
N/A	

12. Tax Status (For completion by nonprofit organizations authorized to mail at nonprofit rates) (Check one)
The purpose, function, and nonprofit status of this organization and the exempt status for federal income tax purposes:
☐ Has Not Changed During Preceding 12 Months
☐ Has Changed During Preceding 12 Months (Publisher must submit explanation of change with this statement)

PS Form 3526, September 2007 (Page 1 of 3) (Instructions Page 3) PSN 7530-01-000-9931 PRIVACY NOTICE: See our Privacy policy in www.usps.com

---

13. Publication Title	14. Issue Date for Circulation Data Below
Surgical Oncology Clinics of North America	July 2012

15. Extent and Nature of Circulation			Average No. Copies Each Issue During Preceding 12 Months	No. Copies of Single Issue Published Nearest to Filing Date
a. Total Number of Copies (Net press run)			548	572
b. Paid Circulation (By Mail and Outside the Mail)	(1)	Mailed Outside-County Paid Subscriptions Stated on PS Form 3541. (Include paid distribution above nominal rate, advertiser's proof copies, and exchange copies)	248	233
	(2)	Mailed In-County Paid Subscriptions Stated on PS Form 3541 (Include paid distribution above nominal rate, advertiser's proof copies, and exchange copies)		
	(3)	Paid Distribution Outside the Mails Including Sales Through Dealers and Carriers, Street Vendors, Counter Sales, and Other Paid Distribution Outside USPS®	87	94
	(4)	Paid Distribution by Other Classes Mailed Through the USPS (e.g. First-Class Mail®)		
c. Total Paid Distribution (Sum of 15b (1), (2), (3), and (4))		▲	335	327
d. Free or Nominal Rate Distribution (By Mail and Outside the Mail)	(1)	Free or Nominal Rate Outside-County Copies Included on PS Form 3541	59	58
	(2)	Free or Nominal Rate In-County Copies Included on PS Form 3541		
	(3)	Free or Nominal Rate Copies Mailed at Other Classes Through the USPS (e.g. First-Class Mail)		
	(4)	Free or Nominal Rate Distribution Outside the Mail (Carriers or other means)		
e. Total Free or Nominal Rate Distribution (Sum of 15d (1), (2), (3) and (4))		▲	59	58
f. Total Distribution (Sum of 15c and 15e)		▲	394	385
g. Copies not Distributed (See instructions to publishers #4 (page #3))		▲	154	187
h. Total (Sum of 15f and g)			548	572
i. Percent Paid (15c divided by 15f times 100)			85.03%	84.94%

16. Publication of Statement of Ownership

If the publication is a general publication, publication of this statement is required. Will be printed ☑ in the October 2012 issue of this publication.   ☐ Publication not required.

17. Signature and Title of Editor, Publisher, Business Manager, or Owner	Date
Stephen R. Bushing —Inventory/Distribution Coordinator	September 14, 2012

Stephen R. Bushing —Inventory/Distribution Coordinator

I certify that all information furnished on this form is true and complete. I understand that anyone who furnishes false or misleading information on this form or who omits material or information requested on the form may be subject to criminal sanctions (including fines and imprisonment) and/or civil sanctions (including civil penalties).

PS Form 3526, September 2007 (Page 2 of 3)

Moving?

Make sure your subscription moves with you!

To notify us of your new address, find your **Clinics Account Number** (located on your mailing label above your name), and contact customer service at:

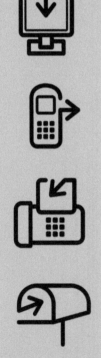

Email: journalscustomerservice-usa@elsevier.com

800-654-2452 (subscribers in the U.S. & Canada)
314-447-8871 (subscribers outside of the U.S. & Canada)

Fax number: 314-447-8029

Elsevier Health Sciences Division
Subscription Customer Service
3251 Riverport Lane
Maryland Heights, MO 63043

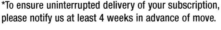

*To ensure uninterrupted delivery of your subscription, please notify us at least 4 weeks in advance of move.

ELSEVIER

Printed and bound by CPI Group (UK) Ltd, Croydon, CR0 4YY

21/10/2024

01777150-0001